Food and Fitness
A Dictionary of Diet and Exercise

Michael Kent

Oxford   New York
OXFORD UNIVERSITY PRESS
1997

Oxford University Press, Great Clarendon Street, Oxford OX2 6DP

Oxford New York
Athens Auckland Bangkok Bogota Bombay
Buenos Aires Calcutta Cape Town Dar es Salaam
Delhi Florence Hong Kong Istanbul Karachi
Kuala Lumpur Madras Madrid Melbourne
Mexico City Nairobi Paris Singapore
Taipei Tokyo Toronto Warsaw

and associated companies in
Berlin Ibadan

Oxford is a trade mark of Oxford University Press

First published 1997

British Library Cataloguing in Publication Data
Data available

Library of Congress Cataloging in Publication Data
Kent, Michael, Dr.
Food and fitness : a dictionary of diet and exercise / Michael Kent.
p.   cm.
1. Nutrition—Encyclopedias.   2. Exercise—Encyclopedias.
3. Physical fitness—Encyclopedias.   I. Title.
613.7'03—dc20   RA784.K397   96-38381
ISBN 0-19-863147-2

Designed by Jane Stevenson, illustrated by Margaret Jones
Typeset in Arial and Swift by Graphicraft Typesetters Ltd.
Printed in Great Britain by Bookcraft Ltd.,
Midsomer Norton, Somerset

Contents

List of Illustrations *iv*

Preface *v*

Acknowledgments *vi*

A–Z entries *1–335*

Appendix 1   Recommended dietary allowances and intakes *336*
Appendix 2   Reference Nutrient Intakes (RNIs) per day for selected
             nutrients *340*
Appendix 3   Composition of selected foods *341*
Appendix 4   Ratings for activities and sports *345*
Appendix 5   Average energy expenditure of various activities and sports *347*
Appendix 6   Benefits of exercises *349*

Thematic index *352*

A–Z index *365*

List of Illustrations

Achilles stretcher 3
adductor stretch 6
agility: Illinois Agility Run 11
alcohol: each of these glasses contains one
    unit of alcohol 13
alimentary canal 13
arm curl 28
arm sprints 28
back care 35
back extensions 36
bench press 42
bent arm hang 43
bent arm pullover 43
bent over row 43
Billig's exercise 45
blind stork test 46
body mass index 51
body movements 52
bone: bone density decreases with age,
    increasing the risk of osteoporosis (brittle
    bone disease) 53
heel raise 62
Canadian trunk strength test 65
catastrophe theory 70
circuit training: a typical circuit 76
contraindicated: four exercises that may be
    harmful 84
curl-up 90
dips 99
foetal stretch 125
food guide pyramid 128
gluteal lift 138
gynoid fat distribution: comparison of the two
    main types of fat distribution 144
half squats 146
hamstring stretcher 147
hexagon test: the footprints indicate where you
    should land 153
iliopsoas stretcher 161
isometrics: two simple exercises 167
knee: three exercise for improving knee
    mobility. They are commonly performed
    after knee injury to minimize the risk of
    recurrence 173

lateral pull-down 177
leg curl: four exercises that can improve the
    strength and mobility of the lower body 178
a lipoprotein 181
low back stretcher 183
lower leg lift 184
military press 195
muscles: front view 199
muscles: side view 200
muscles: back view 201
muscle contraction 203
neck extension exercises 207
osteoporosis: images such as these have
    been used by the National Osteoporosis
    Society (UK) to heighten awareness and to
    encourage women to take preventative
    measures 216
pain cycle 222
PAR-Q: Physical Activity Readiness
    Questionnaire 224
pelvic tilt 227
power clean 235
press up 239
profile of mood states 240
pulse 245
quad stretch 247
Rockport Fitness Walking Test 257
Sargent jump 261
shin stretcher 267
shoulder shrugs 268
sit and reach test 269
sitting tucks 269
skinfold measurements 272
stationary leg change 284
training heart rate 307
training shoe 308
triceps extension 311
trunk lifts 312
upright rowing 316
wrestler's bridge 330
wrist curl 331
yo-yo diet 333

Preface

Experts agree that a balanced diet and regular exercise are the main keys to a healthy life. This book provides the information you need to make sensible decisions about the food you eat and the activities you undertake. The topics covered include diets, food ingredients, sports, and exercises. *Food and Fitness* also describes common disorders related to diet and exercise, and ways in which they can be treated. However, the book is not meant to be a substitute for the medical advice of a doctor or the tuition of a coach (*see* Important health note).

The message of this book is that there is no need to adopt extreme measures to attain fitness and good health. A balanced diet that does not exclude a little of what you fancy, combined with regular, moderate exercise can improve the quality of your life. Healthy living can be fun!

Food and Fitness could not have been written without the help of my wife, Merryn, who played a key role at each stage of the book. Dr Ken Fox, Lecturer in Health at Exeter University, Carol Matta, a State Registered Dietitian; and Dr Nick Smith provided invaluable expert advice. I thank them for their contributions. I would also like to thank Dr David Bender of University College, London, and Professor Clyde Williams of Loughborough University for reading the text and making constructive comments. Their help and encouragement has been much appreciated.

Important health note

This book is not meant to be a substitute for the medical advice of a personal physician, or the expert tuition of a trained coach. The reader should consult a physician in matters relating to his or her health and particularly in respect of any symptoms which may require diagnosis or medical treatment. Exercises, especially those involving the use of weights, should be performed only under the guidance of a trained instructor or coach. If an exercise causes any form of discomfort you should stop immediately. It would be prudent if you have suffered any recent ill health, or if you are over thirty-five, to first see your doctor before embarking on a new diet or a new exercise programme.

Acknowledgments

Thanks are due to the following for permission to use material:

- Health Education Authority: Body Mass Index, Food Guide Pyramid, Balance of Good Health, Height Weight Chart, ©HEA.
- The Controller, Her Majesty's Stationery Office: Appendix 2, Reference Nutrient Intakes (RNIs) per day for Selected Nutrients (HMSO, London 1990).
- National Academy Press: Appendix 1, Recommended Dietary Allowances and Intakes, from *Recommended Dietary Allowances* (10th ed), ©1989 by the National Academy of Sciences.
- *Psychology Today*: Profile of Mood States, from W.P. Morgan, 1980, 'Test of the Champions: the Iceberg Profile', *Psychology Today*, 6 July 91–108.
- The Rockport Company: from *Rockport Fitness Walking Test* and *The Walking Brochure*, ©1986/1987 The Rockport Company.
- Schering Corporation, Kenilworth, NJ: from *Your Back and How to Care For It*.

Adapted material:

- Pelham Books (Penguin Group): *The Flexibility Factor*, Brown, M & Adamson, J, ©1995 Lesley Skates, Bailey.

A

"Anyone can win, unless there happens to be a second entry."
George Ade. Quoted in Esar, E. and Bentley N. *Treasury of humorous quotations.*

....

abdominal contraction
An easy and effective exercise for strengthening the abdominal muscles. It may be performed almost anytime and anywhere, while sitting, standing, or lying down. All you need to do is tense your abdominal (stomach) muscles for a few seconds while breathing out. This causes the muscles to contract without producing any movement of the trunk and hips. Be careful not to overstrain. *See also* **isometrics.**

abdominal hold
An exercise to test and develop your ability to sustain contractions of abdominal muscles.
■ Lie on your back with your knees bent and your lower back pressed gently into the floor. Place your hands in a relaxed position on the top of your thighs. Keep your lower back flat on the floor and slowly curl up to touch your knees with your hands; hold the position for as long as possible: 35 to 60 seconds indicates a good level of endurance. Beginners should not attempt to hold for more than 60 seconds.

abdominal muscles
Four pairs of muscles, often referred to as the stomach muscles, that support and protect the contents of the abdomen and help you to breathe out forcibly. (The technical names for the four pairs of muscles are the rectus abdominis, external oblique, internal oblique, and the transversus abdominis.) Strong and healthy abdominal muscles support the back during lifting by stabilizing the vertebral column. If the muscles are weakened by lack of exercise they become pendulous, forming a 'pot-belly'. Despite claims to the contrary (*see* **spot-reducing**), the only way to develop a flat stomach is

by combining an appropriate diet with regular exercises to strengthen and tone the abdominal muscles. Suitable exercises include the abdominal hold, crunches, and curl-ups.

abduction: *See* **body movements.**

abductor
A muscle that moves a part of the body away from the midline, or causes the fingers or toes to spread apart.

abductor raise
A simple exercise for strengthening the abductor muscles in the groin.
■ Lie on your right side with both legs straight and together. Support your upper body with your right arm. Lift your left leg upwards slowly and smoothly; arch your back slightly so that the leg does not move forwards. Hold the position for a few seconds then gently lower the leg. Repeat the exercise on the other side.
The exercise can be made more difficult by using ankle weights.

abnormal quadriceps pull: *See* Q-angle.

absolute strength: *See* **strength.**

absorption
Absorption is the process by which nutrients in the gut are taken into the bloodstream so that body cells can use them. For a nutrient to be absorbed, it has to be broken down into substances small enough to pass through the gut wall. Despite eating a balanced meal rich in nutrients, a person may still be malnourished if he or she lacks the enzymes required to break down the food into absorbable components (lack of the

enzyme lactase, for example, will result in an inability to digest milk sugar (*see* **lactose**). Malnutrition may also result from damage to the intestinal wall, as happens in people intolerant to gluten (*see* **coeliac disease**), or when one food item interferes with the absorption of another. Absorption of iron and other minerals, for example, may be impaired by drinking tea and coffee, or by eating soya protein, wheat bran, calcium supplements, and fibre. Alternatively, high levels of vitamin C in the diet enhances iron absorption. *See also* **phytic acid**.

acceleration sprint
A special form of sprint-training in which running speed is gradually increased from jogging to striding and finally to sprinting at maximum pace. Each component is usually about 50 metres long. Acceleration sprints are a good form of anaerobic training. They are particularly effective in emphasizing and maintaining the technical components of the sprint action as speed increases. The progressive nature of acceleration sprinting reduces the risk of muscle injury.

acclimation: *See* **acclimatization**.

acclimatization
Acclimatization is the reversible process by which a person becomes adapted to a change in the environment. It requires adaptations to a variety of factors (e.g. temperature, humidity, and atmospheric pressure). Acclimation, by contrast, involves an adaptation to a single factor (e.g. temperature). *See also* **altitude** and **heat acclimatization**.

accommodation principle
A principle which states that training should progress from the general to the specific. According to the principle, your initial concern should be with improving your overall body condition and strength. You should try to improve skills and specific fitness components only after you have attained a good level of general fitness.

acesulfame-K
An artificial sweetener which, like aspartame and saccharin, has no calories and does not cause dental caries. Acesulfame-K is two hundred times sweeter than sucrose. It is now used in more than 2000 products around the world, mainly in conjunction with aspartame. These two sweeteners have a synergistic effect, each boosting the sweetness of the other. *See also* **artificial sweeteners**.

acetylsalicylic acid: *See* aspirin.

Achilles stretch: *See* Achilles tendon.

Achilles tendinitis: *See* Achilles tendon.

Achilles tendon
A large tendon at the back of the ankle which connects the calf muscles (gastrocnemius and soleus) to the heel bone (calcaneus). The tendon is very susceptible to injuries. An Achilles tendon weakened by lack of exercise may rupture if the calf muscle contracts suddenly (for example, when a badminton player suddenly changes from a backward to a forward motion or when a jogger misjudges a curb and lands too far forward on his or her foot). A rupture is often accompanied by a loud crack and victims think they have been struck violently behind the heel. In extreme cases, the tendon may be completely ruptured, leaving the victim incapacitated and requiring surgery. Less severe than a complete rupture, but more common, is Achilles tendinitis. This stress injury is characterized by inflammation, pain, and tenderness in and around the tendon. It is common among runners who train over long distances on hard surfaces, and those who increase their training intensity too quickly. Women distance runners who usually wear high-heeled shoes are at particular risk because these shoes effectively shorten the Achilles tendon over a period of years. When they adopt the more flat footed position during running, their tendons are subjected to more stress than they are used to. Training shoes with high backs or hard heeltabs also increase the risk of injury.

Treatment for Achilles tendinitis usually includes rest, medication (e.g. aspirin) to reduce the swelling, and appropriate physiotherapy. A heel pad to restrict the range of movement may provide some relief. In severe cases, surgery may be required. If not treated properly, an acute inflammation of the Achilles tendon can develop into a chronic condition that is very difficult to resolve. You can reduce the risk of injuring your Achilles tendon by including an Achilles stretch in your warm-up routine (figure 1). Although this stretch may be performed freestanding, it is easier to do against a wall.

Figure 1

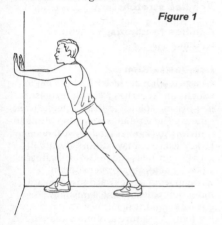

■ Stand upright about one large pace away from the wall with your feet parallel and about hip width apart. Place your hands against the wall, at shoulder height. Move your right leg half a pace forward. Lunge forward on your right leg so that the knee is brought directly above the ankle. Stretch your left leg back as far as is comfortable with the foot remaining flat on the floor. Slowly flex your left leg to stretch the lower calf muscles and tendon. Hold the stretch for about 10 seconds, relax, and repeat on the other leg.

acidosis

The human body functions best when blood and tissue fluids are neither too alkaline nor too acidic. An abnormally high acidity of blood and tissue fluids is called acidosis. It results in chemical reactions taking place less efficiently and can impair muscular contractions which may lead to fatigue.

There are two main types of acidosis: metabolic acidosis and respiratory acidosis. Metabolic acidosis may be caused by loss of bases (chemicals which readily accept hydrogen ions and decrease acidity), ingestion of highly acidic foods, or the production of excessive amounts of acid in the body. Respiratory acidosis results from a failure to exhale carbon dioxide from the lungs as quickly as it forms in respiring tissues. Carbon dioxide accumulates in the blood and tissues where it forms carbonic acids. Heavy or severe exercise may also cause temporary acidosis by producing large amounts of both lactic acid and carbon dioxide. Persistent acidosis is rare and usually associated with disease.

We usually respond to acidosis by breathing very heavily in order to flush out excess carbon dioxide from the body and eliminate excess acids (a process called compensatory hyperventilation). Some athletes use sodium hydrogen carbonate (sodium bicarbonate or baking soda) as a performance enhancer in the belief that it decreases acidity and reduces the risk of acidosis. Research evidence suggests that ingestion of 300 mg of bicarbonate per kilogram of body weight can enhance the performance of all-out, maximal aerobic activities lasting from 1 to 7 minutes.

acquired ageing: *See* ageing.

acquired immune deficiency syndrome (AIDS)

A disease caused by a blood-borne virus (called human immunodeficiency virus or HIV) that disrupts the body's normal immune responses. HIV is transmitted via body fluids, primarily through sexual intercourse, transfusion of infected blood and plasma products, or injections of drugs through contaminated needles. The general medical consensus is that the risk of infection is very low in groups exercising together or participating in a sport. However, the risk is increased during activities in which blood contact may occur (e.g. boxing). Standard common-sense precautions and adherence to basic principles of hygiene should always be followed if any bleeding occurs to prevent infection with HIV or other disease organisms such as the hepatitis viruses. Exercise usually benefits HIV-infected individuals. If started when still healthy, it can play an important role in the management of the disease while improving the quality of life. Diet is also important, with a high energy diet being necessary as the disease progresses.

active rest

A common and effective treatment for many overuse injuries. Active rest involves performing light exercises (often swimming or cycling) that stimulate the recovery process without imposing undue stress on the injured body part. *See also* **rest**.

activity-induced anorexia: *See* anorexia.

acupuncture

An ancient Chinese system of healing in which symptoms are relieved by inserting 3 to 20 thin needles through the skin and muscle at certain points in the body. The points are plotted along the body on lines determined by tradition. Selected points are stimulated by rotating the needle or by passing an electric current through it. The precise mechanism of acupuncture is unknown, but it is thought that the needles act as an external stimulus, encouraging the release of natural chemical painkillers, called endorphins. These are believed to initiate self-healing within the body.

Acupuncture is used in the Far East as an alternative to anaesthesia for some major operations. It is gaining popularity in the West as a technique for the relief of pain and the treatment of ailments such as arthritis, back-pain and depression. If you feel you might benefit from the services of an acupuncturist, choose carefully. Many acupuncturists are not medically qualified. If an acupuncture is not performed properly there is a real danger of infection. Acupuncture has also been used to treat overweight people, and special 'acupressure' ear rings are marketed as weight-loss aids, but there is no evidence that they are effective.

acute injury

An injury with a rapid onset. An acute injury usually responds well to early treatment, but if left untreated can develop into a persistent condition that is much more difficult to treat.

acute muscle soreness: *See* muscle soreness.

adaptation

The process by which a person's body responds positively over a period of time to the effects of exercise so that the exerciser can cope with higher workloads. In a well-designed training programme, it is important to increase the workloads gradually as adaptation takes place to ensure that there is a sufficient stimulus to produce beneficial training effects (see **overload principle**). *See also* **acclimatization**.

adaptation energy

Some scientists believe that each person has a finite amount of energy, called adaptation energy, to cope with different types of stress. Energy expended to cope with one type of stress (such as moving house) results in less being available for other stresses (such as exercise). When adaptation energy is low, a person is more likely to suffer from stress-related diseases and conditions known as burn out and run down.

adapted physical exercise

A number of physical activities have been adapted to enable people with disabilities to participate in competitive sports. The activities may require specially adapted equipment and some specialist medical support, but exercise for the disabled has the same aims and attractions as exercise for the able-bodied.

Athletes with a permanent disability of the lower body (e.g. because of amputations, spinal cord injuries, or poliomyelitis) can participate in wheelchair sports such as road racing, tennis, basketball, archery, softball, and track and field athletics. One of the fastest growing wheelchair sports is quad rugby. This is a highly competitive sport for quadriplegics. It is played on a basketball court. Four players from one team are allowed on the court at a time and their aim is to carry the ball across their opponent's goal line.

Wheelchair sports have similar rules and provide a similar experience to other varieties. They are just as competitive. The winner of the wheelchair New York marathon, for example, has to be totally dedicated to training, and just as aerobically fit as the winner of the able-bodied event. In addition, wheelchair athletes have to master the skills required to manoeuvre and drive the specially designed wheelchair.

The aim of many competitive wheelchair athletes is to take part in the Paralympics. These are competitions, equivalent to the Olympic Games, for athletes with permanent disabilities. The governing body is the International Paralympic Committee, supported and partly funded by the International Olympic Committee. The first Paralympics were held in Rome in 1960, and they have been held every Olympic year since. Activities include archery, athletics, basketball, boccie, cycling, fencing, goal ball, judo, shooting, soccer, swimming, table tennis, and volleyball. Of course, not all disabled people use a wheelchair. Amputees, blind people, those with cerebral palsy, and other physically disabled individuals participate as stand-up participants in many of the activities.

Many disabled athletes train on a daily basis. They train, often with weights, for flexibility, strength, speed, power, endurance, and to develop specific skills. The training principles for the disabled are the same as those for the able-bodied, but disabled athletes have an additional challenge. They must develop an individual style that takes their specific disability into account, but allows them to use their abilities to the maximum.

Sports participation offers disabled people a powerful incentive to become fitter, and plays an important part in both the psychological and physical rehabilitation of the disabled. The vast majority of disabled people do not take part in formal, highly-organized competitive sport. Nevertheless, many acquire the benefits of exercise by taking part in a wide range of physical leisure activities, from low-risk activities such as wheelchair aerobics, to high-risk activities, such as skydiving and mountain climbing. As Dr Frank M Brasile, a physical educator with a special interest in adapted exercise, stated '. . . even the sky is no limit to what the individual can do if he or she wants to participate in a desired activity' (quoted from Mellion, M.B. (1993) *Sports medicine secrets*. p55. Hanley and Belfus Philadelphia.)

adaptogen

An ergogenic aid (performance-enhancing substance) derived from natural plants. Adaptogens include chemicals from the Siberian ginseng (*Eleutherococcus senticosus*). It is claimed that Siberian ginseng heightens resistance to physical, chemical, and psychological stress, enhances stamina, increases resistance to infection, accelerates recovery, and that it is not harmful, even in high doses. Although there are several reports of the effects of Siberian ginseng in Eastern European scientific journals, many Western scientists are sceptical about its beneficial effects and are waiting to see the results of rigorous double-blind, cross-over experiments before they make up their minds.

addiction

A state of physiological dependence produced by habitually taking drugs such as morphine, heroin or alcohol. The term is also applied to a state of psychological dependence on drugs such as barbiturates. *See also* **exercise addiction**.

additive: *See* food additives.

adduction: *See* body movements.

adductor muscles (adductors)

A muscle that moves a body part (e.g. an arm or leg) towards the midline of the body. A strain of the thigh adductors is a relatively common injury of horse riders, fast bowlers, and footballers who make lunge tackles. A simple exercise called the adductor stretch reduces the risk of injury (figure 2). It is also useful for pregnant women and others whose thighs tend to rotate inwards causing backache and flat feet.

■ Sit with your knees apart and legs crossed. Place your hands on the inside of your knees. Contract the adductors in an attempt to raise your knees, but resist the movement with your hands. Hold the contraction for a few seconds, relax, then stretch your adductors as far as possible by

Figure 2 Adductor stretch

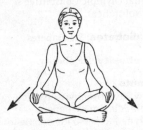

pressing your knees toward the floor. Hold the stretched position for about 5–10 seconds.

adductor stretch: *See* adductor muscles.

adenosine triphosphate
Adenosine triphosphate (ATP) is a relatively simple but remarkable chemical. It is the only compound that the body can use directly as fuel for energy-consuming activities, including movement. Without it, we would die. ATP is a high-energy compound made using the energy derived from the breakdown of food during respiration. Physical activity uses enormous quantities of ATP. An active muscle cell requires about two million ATP molecules per second to drive its biochemical machinery. It has been estimated that more than 75 kilograms of ATP are turned over (i.e. made and broken down) during a marathon. The body has only a small store of ATP (approximately 100 grams in an average person). This would be used up in about 1 second if it were not continuously regenerated by respiration.

adipocyte (fat cell)
A cell containing a glistening oil droplet composed almost entirely of fat. The droplet occupies most of the cell's volume, compressing other components such as the nucleus to one side. Mature adipocytes are among the largest cells of the body. Although they can become plumper by taking up more fat or more wrinkled by losing fat, they are fully specialized for fat storage and have a restricted ability to divide. The number of fat cells within an adult does not usually change, except when a high percentage of the cells are completely full of fat.

However, an appropriate diet and exercise programme can be effective at reducing the size of adipocytes.

adipose tissue
Tissue containing large numbers of fat-storing cells (*see* **adipocytes**) which make up 90 per cent of the tissue. Adipose tissue may develop anywhere, but tends to accumulate beneath the skin where it acts as a shock-absorber and insulator. Women tend to have more adipose tissue than men. *See also* **android fat distribution**; **brown fat**; **gynoid fat distribution** and **obesity**.

adiposis: *See* liposis.

adipostat
A hypothetical mechanism which keeps the level of body fat of most people within a narrow range despite considerable variations in dietary fat intake and physical activity. It is thought that some people may become obese because of a malfunction in the adipostat, but this hypothesis has not gained general support in the scientific community.

Three mechanisms for an adipostat have been proposed. The first proposal likens the adipostat to a thermostat. When fat stores exceed genetically determined limits, the adipostat switches on metabolic processes (called futile cycles) that convert excess fat into heat. Conversely, when fat stores run low, the adipostat switches off the futile cycles. Thus fat stores are regulated by the adipostat increasing or decreasing fat metabolism. The second proposal is that a hormone is released from adipose tissues affecting the appetite control centre in the brain. The third proposal is that the activity of special, metabolically active fatty tissue (*see* **brown fat**) increases when fat stores exceed the normal level, increasing heat output and burning off the excess fat.

adolescence
Adolescence, the period between childhood and adulthood, begins after secondary sexual characteristics (e.g. pubic hair) appear and continues until sexual maturity is complete. It is a period during which bones are still growing and there

is a high risk of skeletal injuries. Rapid physical changes are accompanied by important psychological changes relating particularly to the way the adolescent perceives himself or herself. This can be a turbulent time. Parents and others, especially sports coaches and teachers, who work with adolescents must be very sensitive to both the physical and the psychological changes taking place during this period. It is unwise for adolescents to take part in exercises which put undue strain on the growth regions of their bones. This is one reason why they are usually excluded from taking part in long-distance running events, such as marathons.

It is not unusual for an adolescent to add more than 5 kg in body weight and to grow 10 cm in height in one year. Such rapid growth requires good nutrition. Active adolescent boys may need up to 4000 Calories a day, about twice the normal adult requirement. The protein, vitamin, and mineral requirements of adolescents of both sexes are also higher than for adults. Adequate calcium intake is especially important during adolescence to maximize bone density and reduce the risk of osteoporosis in later life. Eating habits acquired during adolescence are often retained for life. Therefore, adolescents should be encouraged to eat a well balanced diet and not to skip meals.

adrenaline

The so-called 'fight or flight' hormone secreted by the inner part of the adrenal gland. It prepares the body for action by its stimulatory effects on muscles, circulation, and carbohydrate and fat metabolism. Adrenaline increases heart rate, the depth and rate of breathing, and metabolic rate. It also improves the force of muscular contractions and delays the onset of fatigue. Its actions oppose those of insulin. Adrenaline accelerates fat mobilization and encourages the conversion of glycogen to glucose.

Adrenaline and adrenaline-related drugs are sometimes used in sport as stimulants. Although these drugs can improve performance, they may produce harmful side-effects such as heart beat irregularities. Consequently, they are on the International Olympic Committee's list of banned substances.

adult onset diabetes: *See* diabetes.

adult onset obesity: *See* obesity.

advertisements

There are many advertisements, particularly in magazines and newspapers, which are designed to persuade people to invest in slimming aids. A survey in April 1994 by the Advertising Standards Authority (the ASA, the controlling body for advertisements in the UK), reported that almost two-thirds of these adverts flouted the advertising code by making 'miracle' claims guaranteeing weight loss without mentioning the need to diet and exercise. The code states that advertisements should make it clear that the only way to lose weight is by taking in less energy than the body is using. Claims that weight loss can be achieved wholly by any other means than diet and exercise are not acceptable within the code of practice of the ASA.

aerobic capacity

The total amount of work that can be performed using aerobic respiration (i.e. oxygen-dependent respiration).

aerobic dance: *See* dance.

aerobic energy system: *See* aerobic respiration.

aerobic exercise (steady state exercise)

Any repetitive, rhythmical, relatively low intensity exercise involving large muscle groups. Aerobic exercise increases the body's demands for oxygen and adds to the workload of the heart and lungs, strengthening the cardiovascular system and helping to develop endurance. For aerobic exercise to have lasting benefit, it should have the following features:

- FREQUENCY: at least 3 days per week, but no more than 6
- INTENSITY: high enough to elevate the heart rate to between 60 and 80% of its maximum (*see* **training heart rate**)
- DURATION: 20–60 minutes of continuous activity.

Because aerobic exercise is often done slowly and continuously, it is especially suitable for older people, those who have been inactive, or those who are not very fit. However, these groups of people should begin exercising gently and increase the amount gradually as it could be harmful to expect too much too soon. Those with known medical problems should consult a physician to determine appropriate exercise levels. Examples of good aerobic exercise are jogging, brisk walking, cross-country skiing, swimming, cycling, and dance. *See also* **anaerobic exercise**.

aerobic fitness (cardiorespiratory endurance, cardiovascular fitness)
The ability of the whole body to sustain prolonged, rhythmical activity (such as cycling, running, and swimming) of low to moderate intensity. Such activities use the aerobic system of respiration. They depend on the ability of the lungs and heart to take in and transport adequate amounts of oxygen to the working muscles.

aerobic points (Cooper points)
A scoring system, devised in the 1960s by Dr Kenneth C. Cooper, to compare the beneficial effects of different aerobic exercises on the heart, lungs, and circulatory system. Each exercise is awarded points dependent on the type of exercise, its frequency, intensity, and duration. For example, a two mile walk completed in under 30 minutes, performed five times a week, scores 25 points; four sessions of aerobic dance classes per week scores 36 points. Dr Cooper argued that in order to develop cardiovascular fitness and protect the heart a person needs to earn at least 30 aerobic points each week. He popularized his ideas in eleven books selling more than 20 million copies worldwide. In 1970 he established the Cooper Aerobics Center in Dallas for research into the value of exercise and the practice of preventative, diagnostic, and rehabilitative medicine. His top five forms of aerobic exercise are:

- cross-country skiing
- swimming
- jogging
- cycling
- walking.

aerobic power (aerobic work capacity)
The maximum rate at which energy is provided by aerobic respiration. Aerobic power is dependent on the ability of the respiratory and circulatory systems to transport oxygen from the air to the respiring tissues, and the ability of the tissues to use the oxygen to break down metabolic fuels. Aerobic power is usually measured in terms of oxygen consumption. *See also* **maximal oxygen consumption**.

aerobic respiration
The metabolic process that uses oxygen to break down food and release energy. The energy is used to make adenosine triphosphate, the high-energy compound that acts as the fuel for all of the body's energy-consuming activities.

aerobics
Rhythmic exercises performed to music. During an aerobics workout, dance steps are mixed with callisthenics, running and jumping. Ballet, disco, jazz, rock, and other types of music supply the tempo and rhythm for the exercises. A well-structured session works the entire body, and takes muscles and joints through their full range of movement, enhancing flexibility and improving strength. A good workout can also develop stamina and help maintain bone mass, vital for women around the menopause and beyond.

To avoid injury, it is essential to have a good instructor who is properly qualified. Good instructors insist that participants always perform appropriate warm up and cool down exercises to reduce the risk of injury and muscle soreness. They are sensitive to the ability of each member of the class and ensure that the exercise level is neither too low nor too high (many instructors offer graded classes taught at different levels of intensity). Particularly good instructors will expect participants to check their pulse two or three times during the class. They are able and willing to explain how to perform the exercises and the reasons for performing them, and readily correct anyone's poor technique.

An aerobics session may consist of high-impact or low-impact movements, or a combination. High-impact movements include running on the spot and jumping up and down. These can cause stress injuries, such as shin splints and lower back pain, especially if done on a hard floor (concrete floors are worse, sprung floors are best). Low-impact movements are performed keeping one foot on the ground all the time. They have a low incidence of injury but have to be performed at a high intensity to improve aerobic fitness. Low impact aerobic movements are sometimes combined with upper body conditioning in which exercisers use their own body weight (or light hand weights for added resistance) to improve muscle strength and toning.

Many people join aerobics classes to lose weight, but most studies show that, although muscles are toned, there is no significant change in the body weight of the majority of participants.

aerobic training threshold

A rough guide to the training intensity required to produce significant beneficial effects on endurance and cardiovascular fitness of most people. In sports physiology, the threshold is usually expressed as a percentage of a person's maximal oxygen consumption (a measure of aerobic fitness). However, facilities for measuring oxygen consumption are available only to a lucky few, therefore target or training heart rates are used as more convenient measures of exercise intensity. The minimum heart rate required to benefit significantly from aerobic training is about 60 per cent of maximum heart rate. For convenience, it is usually assumed that maximum heart rate per minute equals 220 minus age (in years). Therefore, the heart rates required to reach the aerobic threshold for most healthy adults are as follows:

AGE	AEROBIC TRAINING THRESHOLD (BEATS PER MINUTE)
20	120
25	117
30	114

AGE	AEROBIC TRAINING THRESHOLD (BEATS PER MINUTE)
40	108
45	105
50	102
55	99
60	96
65	93

It should be emphasized that the above threshold is only a rough guide to training intensities. The benefits gained from a particular aerobic activity depend on the initial fitness level of the individual as well as exercise intensity. A completely sedentary person will benefit from any exercise, even gentle walking. However, the fitness improvements will not be sufficient for participation in a race or something more strenuous than gentle walking. Older people or those who have been inactive for a long time, should exercise below the 60 per cent threshold and increase the intensity gradually. Those with known medical problems should consult a physician to determine appropriate exercise levels. The aerobic threshold increases as fitness improves, so a well-trained person may need to exercise at a minimum of 80 per cent maximum heart rate to gain any training benefits.

aerobic training zone

The range of exercise intensities between an individual's aerobic threshold and anaerobic threshold.

aerobic work capacity: *See* aerobic power.

aerobox: *See* boxercise.

aflatoxins

Peanuts, wheat, corn (maize), beans, and rice stored for a long time in a moist, warm atmosphere tend to go mouldy due to the growth of a fungus called *Aspergillus flavus*. This fungus produces complex organic poisons, called aflatoxins, that damage the liver if eaten in large amounts. People infected with the hepatitis B virus are particularly susceptible to the harmful effects of the toxins. In addition, aflatoxins are highly carcinogenic. Stored peanuts are particularly vulnerable to the fungus. Even freshly picked peanuts contain some aflatoxins, but the level is usually too low to be harmful. Most processed nuts are subjected to rigorous controls to prevent contamination. Salt also protects against the mould. However, peanuts or peanut products showing any sign of mould should be discarded. The mould can usually be detected by a white or brownish bloom on the nuts, or by a musty taste.

ageing

As we grow older, we tend to become physically weaker, bones become more brittle and break more easily (*see* **osteoporosis**), reaction times are slower, and fitness declines. The desire and ability to exercise often diminishes, so the tendency to put on body weight (especially in the form of fat) increases. Consequently, the body mass index will also increase. The US National Research Council states that the desirable body mass index range increases with age (from 19 to 24 for a 20-year-old to 24–29 for a 65-year-old). Nevertheless, it is usually difficult for older people to maintain their desirable body mass index because basal metabolic rate decreases as muscle mass declines with age and lack of exercise. After the age of 60 years, metabolism slows down at a rate of up to three per cent a year. Even if activity levels remain the same, energy intake must drop to avoid excessive weight gain. A lower energy intake (and therefore total food intake) makes it more difficult to ensure adequate supplies of vitamins and minerals. Thus, it is very important that elderly people eat a well-balanced diet, rich in these nutrients.

Although you cannot change all of the ageing processes, many authorities believe that several of them are actually caused by other factors, such as inactivity. This type of ageing (called acquired ageing) is not inevitable and can be avoided or delayed by taking regular aerobic exercise, eating a balanced diet, and reducing stress. Gerontologists generally agree that poor physical fitness is one of the greatest problems of the elderly, and that a well-designed programme of exercise could help to reduce the effects of ageing, and improve both physical and mental well-being. Ageing curves of exercisers and sedentary people indicate that

a steady deterioration in fitness occurs with each decade, but the deterioration is much less in active people than in those who are inactive.

You are never too old to benefit from exercise. Regular exercise three times a week, consisting of strength training sandwiched between stretching and cycling for the warm up and cool down, can improve strength by over 90 per cent in men and women aged between 56 and 80. This type of exercise will increase total energy expenditure by up to 15 per cent per day, even if the workout uses less than 250 calories. So, regular exercise can increase the strength and fitness of older exercisers, and enable them to control their weight more easily than non-exercisers. Diet may also affect the ageing process. Laboratory mice and rats kept on a calorie-restricted diet live longer and have less age-related diseases than animals fed on unrestricted diets. The applicability of these results to humans is questionable, but there is a growing body of evidence to support the notion that a well-balanced, calorie-controlled diet can delay ageing. There is also a strong suggestion that many foods are potential carcinogens (even glucose may react with amino acids to form mutagens) and that too much food increases the risk of harmful mutations. On the other hand, foods rich in antioxidants (e.g. vitamins A, C, and E) may slow down the ageing process by mopping up the free radicals that many scientists believe are the underlying cause of ageing.

You cannot halt ageing. It starts at conception and ends at death. But you can increase your chances of maintaining a high level of health throughout your life by taking regular aerobic exercise and eating sensibly.

agility

Agility is the ability to change body position rapidly and accurately without losing balance. It is important in sports and activities in which opponents or obstacles have to be avoided (e.g. slalom events). It is a basic component of physical fitness. Although its exact nature has not been determined, it depends on muscular power, reaction time, coordination, and dynamic flexibility.

Figure 3 Illinois Agility Run

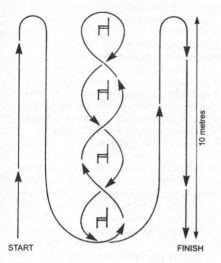

START   FINISH

10 metres

You can use the Illinois Agility Run to evaluate your own agility (figure 3). Mark out two lines 10 metres apart and place four obstacles (e.g. chairs) at regular intervals of 3.3 metres between the lines. Lie prone with your head against the start line and with your hands beside your shoulders. Get a partner to start and time the run. On the command 'go', get up and run as fast as possible, following the course shown in the figure. Use the following table to rate your agility:

TIME IN SECONDS

MALE	FEMALE	RATING
<15.2	<17.0	excellent
16.1	17.9–17.0	good
18.1–16.2	21.7–18.0	average
18.3–18.2	23.0–21.8	fair
>18.3	>23.0	poor

AIDS: *See* **Acquired Immune Deficiency Syndrome.**

aikido: *See* **martial arts.**

Air Force diet: *See* **ketogenic diet.**

air pollutants

Air pollutants include a multitude of substances that reduce the quality of the environment and make it more dangerous. These noxious substances have a cumulative effect. They may affect various parts of the body, but they are particularly damaging to the lungs, reducing the ability to supply oxygen to the body. High pollution levels therefore reduce your ability to exercise.

In many cities, car exhaust fumes create high concentrations of nitrogen oxides, ozone and carbon monoxide. Ozone inhalation can tighten the chest and induce asthma-like symptoms, including nausea, throat irritation, and burning eyes. Inhalation of carbon monoxide reduces the capacity of blood to carry oxygen. Cycling in heavy traffic for half an hour is equivalent to chain-smoking up to 20 cigarettes. Many cyclists in New York, Tokyo, London, and other large cities resort to wearing face masks to filter the air in an attempt to limit the intake of these noxious gases. Runners training in traffic have similar problems, but they can usually escape to nearby parks and wooded areas that have lower pollution levels.

A diet rich in antioxidants (e.g. vitamins A, C, and E) may offer protection against some of the damaging effects of air pollution.

air resistance

Air resistance is the enemy common to all runners and cyclists. Air produces frictional forces which tend to reduce the speed of anyone moving through it. About eight per cent of a runner's energy is expended in overcoming air resistance, but up to 80 per cent of that energy can be saved by drafting (running directly behind another runner). During cycling even greater savings of energy can be made. The larger the group of cyclists and the further from the front the cyclist rides, the greater the energy saved. This is why it is much easier to ride towards the back of the peloton in the Tour de France, than to ride at the head of the race.

alanine

An amino acid involved in the production of glucose and glycogen. Alanine production is increased in exercising muscle, especially in the fasting state. Some bodybuilders and weight-lifters take alanine supplements to increase muscle glycogen levels, and improve their muscular endurance and strength-training ability. Alanine, however, is one of the truly non-essential amino acids. There is no evidence that synthesis from other amino acids is ever inadequate to meet demands, unlike some non-essential amino acids which may be synthesized in inadequate amounts under some conditions. Research on amino acid supplementation shows no beneficial effects on strength, power, or muscle growth.

alcohol

Alcohol (or more precisely ethanol) is a colourless, tasteless, flammable liquid, formed during the fermentation of yeasts. In medicine, it is used as a tincture and antiseptic but its greatest use is in drinks. It is quickly absorbed into the bloodstream from the mouth cavity and stomach. After absorption, it acts as a depressant on the central nervous system. This may have the beneficial effect of reducing feelings of fatigue but it also reduces judgement, self-control, and concentration. Reactions are slowed by alcohol and muscular coordination is impaired. Alcohol also acts as a diuretic, stimulating the kidneys to eliminate more urine which can result in dehydration.

Alcohol can lessen hand tremor and improve performance in 'aiming' sports such as archery, fencing, and shooting, but because of its potentially harmful effects, its use is restricted by some sports federations.

Alcohol and its after-effects decrease aerobic fitness. Tests of rugby players showed that those suffering from a hangover 16 hours after drinking alcohol performed on average almost 12 per cent worse than when they had no hangover.

Alcohol is no great friend to the athlete, nor is it to those on a weight-loss diet. Each gram of pure alcohol provides 7 Calories (7000 calories) of energy. In addition, alcoholic beverages often contain sugar and other nutrients, increasing their calorific value. A single measure of spirits contains about 50 Calories, and one pint of lager contains about 170 Calories. Drinking too much alcohol can lead to obesity because some is converted to fat. Despite its relatively high energy content, alcohol is a poor energy source compared with carbohydrate because it cannot be used directly by muscles, and because of its adverse effects. Before it can be used by heart muscle and skeletal muscle, alcohol has to be broken down in the liver to acetate or acetaldehydes. The breakdown is relatively slow which is why alcohol can remain in the bloodstream for several hours. Alcohol can also inhibit the conversion of glycogen to glucose in the liver. If it is ingested during prolonged exercise it can increase the likelihood of hypoglycaemia (abnormally low blood sugar).

Moderate drinking has not been linked to any significant health problems. On the contrary, several studies have shown that it can be beneficial and may reduce the risk of coronary heart disease by preventing platelets in the blood from sticking together. However, chronic, heavy drinking is a significant health risk: it can shrink the brain; it irritates the stomach and small intestine, resulting in malabsorption and deficiencies of vitamins and minerals; it can damage the liver and cause cirrhosis; and it can adversely affect the cardiovascular system, increasing the risk of heart attacks. Heavy drinking is not compatible with a healthy, active lifestyle.

As a general rule the following alcoholic drinks contain roughly the same amount of ethyl alcohol (about 8 grams):

- a single measure of whisky or other spirit (about 25 ml)
- a glass of wine (125 ml)
- a small glass of sherry or other fortified wine (about 80 ml)
- half a pint of cider, lager or beer (figure 4).

These amounts are often said to equal '1 unit of alcohol'. Although this guide is useful, it can be misleading because some drinks are stronger than others. You can work out exactly how many units are in a drink by the alcohol percentage on the label:

number of units = % alcohol/1000 × volume in ml

For example, a bottle of claret with 12 per cent alcohol has 9 units (12/1000 × 750). Assuming six glasses to the bottle, each glass will contain 1.5 units.

Figure 4 Alcohol. Each of these glasses contains 1 unit of alcohol

| Single measure of whisky (25 mL) | Glass of wine (100 mL) | Small glass of sherry | Half pint of ordinary cider | Quarter pint of strong cider |

The safe maximum amounts per week are:

- 21 units for a man, plus at least 2 days without alcohol
- 14 units for a non-pregnant woman, plus 2 days without alcohol.

It should be remembered, however, that effects of alcohol depend not only on the amount of consumption, but also on the rate. Drinking more than one glass of wine per hour can damage your liver.

A Scottish study showed that there was no adverse effect on the babies of women who drank up to 8 units a week when they were pregnant. Nevertheless, pregnant women, those planning a pregnancy, and nursing mothers are generally advised to take no alcohol because it can pass from the mother's bloodstream to the baby. The risk is greatest during the early stages of pregnancy when the baby's brain is developing.

Alexander technique

A technique that corrects established defects of posture, particularly those related to the back when lying, sitting, standing, or walking. According to its deviser, the Australian therapist F.M. Alexander, the technique promotes relaxation and can help eliminate aches, pains, and other disorders associated with muscle tension and poor posture.

alimentary canal (gut)

A tubular passage extending from the mouth to the anus (figure 5). It has regions specialized for ingestion (the mouth and buccal cavity), digestion (mainly the stomach and small intestine), absorption (mainly the small intestine

Figure 5 Alimentary canal

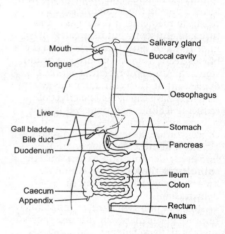

for food and large intestine for water), and egestion (rectum and anus).

alkali (alkalosis; alkalinizer)

An alkali is a substance that has a high pH when in solution and tends to neutralize acids. The amount of alkali available in the body to act as a buffer, moderating changes in pH, is called the alkali reserve or standard bicarbonate (because most of the alkali is in the form of bicarbonate ions). A high alkali reserve is particularly important for those involved in high-intensity activities lasting up to three minutes (e.g. 800 metre run). The bicarbonate ions help to neutralize lactic acid produced during anaerobic respiration. Some athletes boost their alkali reserve artificially by ingesting extra amounts of sodium bicarbonate. This can enhance performance for maximal effort activities of 1–7 minutes duration. When used in this way, sodium bicarbonate is called an alkalinizer. Alkalinizers have also been used by some athletes to avoid drug detection. By raising the pH, they reduce the excretion of metabolic by-products of some stimulant drugs, thereby masking them.

Although a high alkali reserve is beneficial, an abnormally high pH in the blood or tissue fluids (a condition called alkalosis) can be harmful. The excess alkali can make muscles overreact, causing them to go into cramp-like spasms. There are two forms of alkalosis. Respiratory alkalosis usually results from hyperventilation (heavy breathing) which reduces carbon dioxide levels in the body fluids. It can also occur at high altitudes where the air is thin and oxygen levels are low. Metabolic alkalosis often results from ingesting excessive amounts of alkalinizers, or from losing large amounts of acid (for example, by vomiting the acidic stomach contents). *Compare* **acidosis**.

alkalinizer: *See* alkali.

alkalosis: *See* alkali.

allergy

The word 'allergy' was first used in 1906 by a Viennese paediatrician, Baron Clemens von Pirquet, to mean 'altered reactivity'. It was applied to any abnormal response to a substance. This wide meaning has been retained by some people, but in Britain many doctors limit the term to responses which involve an overreaction by the body's immune system. Such responses include the classic allergic disorders of asthma, eczema, hay fever, non-seasonal rhinitis (runny nose) and urticaria (nettle rash). These disorders may be triggered by pollen, house dust, fungi, drugs, air pollutants, and some food constituents. The specific allergy-causing substance (allergen) provokes an immunological reaction in skin-prick tests. In the 1960s, scientists discovered that such reactions involve the production of a specific antibody called immunoglobulin E. This binds to the surface of special large cells (mast cells), stimulating them to secrete histamine, serotonin, and prostaglandins.

These are the chemicals that produce the allergic reactions such as inflammation of the nasal membranes in hay fever or the contraction of the tubes leading to the lungs which causes asthma.

True food allergies involve the release of immunoglobulin E when a problem food is eaten. Allergens occur in cow's milk, eggs, nuts, fish, and shellfish, causing allergic reactions that show up in skin and blood tests. They also produce symptoms such as urticaria and a tight chest that makes breathing difficult. Most reactions are short-lived and relatively harmless, but severe allergic reactions leading to anaphylactic shock and death are not uncommon. These reactions may occur in food allergies (nuts are an especial problem) and in response to bee stings in sensitive people. Very few people (probably less than 1 per cent) suffer a true food allergy but between 20 and 30 per cent may have an adverse reaction to food which is not revealed by skin or blood tests (*see* **food intolerance**).

altitude

As altitude increases, air temperature and pressure decrease and there is less oxygen available for aerobic activities. This lack of oxygen can severely limit the physical performance of endurance athletes and climbers, particularly those accustomed to living at low altitudes. The thin air, however, offers less resistance to sprinters and jumpers, so it is generally easier to perform these activities at high altitudes than at sea level.

High altitudes are potentially dangerous environments. Anyone who ascends too quickly above 2100 metres can become sick. Individuals differ in their susceptibility to altitude or mountain sickness, but nearly everyone suffers above a height of 4900 metres. Twenty five per cent of visitors to the Colorado skiing areas, just 3000 metres above sea level, suffer some form of altitude sickness. The risk appears to be less if you sleep at a lower altitude than the one at which you are active; the mountaineer's advice 'play high, sleep low' appears to be sound.

Altitude sickness is caused by lack of oxygen and is characterized by shortness of breath, feelings of lassitude, muscular weakness, headaches, rapid pulse, loss of appetite, nausea, and sometimes fainting. The symptoms become more severe the higher a person ascends and the faster the ascent is made, but they usually quickly disappear when the sufferer returns to lower altitudes and rests.

It can be fatal to continue climbing when suffering from altitude sickness. Each year several people die in high mountain regions such as the Himalayas. The situation is likely to worsen as more people take to the mountains on organized expedition treks. Altitude sickness is best avoided by ascending slowly, drinking plenty of fluids (non-alcoholic!), and giving your body the opportunity to acclimatize to low oxygen levels.

Altitude acclimatization consists of a number of reversible physiological adaptations. These enable the body to cope with low oxygen levels. In the early stages of acclimatization, breathing and heart rate increase. Major long-term adaptations include the production of more red blood cells, an increase in the haemoglobin content of the blood, and a greater blood supply to muscles. All these adaptations help to improve the ability of the blood to carry oxygen to respiring tissues. Biochemical changes also help the muscles to utilize oxygen more efficiently. Acclimatization to medium altitudes (1829 m above sea level) takes about two weeks, but acclimatization to high altitudes (more than 3048 m above sea level) may take much longer.

Many elite athletes train at medium altitudes to benefit from the effects of altitude acclimatization and to enhance performance in endurance events. Most exercise scientists believe that the training is of significant benefit only to those who intend competing at high altitudes, and that it is of little benefit to sea-level competitors. To be effective, altitude training must take place at least 1500 metres above sea level and for a period of not less than three weeks, with the first week consisting of light exercise only. It is, however, risky to train at altitudes for very long periods because it may lead to loss of muscle and body weight. It takes three to six weeks at sea level to lose all the effects of altitude training and acclimatization.

altitude acclimatization: *See* altitude.

altitude sickness: *See* altitude.

altitude training: *See* altitude.

aluminium

A metallic element that does not appear to be an essential part of the diet even though the body of a 70 kg person contains about 50 mg. Aluminium is toxic and can damage nerve cells. Excess dietary aluminium is normally eliminated in the faeces, but when intakes are very high some aluminium may be retained. Some researchers claim that this retention can contribute to the development of Alzheimer's disease (senile dementia). A study by the Medical Research Council showed that sufferers of the disease have unusual clusters of nerve cells in the brain saturated with aluminium. There is some evidence that vitamin C may help to reduce aluminium levels in the body.

Alzheimer's disease

Alzheimer's disease is a mysterious, progressive degeneration of the brain that shares some of the characteristics of dementia: memory disorders, changes in personality, deterioration in personal care, impaired reasoning ability, and disorientation. It is the fourth biggest killer in the developed world after heart disease, cancer, and stroke. There are millions of sufferers worldwide. The disease can occur at any age but it is more common among the elderly. Unlike some other forms of secondary dementia, Alzheimer's disease is generally regarded as incurable.

Several theories have been proposed to explain the development of the disease. One theory is based on the observation that high concentrations of aluminium may accumulate in the brain. Several groups of research workers have suggested that aluminium taken in the diet over a long period of time may contribute to the development of the disease, but this suggestion has not been generally accepted. Nevertheless, to be on the safe side, aluminium utensils should not be used for cooking acidic foods (e.g. fruits) because the mineral can be absorbed into the food. Some researchers suggest that the disease is due to an accumulation of a protein (amyloid protein) that congests the brain. In 1992, scientists in the United States showed that a genetic defect may stimulate the production of this protein in some sufferers. A recent theory suggests that Alzheimer's disease may be an inflammatory response which can be slowed or even stopped by aspirin-like drugs. These and other suggestions remain controversial. Despite billions of dollars being spent on research and many theories being postulated, no definitive cause is known. It is possible that there are several forms of the disease and that a number of genetic and environmental factors (including diet) contribute to their development.

amenorrhoea

Absence of periods or menses (the flow of blood from the genital tract of women during menstruation). There are many causes of amenorrhoea including pregnancy, stress, weight loss and extreme thinness (amenorrhoea is one of the symptoms of anorexia), and high levels of exercise. The latter condition is sometimes called athletic amenorrhoea. It is relatively common among middle- and long-distance runners, gymnasts, and dancers who tend to have low body weights and a low percentage body fat. There is good evidence that menstruation ceases when the percentage of body fat falls below a critical level, but the relationship between fat levels and menstruation is not simple. Some extremely thin female athletes menstruate normally while others with a higher body fat content are amenorrhoeic. Athletic amenorrhoea is probably due to a number of factors, including the stress associated with regular, intense exercise.

Until recently, athletic amenorrhoea has been regarded as a harmless variation of the female rhythm since it does not affect long-term fertility. However, failure to menstruate over a long period of time is linked with reduced secretions of female hormones, such as oestrogens. These hormones are made in adipose tissue as well as the ovaries; therefore when the levels of body fat are very low, oestrogen production is reduced. Oestrogens

are required for normal mineralization of bone. Low levels of female hormones in young women are associated with a weakening of bones, an increased risk of stress fractures, and osteoporosis. The situation is further exacerbated if the dietary intake of calcium is low. Nevertheless, people of all ages (except young amenorrheic women with low blood oestrogen levels) benefit from exercise, particularly when it is combined with a high calcium diet. It increases bone mineralization and reduces the risk of osteoporosis. *See also* **menstruation**.

American football

American Football is a tough contact sport that dominates the American sporting scene and is gaining popularity in Europe. It is a game requiring all-round physical fitness. Players have to be fast, strong, and proficient in the six basic skills of football: passing, catching, running, blocking, tackling, and kicking. American football has always been associated with a large number of injuries, not surprising when the game commonly involves players in excess of 240 pounds colliding with each other at full speed. In the United States, it is estimated that more than 300 000 high school players, 35 000 college players, and half of the National Football League players are injured to some extent each season. Head and neck injuries are common: there are approximately 250 000 incidents of concussion each year. Some injuries have been fatal or have resulted in players becoming permanent quadriplegics. However, the number of very severe injuries has declined in recent years. This is probably due to rule changes concerning tackling and blocking with the head, and improvements in protective equipment which were introduced in 1976. There has also been a greater emphasis in training on strengthening the muscles of the neck and learning good tackling techniques. This is particularly important in the younger age group.

Protective clothing is an essential feature of modern football, but this makes the players vulnerable to heat stroke. One study reported 12 heat stroke deaths among college and high school football players over a three year period. The victims were all interior linemen, probably the players required to work hardest and longest; most were stricken during pre-season practice so they may have been in poor physical condition; all were dressed in full uniforms which increases workload and interferes with heat loss; and most were not permitted to drink water during practice. Clearly, it is essential that players and officials should be aware of the risk of heat stroke, and ensure that drinking water is available during practice and games.

amino acids

These are the chemicals which form the building blocks of protein. There are about 80 naturally occurring amino acids, but only about 20 are used in proteins. Some amino acids, the essential or indispensable amino acids, can be obtained only from the diet. The other amino acids can be synthesized in the body provided that the total intake of protein is adequate. Amino acids may be used as an energy source during endurance activities, but they probably supply no more than 10 per cent of the body's demands. Some amino acids (such as gamma-aminobutyric acid and glutamate) function as neurotransmitters, acting as chemical intermediaries during the transmission of nerve impulses.

ESSENTIAL AMINO ACIDS

- histidine
- isoleucine
- leucine
- lysine
- methionine
- phenylalanine
- threonine
- tryptophan
- valine

NON-ESSENTIAL AMINO ACIDS

- alanine
- arginine
- aspartic acid
- cysteine (made only from methionine)
- cystine (made only from methionine)
- glutamic acid
- glutamine
- glycine
- hydroxyproline

- ornithine
- proline
- serine
- tyrosine (made only from phenylalanine)

amino acid supplements

Amino acid supplements come in the form of pills, capsules, or powders containing a particular concoction of amino acids. Manufacturers usually claim the supplements have special properties, for example, to cure herpes, strengthen fingernails, cure split ends in the hair, improve sleep patterns, or relieve pain and depression. Dieters may take them to spare their bodies' protein while losing weight. One particular combination of amino acids (which includes arginine, lysine, and ornithine), is sold as a slimming aid, accelerating weight loss. There is little scientific evidence to support these claims.

Most amino acid supplements are sold as anabolic agents to help in bodybuilding; arginine and ornithine are two constituents frequently promoted as 'natural steroids' (a distinctly misleading name since they are chemically very different from steroids). Since amino acids are the building blocks of protein, the main component of muscle, it is not surprising that many people believe that, by taking extra amino acids, they can develop larger muscles. But it is important to note that a muscle grows only in response to extra physical demands placed on it. Excess amino acids not needed for growth or repair of body tissues are broken down and excreted as urea, converted into glucose and used as an energy source, or converted to body fat. There is some evidence to support the use of amino acid supplements when there is a natural stimulus to increase muscle bulk, for example during the initial stages of training. There is no scientific evidence, however, to support claims that amino acid supplements improve strength, power, muscle growth, or work capacity. Most nutritionists state emphatically that a normal, healthy person eating a well-balanced diet does not need amino acid supplements. Overconsumption causes health risks. Unbalanced amino acid mixtures or single amino acids may be toxic. If amino-acid supplements are used as the basis of a high-protein, low fat diet they can be downright dangerous because they can cause abnormal heart rhythms. *See also* **ketogenic diets and tryptophan.**

amphetamines (pep pills)

A group of chemicals belonging to the class of drugs called stimulants. Although their effects are inconsistent, amphetamines act as powerful stimulants on the central nervous system producing feelings of euphoria, aggression, and alertness which may be achieved at the expense of good judgment and self-criticism. They suppress feelings of hunger and were used in slimming pills. But because they are addictive, amphetamines have been replaced by a number of their derivatives (e.g. fenfluramine). Although not as dangerous as amphetamines, these derivatives, in addition to suppressing appetite, may still induce harmful side-effects (e.g. insomnia, depression, and pulmonary hypertension). In 1996, misuse was linked to 15 deaths in the UK. The General Medical Council advise that amphetamine-style drugs should be used only under expert medical supervision to treat certain forms of obesity.

Amphetamines tend to increase metabolic rate, cardiac output, blood pressure, blood glucose levels, and arousal. Claims that they improve the ability to carry out strenuous physical exercise have not been supported by scientific evidence. These drugs are potentially very harmful. Usage may be followed by severe bouts of depression and dependence. Several fatalities have been attributed to the ability of amphetamines to suppress feelings of fatigue, permitting individuals to over-exert themselves to such an extent that they suffer heat stroke and cardiac failure. In 1967, the cyclist Tommy Simpson collapsed during a very long climb in the Tour de France. He died on arrival to hospital. An autopsy revealed that amphetamines almost certainly contributed to his death from heat stroke.

amygdalin: *See* **laetrile.**

anabolic steroids

Anabolic steroids are synthetic drugs similar to the male hormone, testosterone. They are taken as tablets, in powder form, or by intramuscular injection, to improve muscle growth, strength, and power. They can be acquired on prescription for the treatment of a number of diseases including anaemia, breast cancer, and post-surgical muscle wasting. But an estimated 200 000 users in the UK take the drugs to enhance their appearance or strength. Several routes of administration are used simultaneously; a process called stacking. Abusers believe that stacking enhances the effects of the drugs. Anabolic steroids may also increase the ability to train hard because they improve muscle repair and tolerance to fatigue. Until relatively recently, the abuse of anabolic steroids was confined mainly to athletes and adult bodybuilders. Now there seems to be a significant increase in the number of young people, both male and female, taking the drugs. Some estimates place anabolic steroid abuse among young males in American high schools as high as 10 per cent; some are participants in competitive sports but many are not. There is a cultural trend in Western countries for young men to dance at parties with their upper bodies exposed. Many youngsters (some as young as fifteen or less) take anabolic steroids in an attempt to develop well-defined upper body muscles to impress their friends. Young women also take the drug as a short-cut to firm, well-toned bodies low in fat. Users of anabolic steroids may also feel stronger, more aggressive, and more confident. Many law enforcers are seriously concerned that increased aggression associated with steroids (known as 'roid rage') is leading more young people to commit violent crimes. If children and teenagers take anabolic steroids regularly, the drugs can adversely affect their skeletal growth. Adults who take anabolic steroids may be affected psychologically, their livers may become damaged, and they may suffer heart disorders. Numerous investigators report that steroid abuse in males may reduce the size of the testes (reflected by decreased testicular tissue on biopsy) and reduce sperm production. In females, the steroids may cause the development of secondary male characteristics such as growth of facial hair, enlargement of the clitoris, disruption of the menstrual cycle, and reduced breast size. Anabolic steroids are responsible for much of the drug abuse in sport. They are on the International Olympic Committee's list of banned substances.

anabolism

Chemical reactions that take place in the body and are concerned with the synthesis of large molecules from smaller ones. Anabolism is necessary for body-building, growth, and repair.

anaemia

A condition in which the amount of haemoglobin in the blood of an individual, or the number of red blood cells, is below the normal range for a healthy population of comparable age and sex. The standard varies, but in women the haemoglobin concentration is normally greater than 12 grams per decilitre and in men is greater than 13 grams per decilitre. Anaemia may reduce the oxygen-carrying ability of the blood. It is characterized by brittle or ridged fingernails, loss of appetite, abdominal pains, tiredness, shortness of breath, and headaches.

The most common cause of anaemia is iron deficiency. Iron is an essential component of haemoglobin. Iron deficiency may result from lack of iron in the diet; inadequate absorption through the intestinal wall into the bloodstream (coffee, for example, can reduce iron absorption by 40–50 per cent); or excess losses, usually through bleeding (e.g. during menstruation). Iron deficiency affects 10–15 per cent of women of menstruating age, because iron lost in menstrual blood exceeds the iron obtained from food. These women usually require iron supplements. Those on a strict weight-loss or weight-maintenance diet (such as female gymnasts) often suffer from anaemia. Anaemia caused by dietary deficiencies can be rectified by eating plenty of lean red meat, beans, or peas.

Many endurance athletes appear to suffer from anaemia because they have low haemoglobin and red blood cell concentrations. This so-called sports anaemia is usually due to an expansion in blood volume which dilutes the concentration of haemoglobin and red blood cells. Rather than causing the athlete any harm, the increased plasma volume is beneficial to fitness and health by making the blood flow more easily and increasing the efficiency of the heart. This increase more than offsets the fall in haemoglobin concentration as it means that more oxygen can be delivered to muscles. Sports anaemia is not true anaemia but is, in medical terms, a dilutional pseudoanaemia. *See also* **iron**.

anaerobic exercise

An exercise performed at a high intensity and requiring a rate of energy production greater than that supplied by aerobic respiration. A totally anaerobic exercise is an all-out effort of short duration, such as a 100 metre sprint or a clean-and-jerk in weight-lifting. It uses the phosphagen system (sometimes called the ATP-PCr system) of respiration which relies on special high-energy stores. These stores are used as a very quick source of ATP, the chemical required by muscles to contract. The phosphagen system can sustain a maximum effort for only about 10 seconds after which the stores become exhausted. High intensity exercises of longer duration also rely, at least partly, on anaerobic sources of energy. They use a different type of anaerobic respiration, with muscle glycogen as the energy source and lactic acid as a waste product. These exercises can be performed only at submaximal efforts (up to about 90 per cent). A 90 per cent effort can be sustained for a maximum of two or three minutes.

A training programme that includes short bursts of activity is important for many athletes but less important for a personal fitness programme. Such training can be very demanding physically and psychologically. It can harm those not used to strenuous activity. Even a physically fit person must take sufficient rest between sessions of anaerobic exercise so that the body can recover and adapt to the high demands. It is generally advised that anaerobic exercise should be carried out on no more than three days in any one week.

anaerobic threshold

If you start running at a slow pace and gradually increase your speed, there comes a point when the energy supplied by aerobic (oxygen-dependent) respiration is insufficient to sustain your activity. Put simply, you start to get out of breath. This point is known as the anaerobic threshold and reflects your capacity to work at a steady state. It is an important indicator of aerobic fitness. A number of methods have been used to determine this threshold (*see* **blood lactate** and **conversational index**), but none is completely satisfactory. Nevertheless, whichever method is used the anaerobic threshold is higher in those who perform regular, vigorous aerobic exercises than in sedentary people.

anaesthetic

A substance that produces partial or complete loss of sensation either in a restricted area (regional and local anaesthetics) or in the whole body (general anaesthetic). Use of local anaesthetics to treat sports injuries and other ailments is permitted by the International Olympic Committee and most other sports federations, but only under certain conditions.

anal fissure

An anal fissure is a crack-like sore in the anal region. It is the commonest reason for pain in this area. Causes include constipation and the passage of hard stools. As well as being painful, anal fissures may bleed moderately. They can be a particular problem for cyclists and horse riders. The best treatment is scrupulous hygiene, avoidance of constipation by eating a high-fibre diet, and drinking plenty of water. Sometimes analgesic anti-inflammatories are prescribed.

anal itching

Itching of the skin in the anal region often results from faecal soilage, but anal fissures and haemorrhoids are also causes. Itching is exacerbated by sitting on a plastic seat, wearing tight clothes, and the accumulation of sweat in buttocks. Cyclists and horse riders are particularly vulnerable to this complaint because of anal irritation. In most cases of anal itching, simple remedies are sufficient. These include meticulous, gentle cleaning of the affected area with soap and water, followed by thorough rinsing and drying with cotton wool; wearing cotton undergarments; wearing loose clothing; and minimizing exercises which result in anal irritation. In some cases, corticosteroid lotions are prescribed to relieve the itching and allow the skin to heal. Occasionally the condition is caused by infection with an intestinal worm (e.g. threadworms, roundworms, or tapeworms), in which case treatment with a special drug, such as mebendazole (for roundworms and tapeworms) or niclosamide may be necessary.

anaphylactic shock

An immediate over-reaction of the immune system following the administration of a drug or other agent (especially an allergen; *see* **allergy**), in an individual who has been previously exposed to the agent and who has produced antibodies against it. Anaphylactic shock is a potentially fatal form of hypersensitivity (*see* **anaphylaxis**). It is characterized by nausea, lowered blood pressure, irregular heart beats, vomiting, and difficulty in breathing due to a swelling of the larynx. It may lead to coma and death.

anaphylaxis

Hypersensitivity to certain agents, resulting in pain, swelling, and feverishness. A form of anaphylaxis occurs in individuals suffering from nettle rash (urticaria) or asthma, and those who eat foods to which their bodies are allergic (*see* **food allergy**).

A condition called exercise-induced anaphylaxis is triggered in some people by combinations of exercise and particular foods. Typically, symptoms occur five minutes into a bout of intense exercise. Itching is the most common symptom, but others include rashes and difficulty in breathing. The most common food associated with exercise-induced anaphylaxis is raw celery, but other foods including shellfish, peaches, grapes, wheat, and alcohol may increase the risk of an attack. Medications, such as aspirin and antibiotics, have also been linked with the condition. In the USA, there have been over 1000 documented cases of exercise-induced anaphylaxis but no reports of death. However, other forms of anaphylaxis can be more serious (*see* **anaphylactic shock**).

androgen
Any substance that promotes the development of male secondary sexual characteristics (e.g. growth of facial hair and increase in muscle bulk). *See also* **anabolic steroids**.

android fat distribution
The distribution of excess fat, laid down as adipose tissue, predominantly around the abdomen and trunk, and within the abdominal cavity. Fat distribution of this type can result in 'apple-shaped' obesity which carries an increased risk of diabetes and heart disease. It is far more common in males than females.
Although it is not entirely clear why android fat distribution increases the risk of coronary heart diseases, one suggestion is that abdominal fat may be more readily broken down under stress, raising the fatty acid concentration of the blood. This would increase the risk of fat deposition and clogging of the arteries which in turn may lead to high blood pressure and cardiovascular diseases. *See also* **waist-hip ratio**; *compare* **gynoid fat distribution**.

angina (angina pectoris)
A gripping, vice-like pain in the chest which sometimes extends down the left arm. It is induced by increases in physical exertion and relieved by rest. The pain usually lasts about 15 minutes. Angina is a symptom of heart disease. It results from a narrowing of the coronary arteries which reduces the oxygen supply to heart muscle. Pain is produced when the heart muscle does not receive enough oxygen to cope with its workload. A controlled programme of physical activity can benefit angina sufferers, provided it is performed under medical supervision and at a safe level. The appropriate level is usually determined by an exercise test on a cycle ergometer or a treadmill in the presence of a doctor.

anhydrosis (anidrosis)
A condition characterized by the absence or the abnormal reduction of sweating.

Anhydrosis may occur when the normal temperature control mechanisms fail, leading to overheating (*see* **hyperthermia** and **heat stroke**).

animal starch: *See* glycogen.

ankle sprain
Ankle sprain is the most common injury in sport. The ankle forms the area around the joint between the lower parts of the tibia and fibula, and the tarsal bones at the back of the foot. It is a complex joint, criss-crossed by a number of ligaments that can be damaged easily when the foot is turned over. Treatment usually consists of rest, application of ice, compression, and elevation (*see* **RICE**). Non-steroidal anti-inflammatories (e.g. aspirin or ibuprofen) are often taken to relieve the swelling and pain. Ankle sprains are less likely to occur in those with strong and flexible ankles (*see* **ankle stretchers** and **heel raise**).

ankle stretchers
Flexibility of the ankle can be improved by slowly rotating the joint through its full range of movement and by performing the following simple stretching exercises.

- Sit on the floor with your right leg crossed over your left leg so that you can manipulate your right foot. Extend your right foot and stretch the toes. By grasping the top of foot with your left hand and the heel with your right hand, use your hands to stretch the toes a little further.

- Kneel with your hands on the floor to support your body. Slowly lower your buttocks towards and, if possible, onto your heels. Hold the stretched position for about 10 seconds, then relax.

anorexia: *See* anorexia nervosa.

anorexia nervosa
Anorexia nervosa is usually abbreviated to anorexia, and is sometimes referred to as self-starvation syndrome. It is a potentially fatal eating disorder in which there is a loss of appetite or desire for food, leading to severe loss of body weight. Clinical diagnosis is usually based on the following criteria:

- weight less than 85 per cent ideal weight
- intense fear of becoming obese, even when underweight
- disturbance of body image (i.e. feeling fat even when thin)
- in women, cessation of periods for three or more consecutive cycles when not on the contraceptive pill.

Anorexia is often associated with other eating disorders, such as bulimia nervosa. Although it can affect adults, both male and female, it occurs most frequently in adolescent girls. Anorexics are ten times more likely to be female than male.

Anorexia is now recognized as a serious psychological illness and is on the increase in Western societies (one estimate gives a 360 per cent increase over the last 9 years). Anorexics are usually emotionally disturbed and have a distorted body image. They are often convinced that they should be thinner even when their body weight is well below average. They will go to extreme lengths to restrict eating and to lose weight because they have a phobia about becoming obese. This phobia is expressed as an intense fear of gaining weight even when they are dangerously underweight.

There are many suggested causes of anorexia. It has been linked to dietary problems in early life, parental obsessions with food, problems within the family, and rejection of adult sexuality. Some psychologists see the relentless pursuit of thinness as a desire to be autonomous, to have control over one's own body, and to gain an identity. It is also seen as an attempt constantly to please others. Anorexia has been linked with participation in certain types of sports. Gymnasts, distance runners, and dancers are believed to be prone to eating disorders because of the pressure on them to remain slim, but it is generally agreed that these disorders rarely develop into the full condition. Some sport psychologists and sports nutritionists believe that high levels of physical activity can lead to the development of anorexia nervosa. They contend that strenuous exercise can suppress appetite resulting in a reduced food intake and weight loss. Many people who perceive themselves as

being overweight exercise in order to slim. Any weight loss associated with their activity encourages them to exercise even more. This may initiate a cycle of exercise and weight loss that can lead to anorexia. However, although excessive exercise may contribute to anorexia, most experts believe that it is only one contributory factor, and does not explain the majority of cases.

Whatever the cause, the effects of anorexia are dramatic and potentially very dangerous. The persistent anorexic becomes malnourished, may suffer a variety of medical complications (including hair loss, cessation of periods, and cardiovascular abnormalities), and risks death due to starvation. One recent study reported a mortality rate of 6.6 per cent during a ten-year follow-up period.

Anorexia is much more than dieting gone wrong. It requires medical treatment and may respond to psychotherapy. The more chronic the condition, the more difficult it is to treat. If treated early, most of the physical symptoms can be corrected through adequate nutrition and the gradual restoration of normal weight. However, the underlying psychological problems may be more resistant to treatment.

anorexiant drug

A drug that acts on the brain to reduce appetite. Anorexiants are sometimes included in slimming tablets. They should be used only under strict medical supervision. The main anorectic drugs are dexfenfluramine, fenfluramine, diethyl propion, and mazindol. They have been useful in helping some individuals overcome their obesity.

antacid

A medicine that neutralizes an acidic stomach (caused by excessive secretion of hydrochloric acid in the gastric juices). Antacids (e.g. aluminium hydroxide, calcium carbonate, and magnesium hydroxide) are used to relieve the pain and discomfort of digestive disorders such as peptic ulcers and less serious conditions.

antagonist

Muscles usually occur as antagonistic pairs. Each antagonist opposes or reverses the action of its partner. For example, the triceps extends or stretches the arm, and the biceps flexes or bends it. An antagonist may also help to regulate the action of its partner by partially contracting. This resists a movement and reduces the risk of damage from an overload. It may slow or stop an action.

It is important when training to use both members of an antagonistic pair of muscles (e.g. both the quads and hamstrings in the leg) because imbalances increase the risk of injury.

anterior compartment syndrome

A potentially dangerous form of shin splints characterized by feelings of severe pain and burning, inflammation, and hardening of the tissue at the front of the lower leg around the tibia (shin bone). Its exact cause is debatable, but it may result from the expansion of muscle after prolonged training. During exercise, blood flow increases through the compartment. The muscle may swell, pressing blood vessels against the rigid structures of bone and connective tissue. This may reduce the supply of oxygen to the muscle, causing severe pain.

Anterior compartment syndrome requires radical treatment: elevation, compression with bandages, massage, and administration of anti-inflammatory and anti-diuretic drugs to reduce the swelling and eliminate excess fluids. If the condition is very severe, it may be necessary to surgically relieve the pressure on the blood vessels.

anterior cruciate ligaments

The main ligaments in the knee binding the back of the thigh bone (the femur) to the front of the shin bone (the tibia). They stop the shin bone from moving excessively forward in relation to the femur. If they are damaged, the knee becomes unstable and wobbles.

Injuries to the cruciate ligament can be dramatic, incapacitating a person instantly. Falling backwards at high speed is a common cause of such injuries among skiers, especially those who are poorly conditioned. Surgery is sometimes needed to rebind the bones.

Rehabilitation includes special exercises. A typical programme starts immediately after the operation with slow flexion on a passive motion machine. This is followed by several weeks of active bending and straightening of the knee. During this time, more strenuous activities, such as cycling on a stationary bike and exercising in water, are gradually introduced.

anthropometry

Anthropometry is the comparative study of the dimensions of the human body. It involves making precise, highly standardized measurements so that size and shape can be described objectively. Basic anthropometric measurements include those for body mass (weight), stature (height), and skinfold thickness. The procedure for taking the measurements is very strict, as illustrated by the following instructions for measuring height.

■ The individual must stand straight against an upright surface, touching it with heels, buttocks, and back. The heels should be together and on the floor. The head must be oriented so that the upper border of the ear opening and the lower border of the eye socket are on a horizontal line (the Frankfort plane). The individual must take in and hold a deep breath while height is measured to the nearest millimetre.

In many sports, success is often associated with a particular body configuration. For this reason, anthropometry can be used by coaches and trainers to help predict the activity at which an individual is most likely to succeed (*see also* **somatotype**). Anthropometry is also used extensively to monitor health (*see* **body mass index** and **waist-hip ratio**).

antibiotic

A substance secreted by a micro-organism (e.g. bacterium or fungus) that can inhibit or kill other microorganisms. The fungus *Penicillium nodosum*, for example, secretes penicillin that kills some bacteria.

Many people are concerned about the inclusion of antibiotics in animal feedstuffs to accelerate the animals' growth and protect them against disease. Although the antibiotics used in these feedstuffs are not those used in human medicine, some people still fear that antibiotics may be transferred to humans and destroy beneficial bacteria normally resident in the gut. This is not likely.

Indiscriminate use of antibiotics (e.g. not taking a full course) can encourage the development of antibiotic-resistant strains of bacteria. Hence, a particular antibiotic used successfully in the past to treat a disease may no longer be effective.

antigravity muscle

A muscle that contracts to counterbalance the effects of gravity. Antigravity muscles help to maintain posture and are often called tonic muscles.

anti-haemorrhagic vitamin: See vitamin K.

antihistamine

A drug that counteracts the effects of histamine and relieves the symptoms of some allergic conditions, such as hay fever.

antihypertensive

A drug, used in the treatment of hypertension, that reduces blood pressure.

anti-inflammatory

A drug that reduces inflammation. The most commonly used anti-inflammatory is aspirin.

antinutrients

Substances that adversely affect nutrients, for example, by interfering with their digestion or absorption. See also **lectins**; **phytic acid**; **saponins**; and **tannins**.

antioxidant

Antioxidants are chemicals that mop up unstable products of metabolism, called free radicals, which can damage the body. Antioxidants include beta-carotene, and the vitamins A, C, and E. Certain trace elements, such as copper, manganese, selenium, and zinc, also have some antioxidant properties. In addition, phenols (non-alcoholic components of red wine) and many other non-nutrient antioxidants in many plants may act as antioxidants, preventing platelets from sticking together and reducing the risk of blood clots, but this is unproven.

There is strong evidence that the combined antioxidant properties of vitamins A, C, and E provide some protection against certain cancers, particularly those of the bowel and bladder, and against cardiovascular disease. The World Health Organization recommends that we aim for a daily intake of about 450 grams (1 lb) of fruit and vegetables, especially orange and yellow fruits such as carrots, apricots, and oranges, and green vegetables, such as broccoli, and spinach (perhaps the cartoon hero Popeye had the right idea after all!). A variety of nuts, seeds and their oils should also be eaten because they are rich sources of vitamin E. Exercisers tend to consume more oxygen than sedentary people and they may produce more free radicals. Research by sports scientists indicates that consuming extra vitamins C and E may protect muscle fibres from free radical damage.

Some antioxidants, such as synthetic vitamin E (alpha tocopherol), are added to fatty foods (for example, margarine made from sunflower oil) to stop the food from going rancid. See also **free radicals**.

antiperspirant

In hot, humid conditions, exercisers usually drip with sweat as their bodies attempt to dissipate the heat generated by intense activity. Many exercisers, self-conscious of the puddles forming around them, use antiperspirants to reduce the sweating. The active ingredients in most antiperspirants are metal salts, usually those of aluminium. The metals are thought to reduce sweating by seeping into the pores of apocrine glands (sweat glands responsible for body odour) where they combine with proteins and plug the exit from the gland. Deodorants are often added to the metals to mask sweaty smells.

Antiperspirants are mostly innocuous, but some varieties can cause hypersensitive people to develop uncomfortable side-effects. In the USA, antiperspirants are classified as medicines and tested for safety. Common side-effects, such as rashes and skin irritation, are usually minor and easily treated. However, you should not use antiperspirants on broken skin because of the danger of blood poisoning. Contrary to popular belief, most antiperspirants do not seem to affect temperature regulation.

anti-rachitic factor: See vitamin D.

anti-sterility factor: *See* vitamin E.

anxiety

Anxiety produces feelings of apprehension and tension. Two components have been recognized: cognitive anxiety, characterized by distressing thought processes, and somatic anxiety expressed in physical reactions, such as butterflies and sweating. Anxiety may be an enduring personality trait (known as A-trait) or a temporary state (known as A-state). The term is often used synonymously with arousal, but anxiety corresponds only to high arousal states that produce feelings of discomfort. It is also closely associated with the concept of fear, but anxiety is more a feeling of what might happen rather than a response to an immediate fear-provoking situation.

Regular aerobic exercise may reduce general anxiety levels. Habitual exercisers often state that they feel better as a result of engaging in vigorous activity. This may be because exercise stimulates the brain to secrete endorphins, natural chemicals which have characteristics similar to morphine. Relaxation exercises may also reduce anxiety (*see* **relaxation**).

High levels of anxiety can adversely affect sporting performance. This can cause an athlete to enter an anxiety-stress spiral: the poor performance induced by anxiety results in even more anxiety and another poor performance. Anxious performers usually find it more difficult to focus attention, consequently they waste time and energy doing irrelevant tasks. *See also* **catastrophe theory**.

Apgar scores

Measurements of a baby's physical condition and mental alertness evaluated at one and five minutes after birth.

The score is given for each of the signs, so the maximum Apgar score is 10 and indicates that the baby is in an optimum condition. Apgar scores of babies born to mothers who exercise regularly are often significantly higher than those of babies of sedentary mothers.

apocrine glands: *See* sweating.

appendicitis: *See* **appendix**.

appendix

The appendix is a worm-shaped extension of the large intestine. It forms the blind end of the caecum, a pouch at the junction between the small and large intestine.

The appendix is believed to have had an important function in mammalian ancestors of humans, harbouring beneficial bacteria that enabled their hosts to break down the cellulose of plants. The human appendix has lost this function and has diminished in size during its evolution. It is therefore regarded as a vestigial, non-essential organ. One in 100 000 people has no appendix and its absence appears to do no harm.

Despite its lack of function, the appendix is relatively easily infected with bacteria. The infection may cause appendicitis, an acute inflammation causing persistent pain in the lower right abdomen, made worse by pressure, coughing, sneezing, or even slight movements. Nausea is another common symptom. Appendicitis is the commonest reason for emergency abdominal surgery. In Britain, more than 80 000 people who experience these symptoms have their appendix removed surgically. Appendicitis develops suddenly and is potentially very dangerous because the appendix may burst, spreading the infection into the surrounding membranes and causing peritonitis which can be fatal if not treated. Unfortunately, diagnosis is difficult and many of the appendices removed (up to 30 per cent in a recent Swedish study) are found to be healthy. Diagnosis becomes easier as the inflammation develops, but delay in removal increases the danger of an appendix bursting.

Apgar scores

APGAR SCORE	PULSE	RESPIRATORY EFFORT	MUSCLE TONE	COLOUR	ON SUCTION
2	>100	strong cry	active movement	pink	coughs well
1	<100	slow, irregular	limb flexion	blue limbs	depressed
0	0	nil	absent	all blue	nil

Fit people who have undergone surgery for uncomplicated appendicitis can usually return to training within a few weeks of the operation, but should not indulge in very vigorous exercise until a few weeks after that.

appestat

A hypothetical region of the brain thought to control the amount of food intake. Appetite suppressants, such as fenfluramine, probably decrease appetite by interfering with the appestat. *See also* **adipostat**.

appetite

Appetite is a psychological desire to eat and is often related to specific foods. Unlike hunger, it is probably a learned response associated with pleasant tasting and satisfying food. It is an agreeable sensation that aids digestion by stimulating the secretion of saliva and other digestive juices. It also stimulates the desire to eat sufficient food to maintain the body and supply it with enough energy and nutrients to carry out its functions. However, as with other body functions, disorders of appetite occur. Excessive appetite may result in obesity, while diminished appetite is a sign common to many illnesses and may be a manifestation of stress. There is no simple relationship between exercise and appetite, but most experts believe that appetite is likely to increase with exercise only if an individual is normally fairly active and then raises his or her activity even higher. When a sedentary person exercises, appetite may not increase, on the contrary, it may be suppressed (*see also* **anorexia nervosa**).

appetite suppressant

A wide range of over-the-counter substances are marketed as appetite suppressants. Some contain ingredients, such as bran, gums, pectin, and plant fibre, that act indirectly by swelling the stomach and making the consumer feel full. Even that arch enemy of the dieter, sugar, is supposed to reduce appetite if taken immediately before a meal (so those mothers who said that eating sweets ruins your appetite were right after all!). Although some gums reduce appetite

when taken in abnormally high concentrations, tablets containing small quantities are unlikely to have significant appetite-suppressant effects. High intakes of gums are potentially dangerous. In 1989, appetite suppressants containing more than 15 per cent guar gum or locust bean gum were banned in Britain after a number of deaths were linked to their use.

Prescribed appetite suppressants, on the other hand, are effective. They include fenfluramine (a derivative of amphetamines) and related drugs which act directly on the parts of the brain that control appetite. A review of recent studies showed that over a three-month period, slimmers who took prescribed appetite suppressants lost an average of 1.4 kg (3 lb) more than a control group who took placebos (dummy pills). Although the effect of most appetite suppressants wears off after a few months, they may be useful as a short-term measure to encourage dieters. Most doctors prescribe appetite suppressants only to those who really need them (such as the clinically obese), but their effects are also exploited by some members of the slimming industry. An investigation by reporters from the BBC revealed that several slimming clinics prescribed amphetamine derivatives to people who wanted to lose weight, even though there was no medically justifiable reason; the people were not obese nor did they have any other urgent need to lose weight for health reasons. This is a dangerous practice. Slimming drugs are potentially addictive and can have harmful side-effects such as headaches and nausea. Administration and withdrawal can be followed by severe bouts of depression and hallucinations.

Some tablets marketed as appetite suppressants are no more than sugar coated pills. They do no great harm (except to a person's bank balance) but neither do they help to reduce weight. In the UK, new regulations have been introduced to control the use of appetite suppressants and to reduce their misuse. *See also* **slimming pills**.

apple-shaped obesity: *See* **android fat distribution**.

aquarobics

Aquarobics are aerobic exercises performed in water. They have benefits similar to aerobics, but they also have additional advantages. Vigorous body movements create water turbulence which massages the superficial muscles. More importantly, the buoyant effect of water reduces the risk of joint injuries. This makes it a particularly attractive exercise for people who are overweight, or have orthopaedic or back problems. Because body weight is supported, aquarobics does not stimulate bone growth, so it does not protect against the development of osteoporosis. However, it is much better than land-based aerobics for anyone who is already suffering from brittle bones or a bad back. Many land-based athletes train in water when recovering from injuries that would be aggravated by high impact exercises. Recent research has shown that running in water (aqua running) preserves endurance and leg strength, and maintains fitness.

When exercising in water, the heart rate is lower than when exercising at a similar intensity on land. This may be due to water compressing the body and making the blood flow more easily. Whatever the reasons, it seems that the stress on the heart is less in water than on land. Nevertheless, it has been suggested that the average person uses 450 to 700 Calories during an hour of aquarobics, with 77 per cent of the calories coming from fat stores. This helps to reduce fat body mass, while movements performed against the resistance of the water stimulate muscle growth and increase lean body mass.

In 1981, the benefits of aquarobics were recognized in the United States by the President's Council on Physical Fitness and Sports, who recommended an exercise programme for small bodies of water. The programme included standing water drills (e.g. toe touching, side-straddle hopping, and jogging on the spot), pool-side standing drills (e.g. stretching the arms out and pressing the back against the wall), gutter-holding drills (e.g. knee hugs and a variety of flutter kicking), bobbing, and treading water.

Aquarobics is quickly gaining in popularity and manufacturers are responding with a whole range of exercise aids that include aquarobics footwear, buoyancy cuffs and vests, water belts which offer resistance, and peculiar devices called 'woggles'. These are six-foot long, very flexible, sausage-shaped pieces of foam that provide a buoyant weight to push against, and to act as a support when performing muscle-strengthening exercises. At the end of a workout two woggles are often used together, one under the head and the other under the knees, to give a full support for relaxation while floating.

aqua running: *See* **aquarobics**.

archery

Archery develops strength and flexibility in the upper body and arms. People of all abilities, fitness and skill levels can take part. Most injuries associated with archery are due to poor technique or overuse; few injuries are long lasting.

arches

The arches are curved structures, arch-like in profile, which span the foot. There are three arches to each foot: two longitudinal (the medial arch and lateral arch) and one short, anterior, transverse arch. Together, they form a half-dome structure which is essential for efficient load-bearing and locomotion. During standing and walking, the arches distribute half the body weight onto the heel bone, and half onto the tarsal bones in the toes. The shape of the arches is maintained by the combined action of bones, muscles, and ligaments in the foot. Weakening of these structures may lead to biomechanical problems, adversely affecting walking and running. *See* **fallen arches**.

arginine

Arginine is an amino acid that forms creatine, an important constituent of muscles. It is non-essential in adults but may be essential in premature infants. Some people believe that, because arginine is essential for muscle growth in premature infants, it may be advantageous for athletes to take amino acid supplements containing arginine, but there is little evidence to support this belief. *See also* **amino acid supplements**.

Figure 6 Arm curl

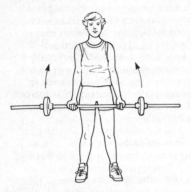 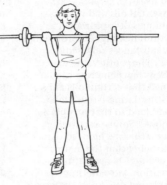

arm curl (biceps curl)

An exercise (figure 6) performed with free-weights to improve arm muscles (biceps and brachialis) and shoulder muscles (deltoids).

■ Stand with your feet shoulder width apart and knees slightly bent. Hold the bar in an underhand grip (i.e. with palms facing upwards) with arms extended. Your hands should be slightly wider than hip width apart. Lift the barbell by bending your arms (ensuring that your elbows are tucked in close to your sides) until the bar just touches your chest. Make sure that you use only the arms to perform the movement, do not permit your body to swing. Hold the position for a few seconds and then lower the barbell slowly to the starting position.

Arm curls can also be performed sitting down, or single-handedly using dumbbells.

arm lift

Two exercises which will strengthen your shoulder muscles (the adductors) and help prevent or correct round shoulders.

■ **Bent arm lift** Lie face down with your head and arms resting on the ground. Your arms should be flexed at 90 degrees with your upper arm extended sideways in line with your shoulders and your hands palm down in line with your head. Contract the adductor muscles between your shoulder blades to lift your arms vertically. Keep your arm flexed at the elbow and shoulder. Hold the position for a few seconds, then slowly lower your arms.

■ **Straight arm lift** Lie face down with your head resting on the floor, your arms extended on the floor beyond your head and held close to your ears. Raise both arms as far as possible without lifting your head. Hold for a few seconds and slowly lower your arms.

arm sprints

Arm sprints are similar to bench stepping, but the hands are used rather than the feet. They are used for strengthening the arms and shoulder muscles (figure 7).

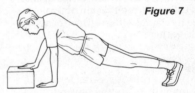

Figure 7

■ With a step or bench immediately in front of you, assume the press-up position, face down with your legs extended. Support the weight of your body on the balls of your feet and your hands. Using each arm alternately in a step-like action, raise your upper body on and off the bench.

arm stretch

A simple warm-up exercise for the upper body, particularly the arms, shoulders, and chest muscles.

■ Stand upright with a straight back. Cross the palm of one hand across the back of the other. With the palms facing forwards, slowly stretch your arms upwards as high as possible and slightly backwards, breathing in as you do so. Hold the fully extended position for about 10 seconds, then return to the starting position.

aromatherapy

The combined use of pure plant extracts or so-called essential oils and various massage techniques. It is promoted as a method of natural healing. According to practitioners, substances released from the oils have a therapeutic value when inhaled or when they penetrate the skin. It is also claimed that certain oils aid slimming by stimulating circulation of the lymph and blood so that surplus body fluids are removed. Some practitioners think that aromatherapy helps to reduce cellulite in the belief that the main cause of cellulite is a sluggish circulation and high fluid retention. Most dietitians dispute these claims.

A bottle of aromatherapy oil containing extracts of fennel (*Foeniculum vulgare*) in spring water is included as part of the 'Revolutionary Three in One Diet', a high protein, high fat, and low carbohydrate diet. The oils are said to act as diuretics, eliminating excess body water. Although there is no rigorous scientific evidence to support this claim, any weight loss associated with fennel would be regained quickly when the dieter started drinking and eating normally again. If fennel does have its claimed effects, there is a risk of dehydration.

arousal

The state of being prepared for action. The intensity of arousal ranges from deep sleep to extreme excitement. Heightening of arousal is brought about by stimulation of the sympathetic nervous system and an increase in secretion of the hormones adrenaline and noradrenaline. As the body becomes prepared for action, the electrical activity of the brain changes; sweating becomes more profuse; muscle tension, heart rate, and metabolic rate all increase; and some blood is diverted from the gut to the skeletal muscle. Exercise psychologists have established that there is an optimal state of arousal above and below which a person underperforms (*see* **catastrophe theory**). Excessive levels of arousal can be very uncomfortable and are better referred to as anxiety.

arrested progress: *See* plateau.

arsenic

Highly toxic in large amounts, some people believe that very small amounts of this metallic greyish element may be essential for health, but no deficiency signs have been described. Total daily intake averages about 90 micrograms, but its role in the body is unknown. It occurs especially in foods such as fish and shellfish. Inorganic arsenic is more toxic than organic forms.

arteriosclerosis

A general term that is applied to a number of problems associated with a thickening and hardening of an arterial wall, and reduced elasticity of blood vessels. Arteriosclerosis is associated with high blood pressure and heart disease. It is more common among people who are inactive and have unbalanced diets, high in fat. The risk is reduced by taking regular, vigorous aerobic exercise.

arthritis

Inflammation of the joints. Arthritis can have a number of causes (*see* **osteoarthritis** and **rheumatoid arthritis**).

arthroscopy

A technique that enables a surgeon to see directly into a joint through a mini-microscope called an arthroscope. A small incision is made in a joint (e.g. the knee) through which the arthroscope can be inserted. A fibre optic lens system allows the surgeon to look around corners and into small crevices for any signs of injury.

artificial colours

A substance added to food to make it appear more appetizing and to restore colours lost during processing. Many added food colours come from natural substances, such as caramel (burnt sugar, E150) and annatto (E160b, a yellowish-red dye from the pulpy seeds of a small South American tree). Some of the most controversial ones are artificial, such as the azo food dyes, which were originally made from coal tar. Some artificial colours have been banned because they are suspected carcinogens or because they cause allergic reactions. In the UK, there are 52 permitted colourings, but baby foods are allowed to contain only three and these are also vitamin sources. *See also* **food additives**.

artificial fats

Fat substitutes that simulate the creaminess and taste of fat, but which have low or zero calories. One 'fat-free fat' called Olestra is made from a type of sucrose polyester that is indigestible and has no calories. Olestra is intended for use in the manufacture of 'fat-free' potato crisps. It is not yet on the market, but is going through the approval process by the Food and Drug Administration in the USA and the Department of Health in the UK. Another artificial fat, Simplesse, is already on the market in extremely low-fat spreads (it has only 5 per cent fat compared with 80 per cent fat in most margarines). It is made from egg white and milk protein. If they pass all the safety tests, many nutritionists would favour the use of these artificial fats if they help to reduce fat intake.

artificial flavours

A synthetic substance added to food to improve its flavour or to restore the flavour lost in processing. They are the most common type of food additive, widely used in savoury foods. As a result of public concern, many manufacturers are replacing artificial flavours with natural ones, such as vanilla and spices.

artificial sweeteners

Substances which increase the sweetness of food. There are two main groups: bulk sweeteners and intense sweeteners.

Bulk sweeteners, such as hydrogenated glucose syrup and sorbitol, are used as flavour-enhancers in many processed foods; they have about the same calorific value as natural sugars. Sorbitol is frequently used as a sugar substitute in confectionery. It is used especially in confectionery for diabetics because it is slowly absorbed and therefore puts less strain on the pancreas than glucose and sucrose. It should be used with care, however, because it has a laxative side-effect with which some people find difficult to cope. European Community directives recommend bulk sweeteners should not be used in food intended for children under three years of age.

Intense sweeteners, such as aspartame and saccharin, have no calories so they are often used as part of weight reducing diets. They produce their sweet taste by triggering specific receptors on the tongue. Some people believe that intense sweeteners disturb blood glucose control, stimulate the appetite, and increase the likelihood of suffering hunger pangs when on a weight-loss diet; there is little scientific evidence for this belief.

New, chemically engineered products much sweeter than current products are being developed and awaiting full approval. Among these super sweeteners are sucralose, 600 times sweeter than sugar, and alitame which is 2000 times sweeter. *See also* **aspartame; acesulfame-K; cyclamate;** and **saccharin**.

ascorbic acid: *See* **vitamin C**.

aspartame

An artificial sweetener 200 times sweeter than sugar. It contains virtually no calories and, unlike some other sweeteners, has no bitter after-taste. It is made of two amino acids, aspartic acid and phenylalanine. It is the most widely used intense sweetener, but it cannot be used in cooking. It quickly loses its sweetness in hot water but is stable for 2–3 months in cold soft drinks. The Food and Drug Administration in the USA says it is safe for a healthy 150-pound adult to consume up to 3.5 grams of aspartame per day. In the UK, the acceptable daily intake is 40 mg per kg body weight (i.e. 2.8 g for a 70 kg adult). There is some doubt about the safety of consuming larger amounts of aspartame. Some people who habitually use the sweetener have reported migraines and headaches, and a few have suffered swelling of the larynx. In addition, it is believed that aspartame may have a toxic effect on the foetal brain. Therefore some people think its use should be avoided by pregnant and lactating women, and young children. People suffering from phenylketonuria (an inborn defect of protein metabolism) are sensitive to phenylalanine, and are generally advised to avoid aspartame.

aspartates
Salts of the non-essential amino acid
aspartic acid that are used in some
ergogenic aids (sports performance boosters) in the belief that they delay fatigue
by accelerating the conversion of ammonia to urea. Experimental results provide
conflicting evidence of their usefulness.

aspartic acid: *See* **aspartates**.

aspirin (acetylsalicylic acid)
A white crystalline powder which has
anti-inflammatory (inflammation-
reducing), antipyretic (fever-reducing),
and analgesic (pain-relieving) properties.
It is widely used to treat headaches.
Aspirin is one of the few effective analgesics not on the International Olympic
Committee list of banned substances.
Consequently, it is frequently prescribed
to athletes and is particularly effective in
the treatment of some injuries and diseases (especially arthritis) involving the
muscles and joints. Aspirin also tends to
increase clotting time, reducing the risk
of thromboses and some other cardiovascular problems. A US physicians' study
indicated that daily consumption of half
an aspirin reduces the risk of cardiovascular disease. Recent research indicates
that aspirin may also offer some protection against Alzheimer's disease. Because
of these many beneficial properties, some
people, including Ron Hill, the famous
British marathon runner, hail aspirin as
a wonder drug and take half or a whole
tablet on a daily basis as a precautionary
measure. However, such routine consumption is not without its risks. One
consequence of the longer clotting time
is that aspirin also increases the tendency
of people to bleed, making it particularly
harmful to sufferers of stomach ulcers.
This effect is exacerbated by the fact that
aspirin irritates the mucous membrane
lining the stomach. Aspirin taken with a
meal also decreases the absorption of
iron, vitamin C, and folic acid (one of the
B vitamins). Therefore, a person taking
aspirin may suffer a deficiency unless
there is a compensatory increase in the
intake of these nutrients.
    Some unfortunate individuals are aller-
gic to aspirin and cannot take advantage
of any of its beneficial properties. If they
take even one dose of the drug they are
liable to go into an anaphylactic shock
similar to a severe asthmatic attack.
Aspirin is not recommended for children
because it has caused liver and brain
damage, albeit rarely, in those with viral
infections (e.g. influenza and chicken-
pox). High doses of aspirin can be poisonous and extremely dangerous, even for
individuals who are not particularly
sensitive.

asthma
A respiratory disorder characterized by
recurrent attacks of difficulty in breathing (described in medical books as
'episodic wheezing'), particularly on
exhalation. It is caused by an increased
resistance to air flow through the respiratory bronchioles (small air tubes leading
to the lungs). Sufferers are hypersensitive
to a variety of stimuli (e.g. house dust
mites; diesel exhaust particulates; and
vehicle exhaust gases, such as ozone and
nitrogen oxides) which cause the airways
to narrow. Asthma may be induced by
exercise (*see* **exercise induced asthma**)
and food allergies. Sports vary in their
tendency to induce asthma, with running having a high tendency, cycling a
moderate tendency, and gymnastics and
swimming a low tendency. Paradoxically,
many asthmatics gain relief from bron-
chospasms by regular exercise, and
exercise is now seen as important in the
management of asthma. Asthmatic
attacks are relieved by a number of
drugs, but competitive sports people
should be aware that some of these are
banned by sports federations because, as
well as controlling asthma, they may act
as artificial stimulants.

atherosclerosis
Atherosclerosis is the accumulation of
fatty materials within arterial walls. This
results in a narrowing of the arteries and
reduction of blood flow which can
encourage the formation of a blood clot
and lead to a heart attack or stroke. The
risk of atherosclerosis has traditionally
been linked to behavioural and dietary
causes, such as eating too much fat (especially saturated fat), not taking enough
exercise, and smoking. Free radicals
(highly reactive chemicals) are thought to

be a major factor in the development of atherosclerosis, consequently antioxidants (e.g. vitamin E) may offer some protection. There seems to be no doubt that too much cholesterol in the blood can line the arteries with plaque, causing atherosclerosis, but several genes have been identified recently that affect the transport and deposition of cholesterol in the body. One of the genes is carried by 24 per cent of the population and may increase their susceptibility independent of the traditional factors. Nevertheless, even those with a genetic predisposition to the disease, can reduce the risk by taking regular, vigorous aerobic exercise and by eating a balanced diet, rich in antioxidants and relatively low in fat.

athlete

An athlete is an individual who, by virtue of special training or natural talent, is fit to compete in a physically demanding sport. The term is derived from the Latin word 'athleta', referring to a person who competed in physical exercises for a prize.

An athlete thought to have a lot of natural talent is often called a 'born athlete'. Such an athlete usually exhibits great proficiency in a range of physical activities, apparently after little practice. Most great athletes are genetically endowed with high athletic potential, but this potential is rarely realized without many years of hard and dedicated training. Great athletes, therefore, are generally made, not born.

athlete's foot

If you have itchy, sore feet and the skin is peeling from between your toes (usually the 4th and 5th), you are likely to be suffering from athlete's foot. This is a contagious infection caused by a fungus, *Tinea pedis*. It may be rampant where there is poor hygiene and communal washing, such as in changing rooms in sports centres. The condition can be avoided by scrupulous care in washing the feet and the application of antifungal ointments, powders, and creams.

athlete's heart

Athletes often have an enlarged heart. When this is a natural, physiological adaptation to regular, endurance exercises, the condition is called athlete's heart. Those with athlete's heart often have a slow heart rate (considerably less than 60 beats per minute). There is no evidence that the condition is detrimental to health. However, when a person's exercise history is not known, athlete's heart is sometimes confused with abnormal, pathological changes associated with some heart diseases. In abnormal enlargements, the changes are not reversible and are accompanied by development of scar-like fibrous tissue (fibrosis) in the heart; athlete's heart is reversible and is not accompanied by fibrosis.

athletic pseudonephritis: *See* proteinuria.

athletics

The central activities of athletics (or track and field events) are running, jumping, and throwing. These are also the core activities of many other sports and are dealt with in a number of separate entries: *see* **jogging**, **jumping**, **sprint**, and **throwing**.

Atkins diet

The Atkins diet (also called 'Dr Atkins Super Energy Diet') is a high-protein, high-fat, low-carbohydrate, weight-reduction diet devised by an American doctor, Robert C. Atkins. The diet appears to contravene most of the generally accepted dietary guidelines for health since it relies on saturated fats as the main energy source.

Atkins recommended that a dieter should eat virtually no carbohydrate in the first week: no carbohydrate-rich alcoholic drinks, bread, fruit, potatoes, pasta, pastries, or sugar. An attractive feature of the diet is that it permits an unlimited intake of fat and protein foods (e.g. meats, poultry, fish, and cheese). After the first week, carbohydrate consumption increases a little, but is still kept at a low level. The low intake of fruit and vegetables could result in vitamin deficiency, except that Atkins prescribed very large vitamin supplements for his dieters.

Atkins claimed that the low level of carbohydrates forces the body to use body fat as a fuel. He suggested that it also stimulates the secretion of a fat mobilizing hormone that encourages the breakdown of fat. (There is no independent scientific evidence to support the existence of this hormone.) Calories are not counted. Instead, the dieter tests the urine with special paper strips which turn mauve-purple in the presence of ketones. Ketones are breakdown products of fat and indicate that it is being burnt off. Despite Atkins' claims to the contrary, they are not a good measure of the effectiveness of a weight-reducing diet.

The diet is unquestionably effective in reducing weight, up to 10 pounds (4.5 kg) in one week. High levels of ketones in the blood suppress the appetite, however it can be very harmful. The ketones create a diabetes-like environment in the body, potentially damaging to the kidneys and allowing blood sugar levels to fall dangerously low.

The Atkins diet is not generally recommended by medical practitioners or dietitians and its introduction provoked strong opposition from the American Medical Association.

ATP: *See* **adenosine triphosphate.**

ATP-PCr system: *See* **phosphagen system.**

atrophy
A reduction in the size or wasting away of an organ or tissue from lack of use or disease. Inactivity results in weakening of both muscles and bones. Space scientists with NASA found that complete immobilization for three days resulted in astronauts losing one-fifth of maximal strength. Early space flights at zero gravity resulted in leg bones becoming thinner and susceptible to fractures. The scientists found that weight-bearing exercises reversed the degenerative changes. They recommended daily exercise, but suggested that three non-consecutive days of programmed activity was sufficient to maintain physical fitness.

The effects of a sedentary lifestyle are not as dramatic as immobilization in space, but the space research supports the notion that 'if you don't use it, you'll lose it'. *See also* **hypokinetic disease.**

atropine: *See* **belladonna.**

Atwater factor
The Atwater factor is the energy value per unit mass of food expressed as kilocalories per gram.

autoconditioning: *See* **biofeedback training.**

autogenic training
Autogenic training is a relaxation technique involving self-suggestion. You learn to associate a series of verbal cues and visual images with feelings of warmth and cold in different parts of the body. At the same time, you train yourself to control certain physiological activities (e.g. heart rate and depth of breathing) in response to the cues and images. Once learnt, these responses can be self-generated when required to reduce anxiety levels.

autoimmunity: *See* **immune system.**

aversion therapy
Aversion therapy is a type of behaviour modification relying on punishment or negative reinforcement. An individual learns that by doing something or behaving in a certain way, an unpleasant consequence can be avoided. Aversion therapy has been used to dissuade people from drinking alcohol, taking drugs, or eating certain foods.

avidin: *See* **biotin.**

azo dyes
Azo dyes are a group of nitrogen-containing chemicals added to some foods. They include amaranth and tartrazine which colour food purple-red and yellow, respectively. These compounds may cause headaches and other unpleasant symptoms in some sensitive people. Azo dyes have also been implicated in causing hyperactivity in some children.

B

"The satisfaction we derive from games is complex. We enjoy struggling to get the best out of ourselves, whether we play games of skill requiring quickness of eye and deftness of touch or games of effort and endurance like athletics. It is not just the desire to succeed. There is the need to feel that our bodies have a skill and energy of their own, apart from the man-made machines they may drive."
Roger Bannister, first man to break the 4-minute mile barrier; he ran the mile in 3:59.4 at Iffley Road, Oxford, 6 May 1954. From Bannister, R. (1955) _The first four minutes_. Putnam, London.

....

backache

Backache is second only to the common cold as a reason for absence from work in the United Kingdom and Europe. Eighty per cent of all Americans will see a physician about backache during their lifetime, and an estimated 75 million Americans have recurring back problems, causing 93 million days of lost work per year and costing an estimated $10 million worth of sickness benefits. Backache has a number of causes. The ache may be associated with an injury, such as a fracture of the spine, prolapsed intervertebral discs, spondylosis or, more commonly, muscle and ligament strains. Most back injuries are the result of poor posture, lack of fitness (including poor flexibility, and lack of strength and muscular endurance), or inappropriate load-carrying techniques, but it is usually due to mechanical stress. As the following table shows, poor posture (particularly while sitting) and poor lifting technique may impose on the back unbearable loads that injure muscles and ligaments:

BODY POSITION	APPROXIMATE PRESSURE ON THE BACK (MM HG)
lying down on back	25
lying down on side	75
standing upright	100
seated, with back upright	140
standing, leaning forwards on hips	150
seated, slumped forward	185

Excess weight, particularly in the abdomen, can contribute to back problems by exaggerating the mechanical stresses.

The majority of backaches occur in the lower back because this is the region that supports most of the weight and is also subject to the greatest strains from activities such as jumping, bending, and twisting. More than 25 per cent of professional golfers suffer from lower back pain caused by the twisting movements of the golf swing. Psychological stress may also cause backache. Highly stressed individuals often tense their back muscles, shortening and tightening them. This can trigger muscular spasms resulting in back pain. In a few cases, a pain felt in the back may be due to diseases in deep-seated organs although the back itself is undamaged; this type of pain is called referred pain.

Most acute backaches could be prevented by performing regular exercises to strengthen and stretch the back and abdominal muscles. It is also important to develop good posture and train the back muscles to move properly and to place the least strain on the back (figure 8). People suffering from, or predisposed to, back problems should avoid exercises that put a strain on the back. It is no good starting a programme of back strengthening and stretching exercises when suffering backache. Sports such as golf and tennis which involve twisting movements, can exacerbate backpain. Running and aerobic dance may also jar the back, but the stress can be minimized

Figure 8 Your back and how to care for it

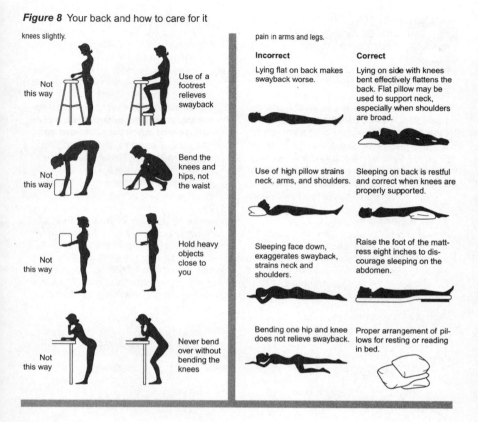

knees slightly.

Not this way / Use of a footrest relieves swayback

Not this way / Bend the knees and hips, not the waist

Not this way / Hold heavy objects close to you

Not this way / Never bend over without bending the knees

pain in arms and legs.

Incorrect	Correct
Lying flat on back makes swayback worse.	Lying on side with knees bent effectively flattens the back. Flat pillow may be used to support neck, especially when shoulders are broad.
Use of high pillow strains neck, arms, and shoulders.	Sleeping on back is restful and correct when knees are properly supported.
Sleeping face down, exaggerates swayback, strains neck and shoulders.	Raise the foot of the mattress eight inches to discourage sleeping on the abdomen.
Bending one hip and knee does not relieve swayback.	Proper arrangement of pillows for resting or reading in bed.

How to sit correctly

A back's best friend is a straight hard chair. If you can't get the chair you prefer, learn to sit properly on whatever chair you get. To correct sitting position from forward slump. Throw head well back, then bend it forward to pull in the chin. This will straighten the back. Now tighten abdominal muscles to raise the chest. Check position frequently.

Relieve strain by sitting well forward, flatten back by tightening abdominal muscles, and cross knees.

Use of footrest relieves swayback. Aim is to have knees higher than hips.

Correct way to sit while driving, close to pedals. Use seat belt or hard backrest available commercially.

TV slump leads to 'dowager's hump', strains neck and shoulders.

If chair is too high, swayback is increased.

Keep neck and back in as straight a line as possible with the spine. Bend forward from hips.

Driver's seat too far from pedals, emphasizes curve in lower back.

Strained reading position. Forward thrusting strains muscles of neck and head.

by wearing the correct shoes. Swimming is the most highly recommended activity for people with back problems.

back and leg stretch

An exercise which stretches and improves the flexibility of the lower back, hamstrings, and buttock muscles. This exercise should not be performed by those with back problems.

■ Stand upright with your knees bent. Gently bend down and grasp your ankles, pulling down a little until you feel the stretch. Hold for about five seconds, relax, and slowly return to the starting position, then repeat.

back extension

A back strengthening exercise, usually performed on an extension bench specially designed to support the hips and which fixes the feet (figure 9). The extension bench isolates the back muscles, allowing the body to bend

safely. If an extension bench is unavailable, the exercise can be performed on a sturdy table and a partner can hold down the legs and feet.

■ Lock your hands on top of your head. Bend your upper body over an extension bench. Slowly lift your trunk upwards to straighten it. Hold for a few seconds, then return to the original angled position. Keep your back straight during the whole routine.

Back extensions increase the flexibility of the latissimus dorsi and trapezius muscles. They also strengthen the abdominals during the lifting phase, and the gluteals and hamstrings when the body is held in the horizontal position. The exercise can be performed with additional weights to improve the definition of back muscles.

back extension test

A test to determine the flexibility of your back. It has also been used as a

Figure 9 Back extensions

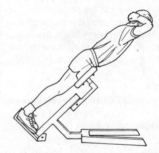
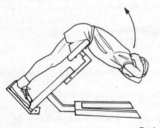

Back extension on extension bench

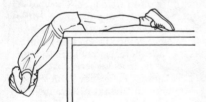
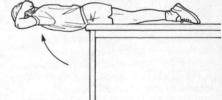

Back extension on table

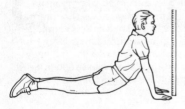

Back extension test

therapeutic exercise for patients with lower back pain.

■ Lie on the floor on your stomach. Place your palms face down on the floor, either side of your head. While keeping your pelvis in contact with the ground, use your arms to raise your head and chest as high as you can without discomfort. Get a partner to measure the distance from the floor to your suprasternal notch (the notch at the top of the chest bone).

Rating: >30 cm, excellent; 20–29 cm, good; 10–19 cm, fair; <9 cm, poor.

back scratcher stretch

A simple exercise, often used in a warm-up routine for stretching the upper arm and shoulder muscles.

■ Standing upright, use one hand to reach behind your neck and touch the area of your back between your shoulder blades; use your other hand to push down slowly and gently on the elbow until you feel a tension but no pain. Hold the position for 10–20 seconds and repeat with the other arm. When you can perform this exercise easily, bend to one side to increase the tension on the lats (latissimus dorsi muscles).

badminton

Badminton is one of the most popular sports in the UK. It can be played at all levels and by all age groups. Great natural ability is not needed to play the game at a recreational level but good skill, agility, and fast reflexes are required to play it at a highly competitive level. An elite player has to be strong, mobile, and flexible to cover the court at speed. Badminton helps to develop all-round fitness: it strengthens legs, arms, and wrists, and improves the flexibility of the trunk, back, and shoulders. Rallies usually consist of short bursts of anaerobic activity but played at a high level, a game can go on for a long time and helps to develop aerobic fitness. If you suffer from a back problem, however, it may not be wise to play badminton because the game involves quick twisting and bending movements. Recreational badminton players who play infrequently are particularly vulnerable to injury unless they incorporate general fitness training into

their schedule and warm up properly before playing a game.

balance

1 The ability to maintain a stable position while either stationary (static balance) or moving (dynamic balance). Balance is achieved by the action of reflexes involving the eyes, the balance organs in the semi-circular canals of the ears, pressure receptors in the skin (particularly on the soles of the feet), and stretch receptors in muscles and joints. Good balance is needed for many sports, especially those requiring sudden changes in movement, such as gymnastics and tennis.

2 The harmonious development of physical, mental, and spiritual aspects of a person. Balance was a philosophical ideal of the ancient Greeks who believed that sport played a key role in its acquisition.

balanced diet

A balanced diet contains sufficient amounts of fibre and the various nutrients (carbohydrates, fats, proteins, vitamins, and minerals) to ensure good health. Food should also provide the appropriate amount of energy and adequate amounts of water. The diet should not contain items that are harmful. In other words, a balanced diet should be both adequate and wholesome. This definition is easy to give, but it is much more difficult to state precisely what constitutes a balanced diet for any particular individual. Government departments, using advice gained from expert committees, provide dietary guidelines that are designed to help us achieve a balanced diet (*see* **Dietary Reference Values**; and **Recommended Dietary Allowance**).

balanced exercise programme

A programme of exercises that improves all the health-related fitness components: aerobic fitness, muscular strength, muscular endurance, flexibility, and body composition. There is no single programme to suit all people. The contents have to be geared to the physical condition and aims of each exerciser, with different components emphasized depending on the type of fitness the exerciser wishes to achieve.

ballistic stretching

Ballistic stretching involves quick, bouncing movements that often take a joint beyond its normal range. Such stretching has been popularized in the workouts of some famous people, but it is potentially harmful because the bouncing movements can result in a protective reflex which causes antagonistic muscles to be torn as they attempt to contract against the direction of the stretch (stretch reflex). Most qualified exercise teachers and coaches advocate static stretching which is a much safer and more effective way of improving flexibility.

balneotherapy

The science of treating disease and injury by giving baths. *See* **baths** and **contrast baths**.

banded gastroplasty

Banded gastroplasty is the medical term for the surgical reduction of stomach size. A drastic method of treating obesity that carries a high risk of harmful side-effects.

Bandura's self-efficacy theory: *See* self-confidence.

banned substance

The International Olympic Committee list of banned substances (performance-enhancing substances subject to doping controls) is generally accepted by the governing bodies of most sports. The Sept. 1994 list includes the following doping classes and methods:

DOPING CLASSES

- stimulants
- narcotics
- anabolic agents
- diuretics
- peptide hormones and analogues

DOPING METHODS

- blood doping
- pharmacological, chemical, and physical manipulation

CLASSES OF DRUGS SUBJECT TO CERTAIN RESTRICTIONS

- alcohol
- marijuana
- local anaesthetics
- corticosteroids
- β blockers

It is not a comprehensive list of individual drugs; the ban applies to all compounds related to those on the list. In addition, individual sports federations may have their own list of banned substances.

barbell

A barbell is a steel bar onto which weights are attached for weight-training. Barbells are usually from 1.2 m (4 ft) to 2.1 m (7 ft) long. The weights are steel or cast iron discs fixed to each end. They are usually added in 2.5 kg (5.5 lbs) amounts to vary the resistance, but equal weights are always added to each side of the barbell. Collars are used to secure the weights in position. They are slipped on either side of the weights and secured by grub screws or lever tighteners. Some exercisers also attach a protective plastic sleeve to prevent blisters and to improve grip.

barbiturates

Barbiturates are a group of drugs derived from barbituric acid. Barbiturates act as depressants of the central nervous system and have powerful sedative and anxiety-reducing properties. They have been commonly used in sleeping pills and to help people to relax. One of their side-effects is to interfere with the ability to perform complex skills. Barbiturates are habit-forming and prolonged use may lead to addiction.

bare foot exercise

Many people enjoy the freedom of exercising without any foot protection, particularly indoors during keep fit classes. Some famous runners, such as Bruce Tulloh and Zola Pieterse (née Budd), ran barefooted outdoors. However, bare foot exercise can considerably increase the risk of injury to those who are not used to it. The majority of exercisers spend most of their waking hours wearing some kind of supportive footwear. Subjecting feet to occasional bursts of activity without any protection can stress them beyond their tolerance limits. It has been estimated that each foot hits the ground more than 1000 times in a 10 minute intensive aerobics workout.

Although some floors are sprung and wooden, many do not offer sufficient cushioning for bare foot exercise. It is important to choose the right footwear; dance and aerobic fitness shoes are specially designed to cushion the foot after vertical jumps while running shoes are designed for shock absorption and motion control as the foot strikes and rolls off the ground. *See also* **training shoes**.

basal metabolic rate (BMR)
The basal metabolic rate is the minimum rate at which the body uses energy at complete rest. It is the minimum amount of energy needed to keep the body alive and is the largest component of an average person's daily energy expenditure. The BMR is usually expressed simply as kilocalories per day or in units of energy per unit surface area (or per kilogram body mass) per unit time. It is very difficult to determine the absolute minimum metabolic rate, but estimates are usually standardized by being made when a person is resting quietly after at least 8 hours sleep and 12 hours since the last meal. BMR for the average, healthy adult is usually between 1200 and 1800 kilocalories per day. It may, however, be less than 700 kilocalories in some individuals. BMR usually remains relatively constant for each individual, but it varies widely from one person to another. Factors which affect BMR include:

- AGE: BMR tends to decrease as we get older because of increased percentage body fat; children have a higher BMR because of the energy cost of growth
- SIZE: BMR tends to be greater in tall, thin people
- BODY COMPOSITION: Those with a high percentage lean body mass (low percentage fat) tend to have high BMRs because muscle is metabolically more active than fat

- BREAST-FEEDING: BMR is higher in nursing mothers than other women, because of the energy cost of synthesizing milk
- DIETING: BMR decreases during a weight-loss diet, fasting, or starvation
- EXERCISE: BMR increases with regular, very strenuous exercise, but is probably little affected by moderate levels of activity
- MALNUTRITION: BMR decreases during malnutrition
- PREGNANCY: BMR increases during pregnancy
- SEX: BMR is higher in males than females even at the same body weight because of their relatively large bulk of muscle
- STRESS: BMR increases during periods of emotional stress
- THYROID ACTIVITY: BMR is regulated by a hormone, thyroxine, secreted by the thyroid gland. It increases if the thyroid is overactive and decreases if the thyroid is underactive
- WEATHER: BMR increases during both very cold and hot weather.

People trying to lose weight often want to increase their BMR as an easy way of burning excess fat. Many manufacturers entice dieters to buy slimming products that claim to increase BMR (*see* **kelp**); most of these claims are not supported by rigorous scientific evidence. Drugs that can increase basal metabolic rate should be taken only under medical supervision.

baseball and softball
Baseball is a physically demanding sport comprised of several specialisms requiring different skills and types of fitness. Running between bases requires good anaerobic fitness, speed, agility, and the strength to stop suddenly after sprinting. Feet-first slides make the ankle, knee, and thigh susceptible to injury; head-first slides may injure the hand, wrist and fingers. Hitting a baseball is one of the most difficult things to do in sport. It requires excellent eye-to-hand coordination, instantaneous reflexes, and the coordinated movements of the hips, shoulders, arms, and wrists. These

movements put a lot of strain on the neck, shoulders, and upper back. Batters therefore require good upper body strength and flexibility. Fielding requires good all-round fitness: fielders have to be able to run quickly and catch a ball (usually with the non-dominant gloved hand) and then throw it accurately. All baseball players have to throw the ball at one time or another, but it is the major function of pitchers. By coordinating the movements of all the muscles of the upper body, a pitcher can release the ball at speeds in excess of 160 km per hour. This imposes tremendous forces on the throwing arm, shoulders, upper chest and abdominal region. Consequently, pitchers must be very well conditioned to avoid injury and must be skilled at minimizing the forces on any one part of the body. Pitchers are often required to throw the ball repeatedly, making them susceptible to overuse injuries (*see* **thrower's elbow**). This is especially true for young pitchers whose tissues are still growing. Sports medicine experts recommend that a growing child who plays baseball should not perform overhand pitching more than 50 times daily or 350 times per week.

Softball can be played in a smaller area than baseball, but it is a faster game. It can be played indoors as well as outdoors. The name is a little inappropriate because it is played with a ball which is actually larger and harder than that used in baseball. In the 1950s softball became one of the biggest participation sports in the United States and it is now played in many different countries. One of its attractions is that it can be played by mixed teams of men and women. There are two versions of the game: slow pitch in which the ball is delivered in an arc from pitcher to batter and not so unreasonably fast, and fast pitch in which the delivery is as fast as the pitcher likes. All pitches are underarm and the pitch distance is shorter than in baseball. Although the slow pitch game is played at a relatively leisurely pace, the fast pitch is action-packed and faster than baseball. The skills and physical demands of softball are similar to those of baseball, and the injuries associated with the game are also similar. It was once thought that the underhand throw of

fast-pitch softball caused less injury than the overhand throw of baseball, but injury statistics are similar for both. Throwing injuries can be minimized by learning sound technique; strengthening the upper body, especially the anterior shoulder, the biceps, and flexor muscles of the throwing arm; and by beginning and ending all activity with appropriate warm-up and cool-down exercises.

baseball finger

An injury resulting from a hard, moving object striking an extended finger and stretching the end joints suddenly, sometimes tearing ligaments. The injury results in swelling, immobility, and pain in the finger. It occurs most commonly in baseball, but also in cricket, volleyball, and other ball games.

base training

All training programmes should start with base training. This consists of high-volume, low-intensity training to improve overall physical condition in preparation for more specific, intensive training. In many sports, base training includes long-slow-distance (LSD) running which improves the cardiovascular system and aerobic capacity. The training is purposely slow to reduce the risk of injury, but the speed and distance are increased gradually as fitness improves. Many coaches recommend between 6 months and 1 year base training for those unused to exercise before they start intensive, anaerobic training.

basketball

Basketball is a physically demanding game requiring high levels of skill and fitness. It involves all muscles involved in sprinting, turning, and jumping, but it is particularly stressful on joints used in landing. The ankle is the body part most frequently injured during basketball. Other common injuries are jumper's knee and bruises on the upper thighs. There is also considerable strain on the chest muscles caused by the overhead arm-stretch movements characteristic of the game. A thorough warm up and good physical condition will reduce the risk of injury. Games tend to be fiercely competitive and basketball requires con-siderable aggression. Basketball is immensely popular in the USA and is one of the most popular spectator sports in the world.

baths
Baths are used as a relaxant after exercise and as a form of treatment for injuries. There are many forms. Contrast baths are commonly used to treat sports injuries, such as a sprained ankle. They involve subjecting a person first to water as hot as he or she can tolerate, then to water as cold as can be tolerated. Alternate use of hot and cold water stimulates the blood supply to the immersed body part and helps to reduce swelling. *See also* **flotation therapy**.

BBC diet
The BBC diet is a low fat, high-fibre diet described in a book by Barry Lynch (Lynch, B. [1988] *The BBC diet*. BBC Books, London). He encourages dieters to reduce their energy intake by eating less fat, and increase their energy expenditure by tak-ing more exercise. He also advises drink-ing plenty of fluids and describes how dieters can adopt sensible eating habits. The book uses conventional nutritional wisdom and the diet plans are sensible.

BCAA: *See* **branched-chain amino acids**.

B complex vitamins
The B complex consists of water soluble vitamins and other related factors that tend to occur together in certain foods (e.g. liver, wholegrain cereals, and brewer's yeast). Vitamins include thiamin (B_1), riboflavin (B_2), nicotinic acid, pan-tothenic acid, pyridoxine (B_6), biotin, folic acid, and vitamin B_{12}. Other factors sometimes included in lists of the B complex vitamins are choline, PABA, pangamic acid, orotic acid, laetrile, and inositol, but these are not strictly vitamins. All, apart from laetrile and pangamic acid, can be synthesized by the body. There is no evidence that laetrile and pangamic acid are dietary essentials.

bee pollen
Bee pollen is a mixture of bee saliva, plant pollen, and nectar. Some people take it in the belief that it has special health-enhancing properties, others take it because they think it acts as an ero-genic aid (performance booster). It has been claimed that bee pollen improves oxygen uptake and helps to accelerate recovery in training. There is no scientific evidence to support claims that bee pollen improves health or physical per-formance. On the contrary, it may con-tain allergy-inducing substances that are dangerous to hypersensitive individuals.

behaviour therapy
Behaviour therapy uses psychological techniques to overcome problem behav-iours. It is used to change the habits of those with eating disorders, whether they are overeating or undereating. Therapists usually achieve this by estab-lishing new attitudes and by focusing, not on the food, but on a person's behavi-our around the food. The therapy uses a wide range of psychological techniques including stimulus control where, for example, a person susceptible to impulse buying, learns to shop only after eating, or shopping only from a prescribed list. Appropriate rewards, such as praise from friends or treats, are used in the therapy to reinforce good behaviour. Subjects learn to control eating behaviour so that they can eat the correct amount of food. Those who should be eating less can learn to put down their knife and fork between mouthfuls of food and to chew food fully.

Setting appropriate goals is an impor-tant part of behaviour therapy. Subjects are discouraged from using words such as 'always' or 'never', and encouraged to set themselves achievable tasks. Physical activity could be increased, even by changing a simple routine, such as by walking to the corner shop rather than taking a car. Continuous feedback forms an essential part of most behaviour ther-apy. Eating and exercise habits are mon-itored by using a food and exercise diary. This enables problems to be identified and good behaviour to be rewarded. Behaviour therapy can be very effective, but it may take a long time to overcome problems. Those with serious eating dis-orders should seek professional help from a clinical psychologist.

Behaviour therapy is also used by athletes who suffer from excessive anxiety before competition. Some competitions, such as the Olympic Games, which are seen by millions of people may invoke a feeling of fear in even the most seasoned athlete. Behaviour therapy uses relaxation techniques and other procedures which enable the athlete to approach such a competition with optimal levels of physiological arousal and minimum anxiety.

belladonna

The poisonous substance extracted from deadly nightshade (*Atropa belladonna*) and from which the drug atropine is obtained. Atropine has powerful effects on the parasympathetic nervous system, blocking nerve transmissions. With the parasympathetic nervous system out of action, the sympathetic system is left to function unopposed. Thus, atropine mimics some of the stimulatory actions of the sympathetic nervous system and adrenaline. Small doses cause the heart rate to increase. Atropine is used in some cough mixtures for the treatment of bronchitis and whooping cough. It is also used to dilate the pupils for eye examination, relieve peptic ulcers, and to relax the smooth muscle of the intestines and stomach before a general anaesthetic.

bench

Weight-training benches are usually tubular or rigid-framed. Most are padded for comfort and can be adjusted to vary the exerciser's position. Some have reclining seats, barbell supports and additional attachments for specific arm and leg exercises. Before using a bench for weight training, ensure that it is sturdy and placed on a firm, flat surface for maximum stability and safety. Make sure also that when you lie on the bench your feet can be firmly planted on the ground and that you can keep your trunk flat on the bench.

bench blasts

Bench blasts, sometimes called Whitney Bench Blasts, are exercises which develop leg power.
■ Stand upright, place your right foot on a bench and your left foot on the floor, then blast (jump) upwards. Switch your feet in mid air so that when you complete the blast your right foot is on the floor and your left foot is on the bench. Continue the blasts, alternating the position of the feet.

bench press

A relatively simple weight-lifting exercise for toning up arm muscles (particularly the triceps brachii), the anterior deltoids in the shoulder, and the pectorals in the chest. It is usually performed with a barbell (figure 10).
■ Lie with your back on a bench and feet flat on the end (or on the floor). Grip the barbell tightly; your palms should face towards your feet, and your arms should be positioned so that you can push vertically upwards. Push slowly against the weights until your arms are fully extended. After holding the extended position, gently lower the weights and return to the starting position. Breathe out when your arms are

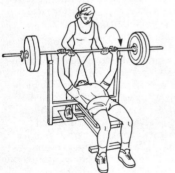
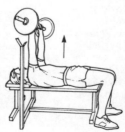
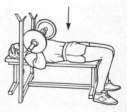

Figure 10 Bench press

straightened and in when they are bent. It is important that your lower back maintains contact with the bench.

benign hypermobility: *See* hypermobility.

bent arm hang
The ability to maintain a bent arm position while hanging from a bar. It is used to test the muscular endurance of the arm and shoulder (figure 11).

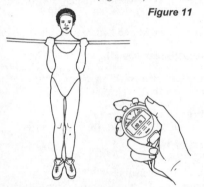

Figure 11

- Hold a fixed bar with palms facing toward your body. Get a partner to lift you off the floor to a position where your chin is above the bar, the elbows are bent, and your chest is close to the bar. Hold the position as long as you can without resting your chin on the bar. Ask your partner to time the hold, stopping the watch when your eyes go below the bar.

Rating: >20 seconds, high; 10–19 seconds, average; <10 seconds, low.

bent arm pullover
A weight training exercise for the chest, shoulder and arm extensors (figure 12).
- Lie on a bench so that your head and upper shoulders are supported. Reach

back to grasp a bar (or dumbbells) placed on the floor close to the bench. With your hands fairly close together, lift the weight over your head and slowly lower it onto your chest. During the lift, your elbows should be tucked in.

bent over row
This weight-training exercise simulates a rowing action and strengthens the shoulder muscles and biceps in the arm. It can be performed with free weights or at a bench press station on an exercise machine (figure 13).

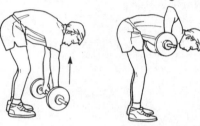

Figure 13

- From a standing position, bend down to the floor to hold a barbell with an overhand grasp (palm down). Your hands should be slightly more than shoulder width apart, your upper trunk parallel to the floor, your knees slightly bent, and your feet apart. Keep your trunk parallel to the floor and pull the barbell directly up to your chest, then return to the start position and repeat the movement.

beriberi
A deficiency disease caused by lack of thiamin (vitamin B_1). Beriberi leads to a decreased appetite; gastrointestinal disturbances; peripheral nerve changes indicated by weakness of legs, cramping of calf muscles, and numbness of feet; heart enlargement; and mental confusion.

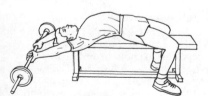

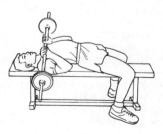

Figure 12 Bent arm pullover

Beriberi is treated with a daily dose of 25 mg of vitamin B_1. Alcoholics often suffer from a form of beriberi called 'alcoholic pseudonephritis', due to poor diet.

beta-blockers

Drugs that reduce anxiety and muscle tension. They are prescribed for some cardiovascular disorders (e.g. angina and high blood pressure). They are also misused by some sports people (e.g. pistol marksmen and snooker players) to reduce muscle tremors.

beta-carotene

A nutrient converted by the body into vitamin A. Beta-carotene is an antioxidant and therefore may offer some protection against certain cancers and other diseases. Foods rich in beta-carotene include orange fruits and vegetables such as apricots, cantaloupes, and carrots, as well as leafy green vegetables such as broccoli and spinach. Beta-carotene is not toxic like vitamin A, but excessive intake may give the skin a yellow hue. *See also* **carotenes**.

beta-oxidation

A biochemical process by which fat is broken down and metabolized so that it can be used as a source of energy in aerobic respiration.

Beverly Hills diet

A high carbohydrate, low protein diet in which specific foods must be eaten in a strict order. For example, in the first week the dieter is allowed to eat only specified fruits, such as pineapples, which are claimed to have fat-burning properties. Most nutritionists and doctors dismiss claims made in the diet as having little scientific basis. Weight loss may occur as a result of water losses associated with the laxative effect of eating large amounts of fruit. It may also occur because the reliance on one type of food produces effects similar to fasting. There is no scientific evidence, however, that weight loss occurs because enzymes from the fruit burn excess body fat. The laxative effects of eating large amounts of fruit are so great that the diet became commonly known as the 'diarrhoea diet'.

Needless to say, the diet is not generally recommended by dietitians.

BHA (butylated hydroxyanisole)

A preservative and artificial antioxidant added to fatty foods to prevent them from going rancid too quickly. It has properties similar to BHT (butylated hydroxytoluene) which is suspected to be carcinogenic in rats. Consequently, some food manufacturers are replacing these synthetic preservatives with natural ones, such as ascorbic acid and vitamin E.

BHT: *See* **butylated hydroxyanisole**.

bicarbonate: *See* **alkali**.

bicarbonate loading: *See* **sodium bicarbonate**.

biceps

A two-headed muscle. The term is often used as an abbreviation for biceps brachii.

biceps brachii

The muscle in the upper arm commonly referred to simply as the biceps. It is involved in movements of the arm and shoulder. Its main action is to bend the arm at the elbow joint.

biceps curl: *See* **arm curl**.

biceps femoris: *See* **hamstrings**.

bile

A greenish-yellow or brownish fluid produced in the liver and stored in the gall-bladder. Its constituents include bile pigments (breakdown products of haemoglobin), salts, and cholesterol. Bile is stored in the gall-bladder and released into the small intestine where bile salts aid the digestion and absorption of fats through their detergent-like action. *See also* **gallstones**.

Billig's exercise

An exercise which stretches the connective tissue around the pelvis, the hip flexors, and the muscles on the inside of the thighs (figure 14). The exercise is reputed to prevent some types of menstrual disorders and to be useful in relieving menstrual cramps.

Figure 14 Billig's exercise

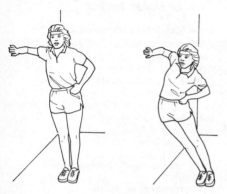

■ Stand upright with your left side facing a wall. Place your left forearm and elbow against the wall at shoulder height. Tilt your pelvis backwards and tighten your buttock and abdominal muscles. Place your right hand on your hip and push your hips towards the wall. Then, without twisting, push with your hips forwards and sideways (at an angle of 45 degrees). Hold the position for a few seconds; return to the starting position and repeat on the opposite side.

binge eating
Rapid consumption of a large amount of food. *See also* **bulimia nervosa**.

binge–purge syndrome: *See* **bulimia nervosa**.

bioelectrical impedance
A method of measuring body composition. Electrodes are placed at four points on the skin to measure the electrical conductance of a weak electrical current. Lean tissue, because of its relatively high electrolyte content, tends to give higher conductivity readings than fatty tissue. The method is probably more precise for measuring fat content than skinfold measurements, but variations in fluid content, electrolyte balance, and skin temperature affect the conductivity readings.

biofeedback training
(autoconditioning)
A technique that can help you to relax. It depends on the subject receiving a continuous and immediate flow of information about one or more physiological functions which indicate stress levels. The most commonly used function is heart rate which usually increases during stress. Reasonably priced, portable heart rate monitors are now widely available. They usually consist of a strap that goes around the chest and a watch-like wrist attachment which displays the heart rate. Biofeedback training teaches you to make a conscious effort to reduce your heart rate (or other physiological functions) as soon as any increase associated with stress occurs. The training enables you to identify when you are under stress. You can then learn to control its physiological effects so that you can become more relaxed.

biomechanics
The application of physics and mechanics to the study of movement. In sport, biomechanics is especially concerned with how the human body applies forces to itself and objects with which it comes into contact, and how the human body is affected by external forces. A sound knowledge of biomechanics equips a coach, athlete, or other performer to choose appropriate training techniques, and to detect and understand faults that may arise in their use.

biorhythm
Cycles of human activity. It is claimed that each person has negative and positive periods within a 23-day physical cycle, a 28-day emotional cycle, and a 33-day intellectual cycle. The physical cycle is said to control a person's energy, strength, aggressiveness, and some other aspects of physical fitness; the emotional cycle influences sensitivity and moods; and the intellectual cycle is supposed to affect mental abilities.

Some competitive athletes compute their biorhythms on specially designed charts to predict when they are most likely to achieve a peak performance and when there is the greatest risk of failure. The correlation between an individual's biorhythm and athletic performance varies greatly. A detailed examination of the biorhythm charts of hundreds of athletes with world or national records showed that the records occurred randomly and were not influenced by biorhythms. *See also* **circadian rhythm**.

biotin

A vitamin of the B complex, also known as vitamin H. Biotin is found in small amounts in body tissues, combined with protein. It plays an important role in many reactions, including the release of energy from carbohydrates, fats, and proteins. Biotin also helps to maintain normal blood glucose concentrations from protein when carbohydrate sources have been exhausted. There is some evidence that biotin is needed for normal vitamin B_{12} activity. Deficiency results in a scaly skin, muscular pain, pallor, loss of appetite, nausea, fatigue and elevated cholesterol levels. Deficiency is extremely rare in adults but it can be induced by consuming too much raw egg white. The egg white contains avidin, a chemical which binds to biotin, preventing it from being absorbed. Avidin is destroyed by heat. Some biotin is synthesized in the gut by bacteria. Dietary sources include yeast extracts, liver, egg yolk, and legumes. Although there are no official recommended dietary intakes, it has been calculated that 10–200 micrograms is a safe and adequate range of intake.

black nail (runner's toe, soccer toe)

Blackening of the toe-nail near its base is quite a common injury among runners and other athletes. It can be very painful and is often accompanied by joint swelling. Black nail is often caused by wearing shoes that are too short or too wide. The foot slides forwards, especially on dry, artificial turf, and jams against the end of the shoe. It may also develop from a direct blow to the toe. The damaged nail, blackened by bruising, dies. The underlying nail grows and displaces the black nail which eventually drops off. Nail injuries can be prevented by wearing well-fitting shoes but if such injuries occur, the pain can be relieved by inserting a heated, sterilized needle through the nail. This creates a hole which releases the blood and reduces the pressure. The procedure should be performed by a medically qualified person!

blind stork test A test of balance

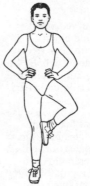

Figure 15

■ With your hands on your hips, stand upright on a firm surface with your weight supported on your stronger leg. Place the sole of the other foot against the knee of your supporting leg. Close your eyes and ask a partner to time how long you can maintain your pose. You may need to sway and shift to maintain balance, but the timing should stop as soon as you move your supporting foot.

Rating: >50 seconds, excellent time; 30–49 seconds, good; 10–29 seconds, fair; <10 seconds, poor.

blister

An injury in which the top layer of skin is detached from the underlying layer; the gap between the two layers becomes filled with a watery fluid from damaged cells. A blister is usually painful because the thick outer epidermis of the skin is lifted away to expose nerve-endings. Blisters are usually caused by friction. Training vigorously in brand new shoes is a common cause among exercisers. The time-honoured practice of applying surgical spirit to harden the feet may reduce the occurrence of blisters. Wearing two pairs of socks may prevent blisters by allowing friction to occur between the socks rather than between the socks and skin. However, if large uncomfortable blisters occur despite precautionary measures, they can be treated by releasing the fluid with a sterilized needle, snipping away dead skin, and then applying a sterile dressing. Small blisters should be left unbroken as long as possible to reduce the risk of infection.

blitz system: *See* body building.

blood

A fluid tissue consisting of red blood cells, white blood cells, and blood platelets (thrombocytes; disc-like structures derived from fragments of bone marrow cells that play an important role in blood clotting) within a liquid matrix called plasma.

An average adult male has about 5 litres of blood. Blood has many functions. It is the main transport medium of the body carrying hormones, nutrients, respiratory gases, and metabolic waste products. It also helps to regulate body temperature by controlling the loss of body heat through the skin. White blood cells and some components of blood plasma play an essential role in the body's defence against disease.

Regular aerobic exercise can significantly change the composition of blood. Exercisers tend to have a higher blood volume, more haemoglobin, more anti-clotting agents, and lower blood cholesterol levels than inactive people.

blood doping

A technique that athletes use to boost their stamina by injecting themselves with extra blood. Blood doping has been used to improve the performance of cross-country skiers, marathoners, and triathletes. Blood doping is carried out in the belief that it increases the oxygen-carrying capacity of the circulatory system and thereby improves endurance. The blood may be obtained from the same individual (autotransfusion) or from another individual.

In autotransfusion, about a litre of blood is extracted usually some time before a competition so that the body has time to replace the lost blood. The blood is frozen for storage to reduce damage to red blood cells. After thawing, the stored blood is returned to the body immediately before competition to boost the red blood cell count. In addition to contravening the ethics of medicine and sport, this procedure carries a number of risks. These include the possibility of increasing the thickness of blood, making it more difficult to pump around the body and imposing an extra strain on the heart. The extra-thick blood may also damage the kidneys. When using donated blood, there is also a very real risk of transmission of infective diseases. Blood doping is banned by the International Olympic Committee. *See also* **erythropoietin**.

blood glucose

It is vital that the blood contains some glucose as it is the only body fuel used by the brain. However, there is an optimal concentration (between 3 and 8 mmol/l). Too much results in hyperglycaemia and too little in hypoglycaemia; both conditions are harmful. The blood glucose level is controlled mainly by insulin (which lowers blood glucose after meals); other hormones involved in its regulation are glucagon, adrenaline, and glucocorticoids (steroids produced by the adrenal cortex), which raise blood glucose in the fasting state or in response to excitement, fear, and shock. *See also* **diabetes mellitus** and **glucose**.

blood lactate

The concentration of lactates (salts of lactic acid, a product of anaerobic respiration) dissolved in the blood. It is used as a biochemical indicator of anaerobic threshold. Normal concentrations are between 0.7 and 1.8 millimoles per litre. *See also* **lactic acid**.

blood platelets: *See* **blood**.

blood pressure

The pressure exerted by the heart and arteries to push blood around the body. The magnitude of blood pressure is determined by the amount of blood being pumped out of the heart per beat (the stroke volume) and the resistance encountered as it passes through the blood vessels (peripheral resistance). Blood pressure is usually expressed as two measurements: systolic blood pressure, indicating the pressure when the heart is actually pumping; and diastolic blood pressure, the pressure when the heart is filling up with blood. Systolic pressure is always the higher and is expressed first. The pressures are measured in millimetres of mercury. Thus a blood pressure of 130/80, or 130 over 80, refers to a systolic blood pressure which will support a column of mercury 130 mm high, and a diastolic pressure which will support a column 80 mm high. Systolic pressure in children is about 100 and in young adults the value is about 120. It tends to rise with age as arteries thicken. A systolic pressure of 180 is not uncommon and it may be as high as 280. The value varies according to a person's position. It tends to drop when you stand up after lying down; this is called postural hypotensive drop. A typical value for diastolic pressure is 80 mm of mercury. Although it is difficult to define precisely what is 'normal' blood pressure, there is general agreement that a desirable blood pressure is less than 140/90. *See also* **hypertension** and **hypotension**.

blue baby syndrome: *See* **nitrates**.

BMI: *See* **body mass index**.

BMR: *See* **basal metabolic rate**.

body awareness
The ability to recognize different parts of one's own body, and their relative positions. It is essential for performing smooth, coordinated movements, and must be well-developed in those aspiring to be top-class dancers, synchronized swimmers, or gymnasts. Body awareness is dependent on being able to perceive and integrate information coming from all the sense organs, including the less well-known ones (proprioceptors) in the muscles and joints, which monitor internal movements. Gymnastics and dance are excellent activities for developing body awareness in children. *See also* **kinaesthesis**.

body building
A routine of exercise and diet designed to make the body appear muscular. Weight-training is used to develop the size, shape, and symmetry of all the superficial muscles in the body so that they are larger, more conspicuous, and better defined. Training routines usually reduce fat levels and, if performed properly, can improve flexibility, particularly of the shoulders, hips, and trunk. When combined with aerobic fitness training, body building can be beneficial to health. However, when the only objective is to obtain a better looking body, the exercises usually have little beneficial effect on fitness and may even be harmful. Body building may, for example, reduce flexibility and mobility if the weight training is performed without using the full range of movements.

One routine, called the 'blitz' system, uses circuits of several different exercises performed on one body part over long periods of time. This enlarges muscles because more blood can be pumped into them, but blitzing does not necessarily strengthen the muscles.

The most controversial aspect of body building concerns the methods used to increase body mass. This can be achieved only if there is a positive energy balance, with food intake exceeding energy expenditure. There are many special food supplements on the market which claim to help body-builders to gain weight. However, a major problem is ensuring that the gain is in the form of muscle rather than fat. Appropriate weight-training exercises can help the process, but only slowly. Many serious body-builders resort to taking drugs, such as androgenic-anabolic steroids, for quick results. This can be expensive, both financially and in terms of health.

Although body-builders require protein, they sometimes over-indulge in protein-rich foods (often in the form of expensive, commercially-packaged supplements) and do not eat enough of the other nutrients. It is difficult to define an individual's exact protein requirements, but the needs of an active body-builder are more than twice those of a sedentary person. Nevertheless, even a 200 lb (90 kg) male body-builder would require no more than 6.5 oz (180 g) of protein per day. Many body-builders eat much more protein than this; the excess is either excreted or turned to fat. *See also* **amino acid supplements** and **pumping-up**.

body composition
The relative percentage of fat, muscle, bone, and other tissue in the body. There are different ways of categorizing body composition. One method assumes that

there are four main components: fat, fat-free water, fat-free mineral, and fat-free protein. Another method, generally preferred because it is easier to measure, divides the body into two components: lean (or fat-free) body mass and body fat. These components contribute unequally to body weight. Fat is less dense than muscle. Consequently, two individuals could have the same body weight but have completely different body compositions and body dimensions.

Body composition has an important effect on physical performance. Generally, the higher the proportion of lean body mass, the greater a person's power to weight ratio. Contact sports (e.g. American football and rugby) favour participants with high body weight. Highly mobile non-contact sports (e.g. gymnastics and distance running) favour those with small body weights. Both groups of sports are usually performed better by those with a high proportion of lean body mass. Regular aerobic exercise and weight training are generally regarded as effective ways of reducing body fat and increasing lean body mass.

body fat

A measurement of the amount of fat in the human body, usually expressed as a percentage of total body weight. Most adult males have between 15 and 25 per cent body fat, and most females have 20–30 per cent; values for athletes and others who exercise regularly and vigorously are usually less. Between 4 and 15 per cent of body fat is contained within muscles. This is the most metabolically active and accessible form of fat. It is sensitive to the 'exercise hormones' (adrenaline and noradrenaline) and is a very important energy source for ultra endurance activities.

Body fat tends to increase with age, but it is uncertain whether this is an inevitable consequence of the ageing process, or whether it is due to a decrease in daily physical activity.

There are a number of ways of measuring body fat, including the rather macabre cadaver (dead body) dissection analysis; hydrostatic weighing (this involves weighing a person under water and in air); skinfold measurements and

the modern techniques of ultrasound analysis; nuclear magnetic resonance; biological impedance; and computerized tomography. One of the easiest ways of determining body fat is by measuring the thickness of the skin at specific points (*see* **skinfold measurements**). *See also* **adipose tissue** and **obesity**.

body fuels

The main sources of energy in the body are carbohydrates and fats. Carbohydrates yield about 4 kilocalories per gram; fat yields more than 9 kilocalories per gram. Protein yields about the same amount of energy as carbohydrates, but, except during starvation or prolonged fasting, only contributes up to 10 per cent of the energy requirements. The energy released from these nutrients during cellular respiration is used to make adenosine triphosphate (ATP), the only chemical that can be used directly by the body as a source of energy. Glycogen stored in muscles is the quickest source of ATP for muscles to use, especially for short bursts of vigorous activity. Fat is a less accessible source of energy. Fat stores in adipose tissue have to be broken down to glycerol and fatty acids, then transported in the blood stream to active muscles before being broken down. Consequently, fat is used mainly when physical activity is relatively gentle and prolonged. Because carbohydrates are the primary source of energy for intense, short bursts of muscular activity, they should constitute at least 50 per cent of the diet of physically active people.

body image (body schema)

The perception, both conscious and unconscious, of one's own body and physical dimensions. Many people who suffer from eating disorders, such as anorexia and bulimia, have a distorted body image and are often convinced that they are fatter than they really are.

body mass

In anthropometry, when scientific measurements of the human body are made, the mass of the human body is measured to the nearest tenth of a kilogram when the subject is nude, or dressed with clothing of known mass so that correction to nude mass can be made. Body mass is commonly referred to as body weight.

body mass index (BMI; Quetelet index)

An index of weight for height, calculated as:

$$BMI = \text{weight in kg}/(\text{height in metre})^2$$

Measurements are for a subject barefooted and without clothes. You can use the above equation to calculate your own BMI (if measurements are made in pounds and inches, divide pounds by 2.2 to convert to kilograms, and divide inches by 39.4 to convert to metres).

The BMI has been used as a guideline for defining whether a person is overweight because it minimizes the effect of height, but it does not take into consideration other important factors, such as age and body build. The BMI has also been used as an indicator of obesity on the assumption that the higher the index, the greater the level of body fat. However, this assumption is not always true. Highly muscular people, such as body-builders, may have a high BMI but low fat content. Nevertheless, for most people, the BMI is a good way of determining a range of acceptable weights (figure 16).

Most authorities use the following guidelines:

BMI	CONDITION
<20	underweight (may need to gain weight)
20–25	advisable range
25–30	overweight (some weight loss may be beneficial to health)
30–40	obese (need to lose weight)
>35	severely obese (urgent need to lose weight; advised to consult doctor)

The risk of developing diseases associated with obesity (e.g. high blood pressure and diabetes), do not appear to occur until the BMI exceeds 27, then there is a gradual increase in risk as the BMI increases. In practical terms, this means that the average woman, 1.63 metres (5 foot 4 inches) in height, should weigh between 52.7 and 67 kg (8 stone 4 pounds to 10 stone 8 pounds), but there is no health risk until she weighs more than 71.3 kg (11 stone 3 pounds). When the BMI exceeds 35, the risk of premature death is doubled.

body movements

The following terms are used to describe body movements (see figure 17):

- ABDUCTION: a movement away from the midline of the body. Abduction also refers to the spreading apart of fingers or toes
- ADDUCTION: a movement towards the middle of the body. It also refers to movements of the fingers or toes when they are drawn closer together
- CIRCUMDUCTION: a complex movement which combines abduction, adduction, extension, and flexion so that a limb, for example, follows a cone-shaped path. Circumduction incorporates all the movements of ball and socket joints (e.g. hips and shoulder)
- DORSIFLEXION: a movement of the foot which brings the toes closer to the shin
- EVERSION: turning the sole of the foot outwards
- EXTENSION: straightening of a joint so that two bones move further apart
- FLEXION: bending a joint so that two bones move closer together
- INVERSION: turning the sole of the foot inwards
- PLANTAR FLEXION: a movement of the foot which takes the toes further away from the shin; pointing the toes downwards
- PRONATION: turning the wrist so that the palm faces downwards (or an inward rotation of the foot)
- ROTATION: movement around the axis of a bone or body part. Movement towards the midline of the body is called medial (or internal) rotation; movement away from the midline is called lateral (or external) rotation
- SUPINATION: turning the palm upwards (or an internal rotation of the foot).

body schema: *See* **body image**.

Figure 16 Chart depicting body weight to height ratio

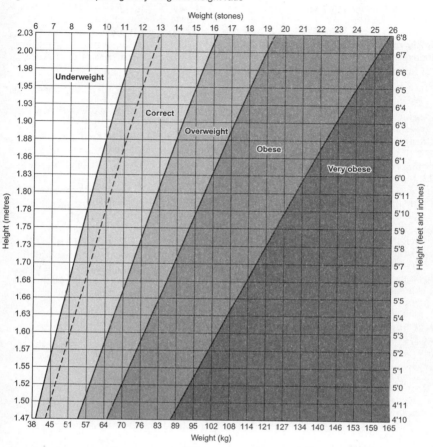

© Health Education Authority 1994, reproduced by permission

Underweight. More food may be needed. In cases of very low weight, a doctor should be consulted.

Correct. The right quantity of food is being eaten to maintain energy balance. If a person falls into the lower end of the weight range, they should maintain their weight and not be tempted to aim for the underweight category.

Overweight. Some loss of weight might be beneficial to health.

Obese. There is a need to lose weight.

Very obese. There is an urgent need to lose weight. It is advisable to consult a doctor or dietitian.

Figure 17 Body movements

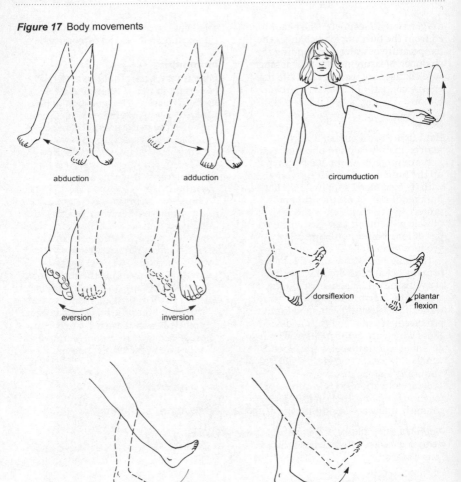

abduction

adduction

circumduction

eversion

inversion

dorsiflexion

plantar flexion

flexion

extension

body size

A characteristic determined by both height and weight. It is often estimated using the ponderal index, the body height divided by the cube root of body weight, i.e.:

$$\text{ponderal index} = \text{height}/\sqrt[3]{\text{weight}}$$

body temperature: *See* core temperature.

body wraps

Some health farms offer body wraps, a form of mud treatment, as a means of reducing weight. It is claimed that wrapping the body in bandages and covering them with mud encourages weight loss by drawing 'toxins' out of fatty tissue. In truth, the body wraps are likely to increase sweating and any weight loss experienced is probably temporary.

bomb calorimeter

A thick-walled container for measuring the energy content of food. The food is placed in a bomb calorimeter filled with oxygen. An electric spark ignites the food which is completely burned in the oxygen-rich atmosphere. The heat liberated from the burning food changes the temperature of water surrounding the chamber. Measurements of the temperature changes are used to calculate the energy content of the food (*see* **Atwater factor**).

bone

Hard tissue consisting of a calcified matrix (mainly calcium phosphate) and fibres of protein. About 200 bones make up the human skeleton. It is living tissue with its own blood supply. Bones have a number of functions: they support and protect soft tissues; they act as levers for muscle movement; and the central cavities of long bones store minerals and produce blood cells.

The long bones and some flat bones contain a central cavity filled with a very active tissue called bone marrow. In adults, the marrow in certain bones (e.g. those of the sternum, ribs, and limbs) produce new red blood cells and destroy those which are defunct. Marrow is also an important source of white blood cells which play a vital role in the body's immunity against disease.

Bone elongation stops in adults, but bones may change their density and strength at any age (figure 18). Bones

Figure 18 Bone density decreases with age, increasing the risk of osteoporosis (brittle bone disease)

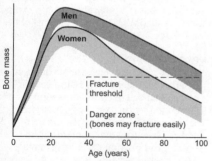

need to be mechanically stressed if they are to remain strong and healthy. They tend to become thicker and denser when exercise intensity increases, but they get less dense and weaker if a person becomes inactive. They also weaken if there is a deficiency of calcium or vita-

min D in the diet, or if calcium absorption is impaired. *See also* **osteoporosis**.

bone injury

Bone is very strong, but it is also relatively rigid so that if it yields at all, it tends to fracture. The sensation of pain is confined to the outer membrane lining the bone (the periosteum). Therefore, unless this part is damaged, some bone disorders may go unrecognized. However, pain is severe if the periosteum is even slightly stretched (e.g. by a stress fracture).

Complete fractures of bone are usually fairly obvious, either from external examination or from an X-ray. Stress fractures, however, are much more difficult to deal with, and often require a bone scan to confirm diagnosis. A bone scan uses scintigraphy to examine the condition of a bone. Scintigraphy is a technique in which a small dose of a radioactive tracer is introduced into the body part to be examined. A scintillation counter helps to produce a picture (a scintigram) of the distribution of the tracer in internal parts of the body.

bone marrow: *See* **bone**.

bone scan: *See* **bone injury**.

bonking

A term used in the USA by long-distance cyclists to describe the disorientation and muscular fatigue resulting from depletion of glycogen stores and abnormally low levels of glucose in the blood (known medically as hypoglycaemia).

bony spur

An abnormal outgrowth of bone.

boredom

A condition characterized by wandering attention, impaired efficiency, and low levels of arousal. It is sometimes confused with fatigue, but boredom usually results from too little stimulation, motivation, and interest. It commonly occurs in those who regularly perform monotonous exercise routines. Unlike fatigue, boredom leads to a lack of desire to exercise, rather than an inability to exercise. Boredom is one of the main reasons why people stop exercising and drop out of sport. It can be avoided if the type and location of exercise is varied, if achievable but challenging targets are set, and if exercise is made more fun.

Borg scale: *See* **perceived exertion.**

born athlete: *See* **athlete.**

boron

An essential mineral for healthy plant growth, boron may also be essential for animals. There is some evidence that, in small amounts, it may reduce calcium loss in post-menopausal women, reducing the risk of osteoporosis, but the evidence is weak and has been challenged.

botulism

A particularly dangerous form of food poisoning caused by a toxin produced by the bacterium *Clostridium botulinum*. The bacterium is common in soil but also thrives in improperly processed foods, especially low-acid canned goods. Extra care should be taken to destroy bacteria during home-bottling. The toxin affects the central nervous system, particularly the cardiac and respiratory centres, and can cause death due to heart and lung failure. The toxin is usually destroyed during cooking.

One authoritative medical book recommends that infants under a year old should not be given home-made honey because it may contain dormant spores of *Clostridium botulinum* which can grow in the immature digestive tract. Honey is safe for older people because it does not contain the toxin and the bacterium cannot survive in the more mature gut.

bouncing breast syndrome

An unpleasant condition experienced by women who run with their breasts not fully supported. Running causes the breasts to bounce, damaging the suspensory ligaments and sometimes resulting in a form of mastitis (inflammation of the breast). The syndrome can be prevented by wearing a well-fitted sports bra.

bovine spongiform encephalopathy (BSE; mad cow disease)

An infectious disease in cattle thought to be caused by a prion, a very small abnormal heat-resistant protein with the unusual property of transforming normal protein into more prions, hence the infectious nature of the disease. The abnormal protein accumulates leading to nerve damage in the brain. Spread between species is possible. Cattle can, for example, contract the disease from feed containing meat and bone-meal from sheep infected with scrapie (the sheep form of the disease). Transfer of the disease has not yet been demonstrated with certainty between cow and man, but it is a possibility if infected offal (specifically, nerve, brains, and spinal cord) is eaten, as it was between 1988 and 1992 in the UK. The human form of the disease is sometimes called Creutzfeldt-Jakob disease or CJD, but, at the time of writing, it is still not known whether or not BSE and CJD are the same disease.

bowel

The large intestine.

bowler's hip

A condition characterized by a chronic hip pain. It is caused by an inflammation of a muscle tendon which attaches onto the front of the femur just below the hip. Bowler's hip may result from any vigorous activity, but it is most common in activities that include repeated hip extensions coupled with twisting actions of the lower back.

bowler's thumb

An injury to either a tendon or nerve at the base of the thumb. It is commonly experienced by tenpin bowlers who attempt to put spin on the ball by keeping the thumb inside the thumbhole until the last possible moment before release. This bowling action puts great strain on tendons and the ulnar nerve. It is usually a transient condition as symptoms subside when bowling stops, but it sometimes results in permanent damage to the nerve. Bowler's thumb can be avoided by widening the thumbhole of the ball, changing technique, or padding the thumb.

bowling

Bowling, whether tenpin bowling with a large, heavy bowl or lawn bowls played with a lighter, wooden bowl, is not a great stamina builder, but it can increase flexibility of arms and shoulders, strengthen legs, and improve coordination. The act of delivering a bowl involves a back swing, forward swing, release, and follow through. These movements involve the coordinated action of muscles in the back, shoulders, arms, and legs. During the delivery, the back may be bent forward and twisted. This imposes considerable mechanical stress on the discs, ligaments, and muscles of the lower back. Consequently, bowling is not recommended for people with persistent lower back problems, and all bowlers are advised to warm up. Gentle mobility and stretching exercises help to reduce the risk of injury.

bowls: *See* bowling.

boxercise (aerobox)

Gleason's Gym in New York, once the training ground of Muhammad Ali and Mike Tyson, is now one of the main locations for a new aerobic activity, boxercise. This activity is quickly gaining in popularity among men and women with many fitness centres across the USA providing classes. Boxercisers perform the same training as professional boxers, including punching balls and shadow boxing, but they do not hit each other. They train not to fight but to improve fitness. In addition to developing power, boxercise also develops grace, coordination, and balance. No doubt one of the additional attractions of boxercise is the opportunity it provides to release pent up aggression. *See also* **boxing**.

boxer's arm

An injury resulting from a direct blow on the arm. The blow detaches a small spur of bone that develops just above the elbow in many boxers and exponents of the martial arts. After extended rest, the spur usually reattaches itself.

boxer's fracture

A fracture of the neck of the fifth metacarpal bone in the hand, commonly resulting from a mistimed punch.

boxer's knuckle

An injury to the soft tissue of the knuckle. It is common in boxers who have their outstretched hands bandaged before a fight. This results in the bandage being too tight when the hand is flexed to make a fist, damaging the underlying tissue.

boxer's muscle

A muscle in the front of the thorax which has the anatomical name serratus anterior. It is the main muscle responsible for pushing and punching movements, hence its common name.

boxing

Boxing is an arduous contact sport requiring very high levels of physical fitness and controlled aggression. There is little doubt that professional boxing is dangerous and can cause serious, even fatal injuries. Many people believe that it is unacceptably hazardous and should be banned. However, supporters of amateur boxing, including some physicians, believe that the amateur code should be considered differently from the professional code. They emphasize that the main aim of amateur boxing is to score points and not to knock out the opponent. Therefore, success depends more on finesse and strategy than brute force. Supporters argue that amateur boxing is much less dangerous than professional boxing (e.g. because of the shorter bouts, more protective gear, heavier gloves etc. in the amateur version). Supporters also cite statistics to indicate that boxing is less dangerous than several other popular contact sports including ice hockey, rugby, and American football. In college and high school American football, for example, three deaths occur per 10 000 participants; in boxing only 1.3 deaths occur per 10 000 participants. Supporters maintain that amateur boxing is a time-honoured way of encouraging young men to develop character and physical fitness, and that it should continue to be a valuable element of the Olympic programme. Nevertheless, many groups of physicians, including the American Medical Association, oppose all forms of boxing because participants suffer repeated blows to the head which have a cumulative effect on the brain (*see* **punch-drunk**

syndrome). These opponents of boxing believe that a sport whose main aim is to inflict damage is repugnant, and that boxing should not be condoned as a civilized sporting activity. *See also* **boxercise.**

bradycardia

A decreased or slowed heart rate, sometimes taken as being less than 60 beats per minute. The significance of bradycardia depends on a person's history. Those who have suffered a heart attack sometimes develop chronic bradycardia that needs to be treated with a pacemaker. A slow resting heart rate is, however, a normal effect of endurance training and is usually taken as a sign of good aerobic fitness. *See also* **athlete's heart**.

branched-chain amino acids (BCAA)

A group of three essential amino acids: isoleucine, leucine, and valine. They may be important in promoting muscle growth and repair, particularly after strenuous training. They are the main amino acids used as fuel by exercising muscle. There are claims that BCAA supplements reduce feelings of fatigue, but these claims are still being tested. A new sports drink incorporates BCAAs. Initial findings suggest that it reduces perceived exertion, but that it has little effect on performance.

breakfast

Breakfast is regarded by many nutritionists as the most important meal of the day, yet it is the one meal that many dieters and exercisers miss: dieters, because they believe that by missing it they can reduce calorific intake and lose weight; exercisers, because their early morning routines often leave them little time to eat. However, food consumed at breakfast seems to be more easily utilized than the same amount eaten at night. In one study, subjects who needed about 2000 Calories per day to maintain body weight, lost weight when the calories were eaten in one morning meal, and gained weight if they ate the same amount at night.

Clearly, to be of any real value, breakfast must be nutritious. Breakfasts vary according to the culture of the country. In Britain and the USA breakfasts often include complex carbohydrates which contain fibre, proteins, minerals, and vitamins, and provide a steady stream of glucose. Equally nutritious breakfasts are provided by salads and soups in Japan, or fish and bread in Norway. There seems to be sound sense in the old adage 'breakfast like a king, lunch like a prince, and dine like a pauper'.

breast-feeding

Breast milk is the perfect food for a newborn baby. It contains a balanced mixture of carbohydrates, fats, and proteins, with adequate amounts of vitamins (except vitamin D) and minerals. During the first two weeks, breast milk is called colostrum or early milk. It contains substances (e.g. immunoglobulins, lactoferrin, and lysozyme) that provide some immunity from infection. Breast-feeding lowers the incidence of food allergies in infants, especially those from families with a history of hypersensitivity.

A study of 926 babies born before the normal 40 week term of pregnancy, found that those fed on breast milk had significantly higher IQs by the time they were 7 years old, than those given formula milk. It was suggested that the effect was due to breast milk containing long chain polyunsaturates, special fatty acids similar to those found in oily fish. These are believed to help the nervous system to develop.

During lactation, the dietary demands of the mother are greater than during pregnancy. A breast-feeding mother has to produce milk continually to satisfy the incessant demands of her child. She has to consume sufficient nutrients for herself and her infant. She can obtain most of these nutrients, especially protein, calcium, magnesium, and vitamin B_2, from cow's milk. (Newborn babies cannot cope with cow's milk because it contains more protein than the infant can deal with and a high mineral content which may damage their kidneys.) Other calcium-rich foods include cheese, yoghurt, soya milk, and dark green vegetables. At least three servings of such foods should be eaten each day.

If the mother's intake of vitamins and minerals is inadequate, the quantity of milk is more likely to be affected than its quality. The baby's supply of vitamins and minerals is usually maintained at the expense of maternal body stores. The American Medical Association is one of several reputable organizations to suggest that multivitamin–mineral supplementation may be beneficial to lactating women.

A nursing mother's milk contains large amounts of water, so she should drink plenty of fluids (at least eight glasses a day) to prevent the supply of milk from drying up.

Anything the mother consumes may affect the quality of her milk. If she smokes tobacco, drinks alcohol, or takes other drugs, the toxins from these substances may seep into her milk and affect the infant.

Lactating mothers often feel overweight, but should not go on a severe weight-loss diet. The mothers need to retain some fat in the breasts and other fat stores for milk production. However, a slow and steady weight loss, no more than 1 kg (2.2 lb) per week, is possible through a sensible selection of low-calorie, nutritious foods. Most fat is lost, anyway, once lactation stops and, in the long term, mothers who breast-feed tend to retain less fat than those who do not.

breast reduction: *See* **mammaplasty**.

breast-stroker's knee
An injury to the inner (medial) surface of the knee, usually caused by the hydrodynamic forces produced by swimmers using a breast-stroke action. It is possible that swimmers who perform whip kicks are more prone to the condition because of extensive movements at the hip. Risk of this injury may be reduced by strengthening the quadriceps and hamstring muscles which act as stabilizers, limiting the amount of abduction and adduction of the lower leg.

breathing
Breathing is a natural act and most people do not give it a second thought unless they encounter difficulty. However, many non-athletes think that there is some magical method of breathing that endows athletes, particularly distance

runners, with greater powers. This is not the case. Arthur Lydiard, one of the gurus of distance running stated: 'There is no set rule for how you breathe. You'll consume a great amount of oxygen when you are running and it doesn't matter how you get it.' Nevertheless, there are coaches who advocate special techniques: many European coaches used to insist that their athletes breathe only through the nose; the Finns, many years ago, introduced an extended rhythm system, beginning with four strides to inhale and two strides to exhale, increasing until there are up to eight strides on inhalation and six on exhalation; and some modern coaches advocate 'belly breathing' using mainly the diaphragm rather than the chest muscles. These techniques may be effective for some, but if they have to be performed consciously they may interfere with the relaxation essential for efficient exercising.

Although not important in aerobic exercises, breathing technique is important for those performing strenuous anaerobic exercises, such as weight training. They should not hold their breath during the complete exercise. This causes an increase in intra-abdominal pressure that might result in dizziness or lightheadedness, which can be dangerous for those with a heart condition. Most coaches train their weight-lifters to inhale as the weight is lowered and exhale as it is lifted. Difficulty in breathing occurs after extreme exertion, but breathlessness after mild exertion may indicate a malfunction of the lungs or heart. *See also* **asthma**.

brittle bone disease: *See* **osteoporosis**.

bromelain
An enzyme extracted from pineapples and used in certain slimming pills. Manufacturers claim that bromelain (with other enzymes in the pills) helps to break down body fat and enables slimmers to lose weight effortlessly. There is no scientific evidence to support this claim. The manufacturers' advertisements state that the pills should be taken as part of a low calorie diet. Users who follow this instruction may well lose weight, but weight loss is probably due

to the low calorie diet, not the pills. Bromelain, like any other protein in the gut, would be digested and have no action.

bronchitis

Inflammation of the bronchioles, restricting air flow to and from the lungs. Acute bronchitis is caused by a viral or bacterial infection and is aggravated by physical activity. Chronic bronchitis may be induced by smoking. Aerobic exercise is generally beneficial to sufferers, particularly those who can give up smoking.

brown adipose tissue: *See* **brown fat.**

brown fat (brown adipose tissue)

A layer of special heat-producing fat cells found mainly around the shoulder blades and kidneys; it is more abundant in infants than adults.

Brown fat cells contain many more mitochondria than other types of fat cells. Mitochondria are sometimes called the powerhouses of the cell because they are the organelles responsible for aerobic respiration. They usually produce the energy-rich storage compound ATP, but in brown fat their activity is diverted to heat production. The colour of brown fat is derived from highly pigmented chemicals (cytochromes) contained within the mitochondria. These cytochromes enable mitochondria to produce heat instead of ATP.

The purpose of brown fat in small mammals and babies is to maintain body temperature. Hibernating mammals metabolize brown fat to re-warm their bodies during arousal. Brown fat is well supplied with blood which can transport the heat to different parts of the body. Unlike other types of fat, it has its own nerve supply which can quickly stimulate it to produce heat when the animal (or baby) gets cold.

There has been a lot of speculation about the significance of brown fat in adults. It makes up less than 1 per cent of the body weight and is generally regarded as unimportant. It is, however, more abundant in lean than in fat animals and some researchers believe that it plays a role in regulating body weight and energy balance, at least in small mammals.

It has also been shown that some forms of obesity and overweight in mice are linked to an inherited lack of brown fat. Some members of the slimming industry have capitalized on these ideas by marketing special clothes with holes in the back and arm pits, which they claim will stimulate the formation of brown fat and help you lose weight effortlessly. The effectiveness of these clothes has yet to be scientifically proven.

bruise (contusion)

A bruise is likely to develop whenever your body collides with another object, so it is a very common injury in any contact sport. A bruise forms from seepage of blood in an internal wound. The blood gradually decomposes, changing colour from red to blue as haemoglobin loses its oxygen, and then to yellow as the haemoglobin is reabsorbed. The accumulation of blood in damaged tissues can be reduced by applying firm pressure for 3–5 minutes immediately after the injury, followed by a cold compress. *See also* **haematoma.**

BSE: *See* **bovine spongiform encephalopathy.**

buffer

A substance that helps to prevent a solution from undergoing a change in pH when an acid or alkali is added. Buffers, such as acetic, carbonic, citric, or lactic acid, are added to foods as acidity regulators. They are commonly used in canned fruits, jams, jellies, and sweets. In the human body, the buffers are chiefly bicarbonate, phosphate, and protein.

bulimia nervosa (binge–purge syndrome)

An eating disorder characterized by sequences of excessive eating followed by purging. Self-induced vomiting is the most common purging behaviour, but others include fasting, excessive exercise, laxative abuse, and diuretic abuse. Individuals who develop bulimia are convinced that they are overweight and that their body shape is abnormal. Bulimics begin restrictive dieting in an effort to lose weight, but this induces hunger and thoughts of food which leads to binge eating. In an effort to undo the excessive eating, the bulimic vomits or purges what he or, more commonly, she has eaten. Bulimia may become chronic if an individual develops a psychological need to binge.

Bulimic behaviour may become a means through which emotional problems are regulated and managed. Binge eating may help to release pent-up emotions and enable the bulimic to be distracted temporarily from unpleasant problems. However, the bulimic then has to purge to remove the feelings of guilt associated with the bingeing.

A number of medical complications can occur as a direct or indirect result of bulimic behaviour. Dental problems, including erosion of tooth enamel and gum disease, may occur if there is frequent vomiting of the acidic contents of the stomach. Gastrointestinal problems are common, including abdominal cramps, constipation and diarrhoea. Laxative abuse may lead to loss of normal bowel function. An imbalance of electrolytes, caused by loss of body fluids, may result in cardiovascular complications. Most of these effects of bulimia are reversible once the sufferer resumes a normal eating pattern.

Bulimia nervosa may occur as a phase of anorexia nervosa, and bulimics often share the same psychological problems as anorexics. Both disorders must be treated seriously and medical advice sought. However, it is not easy to identify bulimics. They may show few symptoms until late in the course of the illness, and, unlike anorexics, they may be of normal weight. In addition, bulimics are very secretive about their condition and usually deny vehemently that they have a problem.

bulk: *See* fibre.

bulking agents

Bulking agents are substances that add to the bulk of food. They are dietary fibres that usually contain no calories and pass through the intestine undigested. Consequently, they are common ingredients of slimming foods. Some so-called slimming pills and tablets contain bulking agents such as guar gum, extracted from the seeds of a tropical Indian member of the pea family, *Cyamopsis tetraglobula*. If taken before a meal, the gum makes you feel full and depresses your appetite. Unfortunately, excessive amounts may block the intestines, so the British government recommends that products should contain no more than 15 per cent of this gum. Other bulking agents, other gums, and cellulose-related substances such as sugar beet fibre, may also block the intestines and cause flatulence if taken in excess.

bungee jumping

An increasingly popular activity in which a person, attached to elasticated ropes, jumps from a considerable height. The jumper goes into a free-fall, broken by the ropes that are secured at the jump-off point. The ropes prevent the jumper from hitting the ground or water. They are elasticated so that the jumper's descent does not come to an abrupt halt and deceleration is at a tolerable rate.

In 1993, there were more than 60 000 bungee jumps in the UK, many for charity. Some of the jumps were made by people with little training. Although there have been few accidents involving collision with the ground or another object, there is concern that the jumps result in a sudden rise in pressure within the eye which may detach the retina and lead to blindness. Prospective jumpers are advised to consult a physician to ensure that they have no medical condition (such as high blood pressure, eye problems, or bone disorders) which might be exacerbated by jumping. In addition, they should ensure that the jump is properly organized. In the UK, the official national body for bungee jumping is the British Elastic Rope Association. It ensures that sites are safe and that jumpers have had sufficient training.

bunion

A deformity at the base of the big toe, relatively common among exercisers who wear training shoes that do not fit properly. The skin over the big toe is thickened and the head of the metatarsal (a bone within the toe) becomes unduly prominent. Treatment may involve simple orthotics, or the use of a soft spongy pad to straighten the big toe. Occasionally surgery is necessary.

burn out

A complex psychological and physiological condition characterized by feelings of anxiety, tension, fatigue, exhaustion, and a loss of concern for other people. It develops as a result of chronic stress, especially among people in very demanding jobs. Burn out has been viewed by psychologists as 'an imbalance between the psychological resources of an individual and the demands being made on these resources'. It leads to mental fatigue and an inability to deal with stressful situations. Anyone can experience burn out but it is particularly prevalent in business middle-managers and professional athletes who push themselves (or are pushed) too hard.

burns

1 Thermal damage to the skin or other tissues as a result of excessive heat. During the performance of vigorous physical activities, heat is generated by friction and the skin can be burned wherever it rubs against another surface. When a burn has occurred, you should avoid activities that risk further friction.

2 A form of weight training designed to increase the size of muscle. The exerciser makes rapid half contractions which produce a burning sensation in the muscle. This is believed to be due to the pumping of blood into muscle. *See also* **pumping-up**.

bursa

A small fibrous fluid-filled sac usually found where soft tissues, such as muscles and tendons, move over bony prominences. Bursae reduce friction during movement and act as shock absorbers. They can become inflamed and blistered internally by repeated mechanical irritation (a condition known as frictional bursitis); by substances formed as a result of inflammation or degeneration of tissue (chemical bursitis), or by bacterial infection (septic bursitis). Frictional bursitis is the most common form suffered by exercisers. Treatment may involve the application of an anti-inflammatory drug or heat therapy. *See also* **housemaid's knee**.

bursitis: *See* bursa.

bute: *See* phenylbutazone.

butterflies

An uncomfortable feeling in the pit of the stomach arising from excessive muscle tension associated with high levels of arousal. Although innocuous, butterflies may be distracting and worrying, and therefore detrimental to athletic performance. They can be controlled by relaxation techniques.

butterfly machine: *See* fixed-weight machine.

butylated hydroxyanisole: *See* BHA.

C

caffeine

Caffeine occurs naturally in about 60 species of plant, including coffee beans, tea leaves, and cocoa nuts. It is a constituent of chocolate bars, coffee, tea, and cola-type drinks and occurs in the following approximate amounts:

	CAFFEINE PER AVERAGE CUP OR BAR (MG)
ground coffee	90
instant coffee	60
decaffeinated coffee	3
tea	40
cola	40
chocolate bar	40

Caffeine is a mildly addictive drug. It acts as a stimulant, increasing blood pressure, and accelerating heart rate and breathing. It also makes you feel more alert and energetic.

High caffeine consumption prior to competition is banned by the International Olympic Committee because it improves performance artificially and it may be harmful if taken in excess. Concentrations above 12 micrograms per millilitre are regarded as positive indicators of doping.

Caffeine may boost athletic performance by improving muscle strength and reaction times. Drinking as little as two cups of coffee may enable athletes of average ability to run the 1500 metres several seconds faster. Coffee may also improve endurance and delay fatigue by mobilizing free fatty acids, making them more readily available as fuel. A high carbohydrate diet appears to nullify this effect.

Excessive caffeine intake can cause sleeplessness, diarrhoea, fluid loss, and stomach irritation. Many researchers have tried to link high caffeine consumption to an increased risk of certain diseases, such as cancer, high blood pressure, and heart disease. As yet, the links have not been confirmed and some of the evidence is contradictory. However, there is a well-established correlation between heart disease and those who both smoke and have high levels of caffeine consumption. Caffeine, when consumed at the same time as other foods, may also interfere with the absorption of minerals, such as calcium and iron. Loss of bone density associated with ageing in adults, may be accelerated by drinking two or more cups of coffee a day. Coffee also acts as a diuretic, increasing urine production by as much as 30 per cent.

Although there is still some uncertainty about the effects of caffeine, the general medical opinion is that between 200–250 milligrams of caffeine a day rarely cause adverse reactions in healthy adults. It also appears that caffeine consumed during exercise (rather than before or after it) has little effect on heart rate, performance, or urine production.

caffeinism

A condition resulting from a very high intake of caffeine and characterized by anxiety, mood swings, sleep disruption, and other physiological and psychological abnormalities. Abstinence following high intake can lead to withdrawal symptoms such as severe headaches. A caffeine intake of more than 600 mg per day may produce depression and other harmful effects. Caffeine intoxification is recognized as a medical condition in the USA. Many doctors believe that young people may be particularly sensitive to the harmful effects of caffeine and want to limit the amount of caffeine in cola drinks (one American high caffeine cola drink has more than 200 mg of caffeine in each can).

calciferol: *See* **vitamin D**.

calcium

A metallic element essential for normal development and health. The average adult contains over 1 kg of calcium, stored mainly as calcium salts in the bones. Calcium is essential for the normal activity of muscles and nerves, for growth of bones and teeth, and for blood clotting.

In the United States, it is recommended that adults take 800 mg of calcium each day; in the UK, the Reference Nutrient Intake (RNI, the amount of nutrient sufficient for almost all individuals) is 700 mg per day. Higher RDAs are recommended for children, adolescents, pregnant and lactating mothers. In the USA, the National Institute of Health recommended that post-menopausal women should consume between 1200 and 1500 mg of calcium per day to reduce the risk of osteoporosis. Some nutritionists believe that this high level of intake after menopause has no benefit. The need for adequate calcium is greatest in adolescents and young adults, so as to maximize bone density. The higher the peak density, the longer the post-menopausal losses can continue without causing significant weakening of the bone. Regular exercise is also important to minimize mineral loss. Good sources of calcium are milk, cheese, yoghurt, legumes, nuts, and wholegrains. Vitamin D aids absorption.

About one-third of the dietary intake of calcium is egested in the faeces. Some is also excreted in the urine with the amount increasing among those on a high protein diet. Long-duration activity and high temperatures increase the amount of calcium lost in urine and sweat. Many sports coaches believe that these losses justify the use of calcium supplements by young women, especially

elite endurance athletes who train at a relatively high intensity for long periods.

Excess calcium depresses some physiological activities associated with nerves and muscles and can lead to the development of kidney stones. Calcium deficiencies can slow down the growth rate of children and cause rickets. Deficiencies in adults may lead to the development of soft, inadequately mineralized bones (osteomalacia) and brittle bones. *See also* **osteoporosis**.

calf raise (heel raise)

An exercise (figure 19) that strengthens the calf muscles (gastrocnemius and soleus).

Figure 19

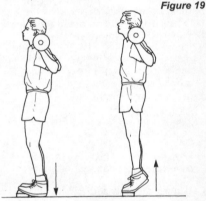

■ Keeping your heels on the ground, place the balls of your feet on a block of wood about 5 cm (2 inches) high. Start with your knees bent and then slowly straighten them so that you stretch your heels. Smoothly and gently, lift up fully on to your toes, raising your heels above the floor. Hold for a few seconds, lower gently, and repeat.

This exercise can be made more difficult by holding a barbell across the back of the shoulders. Alternatively, use a weight-training machine which enables you to apply a weight onto the shoulders only during the lifting phase.

calisthenics

Systematic, rhythmic exercises, such as sit-ups and push-ups, which utilize the weight of the body as resistance. The exercises are usually performed gracefully. They are designed to tone and strengthen muscle, and to promote general fitness. Structured training routines, similar to circuit training, have been formulated using timed calisthenics. Exercise intensity is controlled by varying the number of repetitions performed in a given time. As fitness improves, you can increase the number of repetitions and circuits. However, once you can perform a certain number of repetitions (approximately 25), additional repetitions will only improve your muscular endurance, not your strength. To develop strength, you can add weights or change your body position to increase the resistance. For example, you can wear a weighted vest or elevate your feet while doing push-ups. Exercises in a calisthenics routine should be chosen carefully so that all the major muscle groups are worked. A typical routine might consist of seven exercises: burpees, curl-ups, push-ups, treadmills, running on the spot, star jumps, and chin-ups. Each exercise lasts a predetermined time depending on fitness level, and is separated from the next exercise by a 10 second rest period. Exercisers usually walk for two minutes between circuits to hasten recovery.

caloric balance: *See* energy balance.

caloric equivalence: *See* heat equivalence.

calorie

Despite an international convention which agreed to use the joule (J) as the standard unit for energy, work, and heat, the calorie is the unit most commonly used in written work about nutrition. One calorie is the amount of heat required to raise the temperature of 1 g of water through 1°C (more precisely, from 14.5°C to 15.5°C). It is easy to convert calories into joules, as one calorie equals 4.2 joules (more exactly, 4.184 joules). These units are very small in relation to the energy used by a person, so it is usual to use units 1000 times larger. These should be called kilocalories (often written as Calorie), but most diet and exercise books use 'calories' to mean kilocalories; so a 1000 calorie diet is really a diet that provides 1000 kilocalories a day.

calorie counting

An awareness of the calorie content of foods is healthy, but an obsessive preoccupation with the exact number of calories you eat in any one day can be both unhealthy and ineffective. It can be unhealthy because the calorie content gives no indication of the nutritional value of the food, only its energy content. It can be ineffective because once those on a calorie controlled diet overshoot their daily target they often eat without restraint. Calorie awareness should include the fact that all foods contain calories (even a piece of celery!), but that it is really only worth considering calorie consumption and expenditure in hundreds of calories; many drinks, especially alcohol, have a significant calorie content; and that fats and sugars are the most calorie dense foods (25 g of butter, for example, has more calories than 275 g of potatoes). Most dietitians and nutritionists agree that it is better to understand the basic principles of nutrition so that you can eat a balanced diet containing all the main food groups in their correct proportions, than blindly follow a set of calorie-counting rules. Nevertheless, simple calorie counting does provide a way of controlling energy intake and losing weight.

calorimetry

Measurements of energy expenditure and energy consumption in terms of heat units, usually expressed as kilocalories. There are two main types of calorimetry: direct and indirect.

Direct calorimetry is based on the premise that energy expended by an individual doing any kind of work is ultimately converted to heat. To measure this heat, a person is placed in a specially designed, insulated chamber (called a calorimeter) supplied with air and surrounded by a jacket of circulating water; the heat production (or energy expenditure) is estimated from changes in the temperature of the surrounding water.

Indirect calorimetry uses oxygen consumption as a means of estimating energy expenditure. Oxygen is required to release from food the energy needed for activity. The more energy expended, the more oxygen is consumed. To convert values of oxygen consumption to kilo-calories of energy expenditure, it is necessary to know what type of food is being used as the energy source. This is because a litre of oxygen will release different amounts of energy from fats, carbohydrates, and proteins.

A new method for measuring energy expenditure has been devised. This entails drinking heavy water (it has the formula $^2H_2{}^{18}O$; normal water has the formula $^1H_2{}^{16}O$). Oxygen-18 and deuterium (hydrogen-2) are two stable, harmless isotopes that can be detected in liquids or in air. Some of the oxygen-18 is exhaled as carbon dioxide (the waste product of respiration), and some is excreted in urine along with some of the deuterium. Deuterium is lost from the body only in water. The difference between the rate of excretion of deuterium and oxygen-18 in the urine over a reasonable length of time (usually a day or more) can be used to estimate energy expenditure. The estimates can be made using daily urine samples and do not affect performance. The method has been used to gain valuable information about true energy expenditure under natural, as opposed to laboratory, conditions. Dual-labelled water was used to show that Sir Ranulph Fiennes and Dr Mike Stroud expended more than 8000 Calories a day during their polar expedition. This is three to four times an average person's daily energy expenditure and double the amount used by riders in the gruelling Tour de France.

Cambridge diet

A supervised, very low calorie diet first introduced in 1984. The original diet was criticized because it did not provide sufficient calories and protein, so it was reformulated. The new Cambridge diet (now part of the Cambridge Health Plan) uses specially formulated meal replacements to provide the vitamins, minerals, and fatty acids needed to maintain health. The reformulated diet provides the calories and protein recommended by the 1989 report of the Committee on Medical Aspects of Food Policy (COMA). The diet is designed to provide full nutritional needs with minimum energy. It is available only from trained counsellors

who check that prospective users have no medical problems and ensure that the diet is not taken for too long.

campylobacteriosis

A form of food poisoning caused by eating food contaminated with the bacterium *Campylobacter jejuni*. Sources of infection include raw or undercooked meat and poultry, untreated milk, shellfish, and untreated water.

Canadian home fitness test

A simple self-administered test that gives a rough guide to fitness levels. Its main purpose is to motivate exercisers by enabling them to monitor their own performance easily.

After warming up, exercisers climb two steps of a standard staircase (each step 8 inches or 20.3 cm high) at a rhythm set according to their age and sex. The stepping continues for one or two periods of 3 minutes each at a stepping rate approximating to 70 per cent maximum aerobic capacity. A fitness score is computed from the duration of the exercise and from changes in heart rate. Although the test is described by its authors as 'safe', they recommend that exercisers should complete a questionnaire prior to taking the test, to ensure basic fitness and health.

Canadian trunk strength test

A test of the muscular endurance of the abdominal muscles (figure 20).

■ Lie on your back with the knees flexed at 90 degrees and your fingertips touching a strip of masking tape placed perpendicular to your body. Perform a slow, partial curl-up by flattening out your lower back, then curling up your upper spine until your fingertips touch a second strip of masking tape, 8 cm from the first strip. Return to the start position and repeat as many times as you can at a rate of 20 curl-ups per minute, up to a maximum of 75.

cancer

A group of diseases characterized by the uncontrolled growth of abnormal cells which have the ability to spread throughout the body or body parts. Cancers are

Figure 20 Canadian trunk strength test

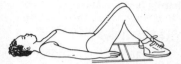 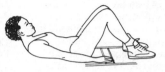

among the most insidious and feared diseases. There have been great advances in our understanding of cancers in recent years, but much remains unknown. Nevertheless, cancer research is a very active field and new knowledge is gained every day enabling doctors to establish the causes for the diseases and design new treatments. Unfortunately, a lot of this is pioneering research and sometimes claims are made prematurely or are exaggerated.

Diet has featured strongly in cancer research. Results are often inconclusive, but there are clear indications that some diets can affect the risk of contracting cancer. Scotland has a diet with one of the lowest levels of fruit and vegetable consumption in the world, and a particularly high incidence of bowel cancer. Some doctors believe that up to 1563 deaths a year, 90 per cent of the total caused by bowel cancer, could be avoided if people changed their diet. It is believed that high fibre diets with plenty of fruit and vegetables give some (but not complete) protection against bowel cancer, and a substance in garlic (diallylsulphide) may reduce the risk of stomach cancers. Animal research has shown that certain fish oil derivatives may halt the growth of some tumours. It is claimed that gamma-linoleic acid (GLA), found in evening primrose oil, has powerful anti-cancer properties; and there is a catalogue of claims about the effects of antioxidants, with the vitamins A, C, and E gaining most attention recently. Cancers of the pancreas, prostate, bladder, breast, cervix, womb, ovary, small intestine, and rectum have at some time been linked with obesity and unhealthy diets. These are just a few examples of the possible relationship between foods and cancers, and it is important to emphasize that many of the claims are not fully substantiated. In January 1993 the European Prospective Investigation of Cancer was

set up to examine links between diet and cancer. Detailed diet diaries and health records of 250 000 people across Europe are being studied over a ten-year period. The results will allow researchers to examine the diets of apparently healthy patients who later develop cancer.

The relationship between exercise and cancers has been studied in less depth. The general consensus, although tentative, seems to be that there is an optimum amount of exercise that activates the immune system and reduces risk of tumour development; regular exercise above and below this level may weaken the immune system and increase the risk of certain cancers. One study undertaken in 1977 examined the exercise habits of 17 000 Harvard graduates. Those who burned at least 1000 extra Calories a week exercising had half the incidence of colon cancer compared with sedentary people within the same age group. It was suggested that exercise may reduce the intestinal transit time (the amount of time food remains in the gut) and the exposure of the gut wall to carcinogens. The results, however, may be due to differences in diet between exercisers and non-exercisers.

candida

A group of yeast-like fungi that lives in moist areas of the body, including the alimentary tract and vagina. Normally, the populations of candida are kept in check by beneficial bacteria in the body, but sometimes they grow beyond tolerance levels and the infected person suffers a disease called candidiasis or thrush. In the vagina, thrush causes a white discharge and is accompanied by itching and soreness. Some doctors believe that heavy infections of candida in the gut can contribute to a wide range of different disorders, including abdominal discomfort, disturbed bowel function, soreness, and itching.

Some nutritionists believe that the

incidence of candidiasis is affected by an individual's health and diet. The fungi are thought to thrive on simple sugars, bread, and biscuits, as well as fermented foods such as yoghurt, cheese, and alcohol, which form a large part of the modern diet. A person in good health can usually keep candida under control, but if the immune system is weakened by illness or stress, or if friendly bacteria are killed off (for example, by antibiotics) the opportunistic fungus grows rapidly. People suffering from candidiasis often have cravings for sweets and yeast-containing foods and drinks, which makes weight control very difficult. Candidiasis can be treated with a special diet that emphasizes the avoidance of yeasty foods and the foods on which candida thrive, but doctors often use anti-candida drugs, such as nystatin.

candidiasis: *See* candida.

canoeing and kayaking

Performed correctly, canoeing and kayaking use every major muscle group in the body and are very good for developing aerobic fitness. Competitions require a lot of practice time and high levels of cardio-respiratory endurance. Recreational canoeing and kayaking are suitable for people over a wide range of age and fitness. Even if pursued solely as recreation, these activities have definite training effects improving stamina, firming muscles, and increasing shoulder and wrist flexibility. Despite their attractions, canoeing and kayaking share the same dangers as most water sports. To minimize these dangers, participants should be trained by well-qualified instructors, life jackets should always be worn and other water-safety guidelines followed.

carbohydrate addict's diet

A diet that appeals to the chocaholic has been described in the book *The carbohydrate addict's diet*, written by Drs Rachael and Richard Heller (1994, Mandarin, London).

Users of this diet are allowed three meals a day, two of which must contain no carbohydrates (no pasta, potatoes, fruit, sweets etc.). The Hellers recommend that the third meal should be balanced to include all the food groups, but it allows the dieters to have whatever they want, as long as it is consumed in less than one hour. This third meal is regarded by dieters as being a reward, and some use it as an excuse to satisfy their cravings for rich, chocolate-laden foods.

The theory behind the diet is that, by restricting most of the carbohydrate intake to one meal, hunger pangs are less likely to occur. High blood glucose levels stimulate insulin secretion which, in turn, causes the glucose to be converted into the storage carbohydrate, glycogen. Insulin production is believed to be linked to the development of hunger pangs. The Hellers claim that thousands of people have been helped to lose weight on this diet, through the Carbohydrate Centre they set up.

Helen Kon, a self-confessed chocaholic, reported in the *Independent* newspaper (16 August 1994) that she neither lost nor gained weight on the diet. However, although she was unsure of its nutritional benefits, she reported that she was going to keep to the carbohydrate addict's diet because she was having so much fun during what she called her 'happy hour'! *See also* **chocoholic**.

carbohydrate loading (carboloading; glycogen overshoot; muscle glycogen loading)

A classic experiment showed that a high carbohydrate diet can triple an athlete's endurance. It compared fuel use during exercise among three groups of runners. One group consumed a normal diet (about 55 per cent carbohydrate); one group consumed a high carbohydrate diet (83 per cent carbohydrate); and the third group consumed a low carbohydrate, high fat diet (about 94 per cent fat). The high carbohydrate group sustained activity for an average of 167 minutes, those on a normal balanced diet for 114 minutes, and those on a high fat diet for only 57 minutes. This study encouraged athletes to increase the carbohydrate stores within muscle artificially to improve their endurance capacity; a procedure called carbohydrate loading.

There are two main methods of carbohydrate loading. The traditional method is a combined diet and exercise regime that artificially raises the muscle glycogen (the main carbohydrate storage molecule in muscles). It is based on the assumption that depleting the muscle of its glycogen stores stimulates the body to take up and store more glycogen than normal. A typical carbohydrate-loading procedure for a marathon runner starts seven days before a race when the athlete depletes the muscle of its glycogen by running a long distance, usually about 20 miles (32 km). For the next three days (the depletion phase), the athlete eats a high protein, low carbohydrate diet and usually continues exercising to ensure that glycogen stores are completely depleted, and to sensitize the physiological processes which manufacture and store glycogen. For the final three days before a race, the athlete eats a high carbohydrate diet and takes little or no exercise. In the second method, training is tapered during the week before exercise and then the carbohydrate content of the diet is increased for the three days before the event. The second method has generally replaced the traditional method because it is simpler to follow, achieves the same muscle glycogen concentrations, and avoids the side-effects (diarrhoea, dehydration, and insomnia) sometimes experienced during the depletion phase of the traditional method.

Both methods of carbohydrate loading can more than double the glycogen content of muscle. However, the procedures are not without risks. Carbohydrate loading causes more water to be stored in the body (each gram of carbohydrate stored requires an extra 2.7 grams of water). This sometimes makes the athlete feel heavy and stiff. Some body-builders take advantage of this effect by carbohydrate loading before competition to 'pump' up their muscles. If used repeatedly, carbohydrate loading can lead to the presence of the red muscle pigment, myoglobin, in the urine (myoglobinuria), chest pains, and heart irregularities. A lot of the harmful effects of carbohydrate loading are linked to the depletion phase. Most sports nutritionists believe this phase is unnecessary and that an athlete needs only to load up on carbohydrate to benefit from it. It may be less risky to maintain a high muscle glycogen content by ensuring a good, regular daily intake of carbohydrates rather than by having a short period of carbohydrate loading.

carbohydrates

Carbohydrates are the most accessible and most used form of fuel in the body. One gram yields approximately 4 Calories of energy (about 16.7 joules).

Simple carbohydrates include the sugars (monosaccharides and disaccharides) found in jams, confectionery, cakes, biscuits, pastries, and table sugar. Complex carbohydrates include starches and fibres found in unrefined foods (e.g. bread, potatoes, rice, pasta, cereals, and nuts). Most carbohydrates (but not fibre) are broken down during digestion to glucose and other monosaccharides.

Although the precise figures differ, most nutritionists and dietitians recommend that carbohydrates (mainly complex carbohydrates because they contain other nutrients and fibre) should be the prime source of energy for everyone (*see also* **glycaemic index**). A typical recommendation is that 55–60 per cent of daily calories should come from carbohydrates, of which 85 per cent should be complex carbohydrates. The figure should be even higher (about 70 per cent of daily calories) for those who are regularly engaged in strenuous endurance activities. This means that an adult male exerciser in hard training and requiring about 4000 Calories a day, would need to eat about 500 grams of carbohydrate; a large plateful of pasta supplies about 110 grams of carbohydrate.

The ability of the body to store carbohydrate is limited, but relatively small amounts of glycogen can be stored in the liver and muscle (about 2000 kcal of energy, or the equivalent of the energy needed for about 32 km of running). Diets rich in carbohydrate help to replace muscle glycogen which is the main fuel used during exercise. There is also some evidence that carbohydrates are less easily converted to body fat than is dietary fat. *See also* **carbohydrate loading** and **glucose**.

carboloading: *See* **carbohydrate loading**.

cardiac arrest

The cessation of the effective pumping action of the heart. The heart may be beating rapidly without pumping any blood, or it may have stopped beating entirely. Cardiac arrest is marked by an abrupt loss of consciousness, and the absence of breathing and pulse.

cardiac arrhythmia

Any deviation from the normal rhythm of the heartbeat. Arrhythmias include palpitations and ectopic beats (extra beats outside the normal rhythm of heartbeats). They may be the result of heart disease, or have no apparent cause. Anyone experiencing cardiac arrythmias should consult a physician before performing vigorous exercise.

cardiac hypertrophy

Increase in the size of the heart. In endurance athletes, it is characterized by a larger, more efficient heart (see **athlete's heart**) and is a result of regular aerobic exercise. In non-athletes, cardiac hypertrophy may be the result of a number of pathological conditions, including heart valve disease. In these cases, the heart enlarges in an attempt to compensate for an inadequate supply of oxygenated blood. Cardiac enlargement is also associated with prolonged alcohol abuse. This is possibly related to vitamin B_1 deficiency due to alcoholism.

cardiac muscle

Special muscle found only within the heart. It can contract rhythmically without any external stimulation from nerves or hormones, as long as it is supplied with sufficient nutrients and oxygen. Unlike other types of muscle, cardiac muscle does not fatigue. However, it will stop contracting if its oxygen supply is interrupted.

cardiac output

The volume of blood pumped by the left ventricle of the heart in one minute. Cardiac output is the product of the stroke volume (the volume of blood leaving the left ventricle after each beat) and heart rate. The average cardiac output at rest is 5–6 litres per minute.

Regular aerobic exercise strengthens heart muscle and enables it to increase its stroke volume. A typical value for a sedentary man at complete rest is only 75 ml per beat; a typical value for a trained endurance athlete at rest is 105 ml per beat. A well conditioned person usually has a lower heart rate than a sedentary person for the same cardiac output. The high stroke volume of endurance athletes enables them to have a cardiac output of more than 30 litres per minute during exercise.

cardiac rehabilitation

A programme of activities designed to help patients who have suffered from heart disorders to return to normal activity without additional heart problems. The programme usually includes carefully controlled aerobic exercises; anaerobic activities are generally avoided.

cardiorespiratory endurance: *See* aerobic fitness.

cardiovascular disease

Diseases of the heart and blood vessels. The risk of suffering from a cardiovascular disease is increased by a number of factors including high blood pressure, obesity, smoking, psychological stress, and lack of exercise. *See also* **atherosclerosis** and **coronary heart disease**.

cardiovascular fitness: *See* aerobic fitness.

cardiovascular system

The body system, consisting of the heart and blood vessels, which circulates blood around the body.

carnitine

A compound found mostly in muscles where it plays an essential role as a transporter of the fatty acids used in energy production. Carnitine is synthesized in the body from two amino acids, lysine and methionine. The synthesis requires iron and certain vitamins (B_6, C, and niacin).

Two forms of carnitine exist: D-carnitine and L-carnitine, but only L-carnitine is physiologically significant. There is speculation that an extra dose of L-carnitine can boost long-term energy supplies and reduce body fat because it accelerates fat metabolism, or fat burning. Manufacturers of special diet foods containing carnitine claim that they boost athletic performance and help people to lose weight.

It is widely agreed that carnitine supplements are necessary for those who have a deficiency, but there is less agreement about its general use. Over-the-counter products were banned in the United States because there was no rigorous proof of the manufacturers' claims. In 1993, France stopped the sale of dozens of products containing carnitine because a government investigation concluded that carnitine neither enhances athletic performance nor helps people lose weight. *See also* **amino acid supplements**.

carotenes

A group of yellow substances, designated alpha-, beta-, and gamma-carotene, which are converted in the intestines and the liver into vitamin A. Beta-carotene is the best source of vitamin A. Carotenes are destroyed by heat, oxygen, and light. Excessive intake can make the skin appear yellow, simulating jaundice. However, the condition is harmless and reversible. Carotenes are important antioxidants. It has been claimed that carotene offers some protection against lung cancer induced by tobacco smoking. Research in the USA also suggests that beta-carotene may reduce several other types of cancer and coronary heart diseases. However, a study carried out in Finland in 1994 of 10 000 people showed that more lung cancer deaths actually occurred in those given carotene supplements, so the value of supplementation is unclear. Carotenes are present in a wide range of foods, but concentrations are especially high in carrots, parsley, and green leafy vegetables.

carotid artery

The main artery supplying oxygenated blood to the head. There is one carotid artery on each side of the neck. If the fingers are pressed gently against one of the arteries, the pulse (called the carotid pulse) can be felt. Simultaneous pressure against both carotid arteries is dangerous

as it may stop blood flowing to the brain. Within the wall of each carotid artery is a swelling (the carotid sinus) which contains nerve-endings sensitive to pressure changes in the blood. Pressure against the sinuses (e.g. in a wrestling stranglehold) causes a reflex lowering of the blood pressure and slowing of the heart, which may result in loss of consciousness.

carotid pulse: *See* carotid artery.

carotid sinus: *See* carotid artery.

carpal tunnel syndrome

A condition characterized by pins and needles, pain, and numbness in the thumb and first three fingers of the hand. It arises when a nerve in the carpal tunnel is compressed. The carpal tunnel is a narrow tunnel at the base of the palm, through which tendons and a major nerve (the median nerve) pass from the wrist to the hand. Carpal tunnel syndrome is quite common among middle-aged and pregnant women. It is also probably the most common over-use sports injury involving the wrist. Long-distance cyclists who maintain a constant grip on the handlebars, weight-lifters, racket players, and golfers are all susceptible. The first step in treatment is to remove the cause. Most cases respond well to rest and hydrocortisone treatment, but sometimes surgical relief is needed. In the case of cyclists, wearing padded cycling gloves and regularly changing the grip on the handlebars can prevent the condition from arising.

catastrophe theory

A mathematical model developed by the French mathematician, René Thom, to show how the interaction of varying factors produce sudden, dramatic changes. Sports psychologists use catastrophe theory to explain why athletes subjected to a critical level of stress experience a huge and sudden loss of performance.

Among athletes, two main factors are associated with stress: physiological arousal (changes in heart rate, sweating, adrenaline secretion etc.) and cognitive anxiety (i.e. mental anxiety). The relationship between these two factors and the performance of an athlete can be depicted in a 3-D graph, with the surface shape representing performance (figure 21). The

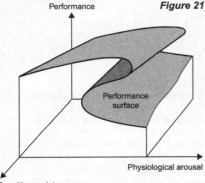

Performance

Figure 21

Performance surface

Physiological arousal

Cognitive anxiety

graph shows that when stress increases up to a critical level, performance improves. At the critical level, the surface folds so that more than one level of performance can occur; an athlete's performance can leap unexpectedly from one level to the other. Beyond the critical level, further increases in stress result in poorer performances.

CAT scan: *See* **computerized tomography.**

cat stretch

An exercise which tones and strengthens the body as a whole, but has a particularly beneficial effect on the back and abdominal muscles.

■ Assume a kneeling position, resting on the balls of your feet and the palms of your hands. Slowly and smoothly raise your buttocks as high as possible and drop your head between your arms. Hold the raised position for a few seconds, then slowly lower yourself back to the starting position. Gently thrust your head back, push up with your arms, and push down with your buttocks to hollow the spine. Repeat about ten times.

If performed too enthusiastically and forcibly, this exercise can do more harm than good. Remember to move slowly and smoothly; never bounce into the end positions. Stop when you feel resistance or at the first signs of pain or real discomfort (*see* **stretch stress**).

cellulite

A term adopted by the diet industry to describe the bulged, rippled, and waffled appearance associated with subcutaneous fat on hips, thighs, and buttocks. It occurs almost exclusively in women. Cellulite is less common in men because they have a different fat distribution; the connective tissue around their fat cells is stronger, and their skin is thicker.

The general consensus of medical opinion in Britain and the USA is that cellulite is merely an effect created by weakened connective tissue and cells filled with fat, and that it can be reduced by regular exercise and dieting. Typically, treatment consists of:

● a low fat, high fibre diet with plenty of fruit and vegetables

● regular, vigorous exercise, such as brisk walking for 30 minutes, three times a week

● drinking plenty of water (about eight glasses a day).

Many doctors on the European mainland have a different opinion. They believe that cellulite is a medical problem requiring medical treatment. Some European researchers suggest that an oversensitivity to oestrogen may disturb the normal pattern of fluid and fat storage. They called cellulite 'localized hydrolipodystrophy'. They believe that the bulging fat cells of cellulite harden if left untreated and recommend mesotherapy. This is a treatment used on a wide range of medical conditions including osteoarthritis and some sports injuries. It consists of injecting minute quantities of drugs under the skin in areas of tenderness associated with cellulite. Mesotherapy should be administered only by those medically qualified. In 1994, only one specialist in Britain provided this treatment.

cellulose

A fibrous, complex carbohydrate. It is the main component of plant tissues. Roughage or fibre in a diet is mainly cellulose. Humans and most other animals lack cellulase, an enzyme needed to break down cellulose to its constituent molecules of glucose.

cerebrotonic trait: *See* **somatotype.**

chafing (intertrigo)

Abrasion caused by mechanical friction where two areas of skin rub together (e.g. in the groin) causing reddening and tenderness. Chafing is particularly common among obese people. Sweating may exacerbate the condition and increase the risk of bacterial infections. Chafing resulting from exercise can be reduced by applying petroleum jelly to areas which are likely to rub against each other (e.g. the inner thighs or nipples of runners).

cheating

A weight-training technique that enables a trainee to lift loads which he or she could not otherwise lift. The ability to lift a weight at constant speed depends mainly on the strength of the muscle at its weakest point, commonly called the sticking point. Cheating is a slight assistance movement, such as bouncing the barbell and raising the hips during a bench press. This accelerates the bar and carries the weight beyond the sticking point.

chest pain

Discomfort and soreness in and around the chest. Pain may result from a wide range of causes including physical overexertion and muscle strains. A long-lasting pain in the centre or left side of the chest (especially if it extends down into the arms and around to the back and neck) requires medical attention. It is even more urgent if the pain is accompanied by shortness of breath, cold sweat, and fatigue. Such pains may be associated with a heart disorder (e.g. angina) which precludes vigorous physical activity. A stabbing pain in the chest may be caused by lung infection. More often, the pain is due to indigestion (dyspepsia) or reflux of the acid contents of the stomach into the oesophagus. Nevertheless, anyone suffering from a persistent undiagnosed chest pain should seek medical advice.

chest stretch

A simple warm-up exercise for the chest muscles.

■ Interlock the fingers of both hands behind your back. Gently and slowly lift your arms behind you with your shoulders pushed

back, and chest stuck out. Stop when you feel a reasonable resistance, before you feel any pain, and hold for about 10 seconds.

childhood

The period between infancy (about 1–2 years) and pubescence. Most of the physical and mental development of a person takes place in childhood. It is the critical period for establishing good habits of both exercise and nutrition which can last a lifetime. By the age of seven, nearly all of the motor control mechanisms in the brain are present and the child is rapidly developing motor skills. During the major growth spurts (usually experienced by girls between the ages of 9 and 12 years, and by boys between 11 and 14 years) reasonable exercise encourages growth of muscles, tendons, and bones, but excessive exercise can permanently damage bones and joints. Most experts agree that, although exercise during childhood is important, the emphasis should be on fun. There are both physical and mental dangers if children are forced into activities for which they are not ready. Parents should work with expert coaches and the child, to ensure that exercises are appropriate and carry little risk of permanent injury.

childhood onset obesity: See obesity.

Chinese restaurant syndrome

A disorder experienced by some people after eating Chinese food. It is characterized by headaches, thirst, tightness in the chest, palpitations, and numbness in the hands and neck. The syndrome has been attributed to monosodium glutamate (MSG) contained in highly flavoured foods and sauces (especially the soy sauce which is offered as an accompaniment to many Chinese meals).

MSG adversely affects certain susceptible individuals but it may not be entirely responsible for the syndrome. Some victims of Chinese restaurant syndrome have a low vitamin B_6 status which is thought to increase their sensitivity to MSG. When given vitamin B_6 supplements, most of these victims quickly recover. In double-blind experiments comparing the effects of MSG and a placebo, the percentage of those who experienced unpleasant symptoms was not significantly different between the two groups. This suggests that some other factor, such as histamine, may be involved in the syndrome. Certain foods contain histamine (interestingly, soy sauce when fermented produces this chemical). Histamine is also released by the body during stressful situations.

chinnies

An exercise for strengthening the abdominal muscles.

■ Lie flat on your back. Slowly sit up and at the same time rapidly bring one knee to make contact with your chest while twisting your body slightly towards that knee.

chinning: See **chin-up**.

chin-up (chinning; pull-up)

An excellent exercise for developing and strengthening muscles in the back, shoulders and upper arms, and for improving upper body posture.

■ Grasp a horizontal bar with the palms of your hands towards your face. From a hanging position, pull yourself up until your chin is raised above the bar. Hold the position for a few seconds then gradually lower your body to the starting position.

If you wish to use chin-ups to test your muscular endurance, record the maximum number of chin-ups you can do. Rating: >9, good; 3–8, average; 0–2, poor.

To chin-up successfully, you need to use the muscles of the middle and lower back, as well as the biceps. Failure or poor performances often result from using only the biceps.

chiropractic

The treatment and correction of bodily ills (including sports injuries) by mechanical means. The spine is regarded by many chiropractors as the control centre of the body so that many ailments, such as headaches, can be treated successfully by correcting a faulty alignment of the backbone. The established medical profession in many Western countries has expressed reservations about chiropractic treatment.

chocoholic

A slang term applied to a person who frequently consumes large amounts of chocolate and has an insatiable craving for chocolate products. In 1991, each Briton consumed an average of 7.3 kilograms (16 lb) of chocolate.

Chocolate contains high levels of magnesium and there might be a link between chocolate cravings and the body's need for this element. Some scientists believe that the cravings are linked to two other chemicals found in chocolate: phenylethylamine (PEA) and theobromine. PEA produces feelings of euphoria described as being similar in kind, if not intensity, to a sexual climax. Levels of PEA in the brain increase when people fall in love, and decrease when they fall out of love. Theobromine is related to caffeine and has similar stimulatory effects.

Recent studies question this link between cravings for chocolate and chemicals. When self-confessed chocohoiics were given capsules of cocoa powder, chocolate with the flavour removed, or unadulterated chocolate, only those eating real chocolate satisfied their cravings although all consumed EPA and theobromine. These chemicals may have stimulatory effects, but it appears that chocoholics crave chocolate primarily because they like the taste.

Some psychologists and nutritionists believe that overindulgence in chocolate is due to emotional and social conditioning in early life when chocolate is often given as a sign of social approval. It is suggested that we get addicted to chocolate because it makes us feel better and because it provides a satisfying amount of calories. See also **carbohydrate addict's diet**.

choking

1 Difficulty in breathing because of blockage or partial blockage of the airway. Choking may have internal causes, such as emotional distress, as well as external causes, such as a direct blow to the throat.

2 Colloquially applied to athletes whose performance deteriorates under stress. Such athletes may feel as if they are physically choking because of tightening of the bronchial muscles around the airway. An athlete who chokes may be one who, through poor pacing or excessive enthusiasm, makes too much effort too early in a competition (e.g. a runner may go off too fast at the start of a race). The resulting accumulation of lactic acid induces hyperventilation and an uncomfortable tightening of the airway. The fear of competition may also induce excessive hyperventilation.

cholecalciferol: *See* vitamin D.

cholera

A disease caused by the bacterium *Vibrio cholerae*. Cholera is contracted by eating food or drinking water contaminated with infected faeces. Outbreaks are very rare in good sanitary conditions, but anyone eating fish or shellfish grown in water polluted by sewage is at risk. Symptoms range from mild to severe diarrhoea and abdominal pain that can lead to shock. The diarrhoea can cause dehydration which may be fatal if untreated. Treatment usually includes a course of tetracycline antibiotics and intravenous fluid replacement.

cholesterol

A white, waxy substance, related to fats. It occurs naturally in most animal tissue. Foods particularly rich in cholesterol include eggs and offal.

Many people are surprised to learn that cholesterol has a number of essential functions in the human body: it is used in tissue repair; for strengthening cell membranes; and for the manufacture of bile salts, steroid hormones (including the sex hormones, oestrogen and testosterone), and vitamin D. There is little danger of cholesterol deficiency because it can be manufactured in the liver from fats, carbohydrates, and proteins.

The problems associated with cholesterol arise because modern diets in northern Europe and North America often result in over-production. A lot of cholesterol is not used but is deposited in the walls of blood vessels where it increases the risk of coronary heart disease and atherosclerosis. The most influential factor in raising blood cholesterol levels is eating foods high in saturated fat. Nicotine increases deposition of cholesterol in the walls of blood vessels. Hereditary factors are also important determinants of blood cholesterol levels.

A good diet can decrease blood cholesterol levels. Soluble fibre, polyunsaturated fat (especially fish fats which contain omega-3 fatty acids), and monounsaturated fat (such as olive oil) may all lower cholesterol levels. Regular aerobic exercise helps to reduce deposition of cholesterol in blood vessels.

Blood cholesterol levels vary considerably and there is no universally accepted safe level, but the following are guidelines used by most doctors:

	CHOLESTEROL LEVELS
desirable levels	<5.2 mmol/l (<200 mg/dl)
slightly raised	5.2–6.4 mmol/l (200–250 mg/dl)
high	6.5–7.8 mmol/l (251–300 mg/dl)
very high	>7.8 mmol/l (>300 mg/dl)

Some people with cholesterol levels just below 200 mg/dl may also be at risk of cardiovascular diseases because of the type of lipoprotein they possess (lipoproteins carry cholesterol and fats in the blood; *see* **lipoprotein**).

Several cholesterol test-kits can be bought over the counter. If used properly, these can give quite accurate readings, but interpreting the results is not easy, and the results may make a person unnecessarily anxious. A number of factors can affect blood cholesterol levels temporarily. Exercising or eating before the test can raise levels by more than 15 per cent. It is normal for cholesterol levels to fluctuate, so at least two tests, separated by one or two months, are needed to give a reliable average. People who are worried about their cholesterol level should have it checked properly by a doctor.

Although many people with high cholesterol levels have an increased risk of coronary heart disease, the effects of treatment are not straightforward. Treatment has been linked to increases in deaths from other causes (notably violent deaths). Cholesterol testing may be advisable for those at greatest risk (such as those with a family history of high cholesterol levels or coronary heart disease) and who are prepared to change their lifestyle. But many doctors believe that automatic screening and self-testing may turn healthy people into patients chronically anxious about their cholesterol levels. As one medical textbook states 'It may be healthier not to know'.

cholesterol-lowering drugs

Drugs that reduce the level of blood cholesterol. They are sometimes prescribed to individuals who cannot reduce their high cholesterol levels by special diets or exercise. There are a number of cholesterol-lowering drugs, some of which have unpleasant and potentially dangerous side-effects. Drugs containing niacin have gained particular notoriety. Niacin (specifically, one form called nicotinic acid) may reduce cholesterol levels, but large doses can cause irreversible liver damage. Clearly, no one should take any cholesterol-lowering drug without medical advice. The patient should also be monitored to ensure that the drug is effective and does not cause any harmful side-effects. *See also* **laxative**.

cholesterol-testing kits: *See* cholesterol.

chondromalacia patellae

Deterioration and softening of the articular cartilage of the kneecap in adolescents and young people. It can lead to osteoarthritis. The condition may occur as an overuse injury in exercisers, and is associated with recurrent swelling. Pain is felt after exercise, during exercise, or after sitting for prolonged periods. Often, the knee gives way unexpectedly. Chondromalacia patellae has become, in the words of one eminent specialist of sports injuries, a 'wastebasket' term applied to any syndrome characterized by pain and a crackling sound around the front of the knee. The term should be restricted to those conditions in which there is actual damage of the articular cartilage. *See also* **patellofemoral malalignment**.

chromium

A metallic element essential in the diet for efficient carbohydrate metabolism. It improves the ability of insulin to convert glucose to glycogen (the main energy store in muscles).

Some body-builders use a salt of chromium (chromium picolinate) as an anabolic agent. They claim it burns fat and increases lean body mass by accelerating protein metabolism. They also claim that it may reduce the risk of cardiovascular diseases by increasing the proportion of high density lipoproteins in the blood. Studies in the USA have recently disproved these claims. Obesity experts state that chromium supplements do not speed up metabolism or burn fat. Nutritionists generally advise that you should get enough chromium from a well-balanced diet. Good sources of chromium include liver, meat, cheese, wholegrains, brewer's yeast, and wine.

chymotrypsin

An enzyme involved in protein digestion in the small intestine. Chymotrypsin has been used to accelerate the repair of soft-tissue sports injuries, such as sprains and internal bruising of muscles. However, the treatment has not always been successful, and chymotrypsin may be toxic to some hypersensitive people.

circadian rhythm

Circadian rhythms are cyclical changes that recur regularly over an approximately 24-hour cycle. They are a type of biological rhythm affecting many aspects of human life and should not be confused with 'biorhythms', a theory which has little scientific support.

Circadian rhythms ranging from cellular and tissue processes to whole-body functions, have been demonstrated in volunteers kept in experimentally controlled conditions (e.g. constant temperature and light). One of the best known circadian rhythms is the daily change in body core temperature. We tend to be at our coolest in the early morning and at our warmest in the late afternoon and early evening. Other circadian rhythms include arm and leg strength, heart rate, metabolic rate, wakefulness, and flexibility. It is not surprising, therefore, that the ability to perform many physical activities also follows a circadian rhythm. Several studies show that runners, cyclists, and swimmers perform best in the afternoon and early evening. In most cases (but by no means all) they performed better in the late afternoon (4.30 p.m.–5.30 p.m) than in the morning for both aerobic and anaerobic exercises of short to moderate duration. The peak probably corresponds to the time when body temperature is highest since muscles work better when warm. Although the variations in performance were usually small (3 per cent either side of the average), they can make a difference between the success and failure of athletes attempting to break records. Not all sports share the same circadian rhythm. Fencers, for example, seem to perform better in the middle of the day, perhaps because their sport demands mental skills which peak around noon. The results on endurance exercises have been less clear. Some studies have reported that peak performances occur later in the day, but others have shown no clear association between time of day and performance.

Circadian rhythms may be affected by personality and altered by environmental factors such as sleeplessness and travel. Introverts tend to perform better in the morning than extroverts. In addition, the circadian rhythms may be modified by the way people phase their normal habitual activities. Those who prefer to work in the morning (so-called 'larks' or morning types) may perform better early in the day than those who normally prefer to work in the evenings ('owls' or evening types). Long-distance travel to different time zones can alter circadian rhythms and impair sporting performance. Pistol shooters travelling from Britain to New Zealand took eight days to regain form. The following advice is given to athletes travelling to compete in a new time zone:

- ensure that there is plenty of time to adjust to the new time zone
- start the process of rhythm adjustment on the aircraft by resting and being active at times which match those at the destination

- on arrival, sleep properly so that the rhythm can be reset quickly.

circuit training

Circuit training is an intensive form of fitness training in which a group of exercises are completed one after the other. Each exercise is performed for a specified number of repetitions or for a prescribed time before you move on to the next exercise. Whether you are a swimmer, cyclist, rower, racket player, or runner, circuit training will improve your mobility and stamina, enabling you to move more powerfully.

Circuit training using weight machines improves aerobic fitness, flexibility, and strength. Each machine in the circuit is designed to exercise a different group of muscles. Individuals move from machine to machine completing a set of exercises, usually in a predetermined time. Generally there are between 6–15 stations to complete in a time of 5–20 minutes. Aerobic benefit is gained by moving swiftly between machines and completing the circuit as a continuous flow of activity. This keeps the heart rate at a steady and fairly high level.

Circuits without weights or with free standing weights usually consist of eight to ten exercises chosen from a large number of possible ones, such as pattering or running on the spot, press-ups, abdominal curl-ups, free squats, squat thrusts, step ups, and arm curls (figure 22). Each session should start with a warm-up and mobility exercises, and end with cooldown exercises. The circuit should be designed so that the same muscle groups are not worked in consecutive stations. In the following circuit each part of the body is worked twice:

1 total-body exercise: e.g. ski-jumps
2 upper-body exercise: e.g. press-ups
3 lower-body exercise: e.g. bench step-ups
4 trunk exercise: e.g. sit-ups
5 total-body exercise: e.g. squat thrusts
6 upper-body exercise: e.g. chin-ups
7 lower-body exercise: e.g. free squats
8 trunk exercise: e.g. back extensions.

A complete session (warm-up, stretching, circuits, and cool down) should take about one hour. Generally, you should

Figure 22 A typical circuit

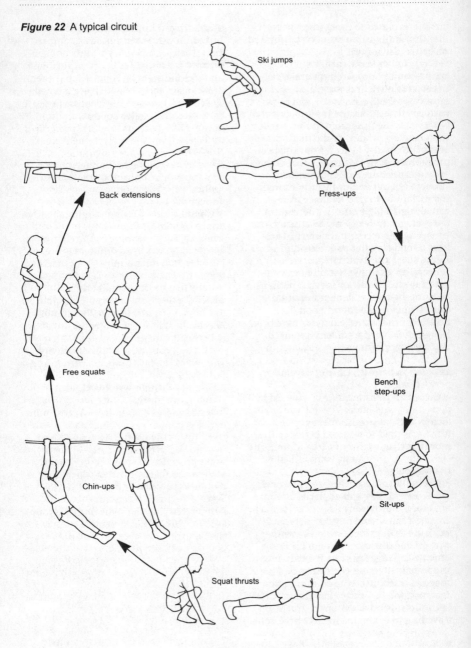

circuit train two to three times per week; circuit training should not be performed on consecutive days.

Circuit training is excellent for developing overall body strength and aerobic fitness. However, it is essential that the correct weights, repetitions and positions are established to avoid injury and to achieve all the fitness objectives. For serious athletes, the aim of the first training session is usually to establish the maximum number of repetitions that can be completed for each exercise, either to a point of exhaustion or in a given time. Each score is divided by three to determine the training rate for the exercise. At subsequent training sessions the athlete performs three circuits of all the exercises at the training rate. This rate can be adjusted as the athlete improves. Stage training is a variation of circuit training. Individuals perform exercises in sets, repeating the same exercise a number of times, before moving on to the next exercise. It tends to make more demands on the lactic acid system than traditional circuit training.

circumduction: *See* **body movements**.

cis: *See* **unsaturated fat**.

citric acid cycle: *See* **Krebs cycle**.

clavicle: *See* **collar bone**.

clenbuterol
A drug that has stimulatory effects similar to adrenaline and anabolic effects similar to steroids. As a stimulant, it is used to treat asthma, but it is sometimes misused to improve sporting performance. Because of this and its possible harmful effects (for example, clenbuterol is known to damage the hearts of laboratory rats) clenbuterol is on the International Olympic Committee list of substances banned during competition. There is growing concern, however, that it is still being misused outside competition periods to promote muscle growth and repair artificially. In the 1992 Barcelona Olympics, two British weightlifters, Andrew Davies and Andrew Saxton, tested positive for clenbuterol and were sent home accused of drug

abuse. They admitted taking the drug, but only outside the period of competition. They argued that this was not contrary to the IOC rules because, although an anabolic agent, it is not related chemically to the steroids, which are banned. They were subsequently cleared. The case illustrates the confusion surrounding the use of drugs in sport.

climbing
An activity gaining in popularity both as a recreation and a demanding sport. Outdoor climbing improves aerobic fitness and all-over body strength, but is particularly good for developing muscles in the hands, forearms, and shoulders. Good technique and flexibility can compensate for lack of strength. Some women, despite their relatively low strength, are outstanding climbers. In addition to its physical benefits, climbing also helps to develop courage and self-confidence. Apart from bruises, bumps, and scrapes, few injuries occur during outdoor climbs as long as climbers have the appropriate safety equipment and instruction.

Climbing has become accessible to many more people since the introduction of climbing walls at many sports centres. Unlike outdoor climbing, indoor climbing emphasizes anaerobic fitness. Usually the aim is to climb a wall as quickly as possible. This requires powerful bursts of activity and good upper body strength. Indoor climbing is used as training by outdoor climbers, by exercisers as part of a general fitness training programme, and to relieve stress. Many people in managerial positions find the total concentration required for a quick climb blocks out all their worries. They also find the physical effort and excitement invigorating. There is even less risk of injury in indoor climbs than outdoor climbing. It is rare to have a fall because climbers should be roped at all times. The most common injury is a strained finger tendon.

clothing
Exercise has become extremely popular and sports clothes manufacturers have been quick to respond to consumer demand. Each sport has its own specific clothing requirements, but the most

important consideration for the general exerciser is that clothes are comfortable, that they allow the body to breathe normally, and that they stretch to allow maximum freedom of movement. There is no need to buy expensive designer sports clothes, some of which are more suited to the poser than the exerciser. Loose-fitting cotton T-shirts, high-cut elasticated shorts, and one-piece leotards with tights which fit snugly over the legs are popular and fulfil the basic requirements. It is also important to wear a tracksuit or shell suit at the start and end of an exercise session to prevent chills. If the temperature is very low, the best way to keep warm is by wearing two or more layers of clothes. The inner layer should allow sweat to escape so that you will not get wet. The outer layer should be wind-resistant, waterproof, and ideally should also let sweat escape. Up to 40 per cent of body heat can be lost through the head, so you should wear a hat in cold weather. You should not overdress or you might overheat during exercise. It is a good idea to wear an outer layer which can be zipped open for quick cooling off.

Gloves are a very useful accessory for several sports. Weight-lifters use finger-less gloves to improve grip and to prevent blisters forming; cyclists use padded gloves to reduce the risk of injuring the delicate structures in the palm of the hand when gripping handlebars for long periods; and runners often put on thin woollen gloves to keep their hands warm in cold weather.

Probably the most important parts of the body to clothe properly are the feet. Padded socks made from cotton or a cotton–wool mixture absorb sweat and help protect the feet from blisters and other injuries. A wide range of footwear is available, but it is important to obtain shoes specifically designed for your activity and which suit your own requirements (*see* **training shoes**).

Those exercising as part of a weight reduction programme should avoid rubberized or plastic suits as they prevent heat loss and can be very dangerous. Despite claims to the contrary, these suits do not accelerate fat loss. *See also* **clo unit**.

clo unit

The basic measurement of the thermal properties of clothing. One clo unit is the thermal insulation required to keep a resting person comfortable at 21°C where relative humidity is less than 50 per cent and air movement is less than 6 metres per minute. It equates to a man wearing a three-piece suit and light underclothes. At −40°C, 12 clo units are required; light activity lowers this to 4 clo units.

coach (instructor)

Most top-class sports people and serious exercisers have a coach or instructor to help them improve their performance and reach their full potential. Good coaches act as motivators and teachers. Ideally, they should be able to convey both theoretical understanding and practical instruction, and they should be sympathetic to the requirements of those they coach.

The way a coach or physical fitness instructor works varies greatly. It usually reflects the coach's personality, ability, and experience, as well as the nature of the work, and the aspirations and personalities of those being coached.

The popular image of the coach, stereotyped in fiction and films, is often of a person who strives for excellence and fitness, and who presents a tough inflexible front to his charges. Some studies by sports sociologists have supported this image that many coaches are dominant; they are able to express aggression easily; they are not very interested in the dependency needs of others; and they are autocratic, often requiring unquestioning obedience. However, it is unclear whether this pattern of behaviour is a true reflection of personality or an attempt to act out the role imposed by society. Other studies have shown that coaches do not differ from other people in the way and extent to which they exploit situations and people. These studies showed that coaches exhibit a whole spectrum of behaviours, ranging from the autocratic described above, to the democratic, maintaining an open dialogue with their athletes about all aspects of their coaching.

Whatever behavioural style the coach adopts, most sports psychologists agree that compatibility between coach and athlete is a critical factor in the success and satisfaction of the athlete, so it is important to choose a coach who suits you.

cobalamin: *See* vitamin B₁₂.

cobalt

An essential trace mineral. Cobalt is found in all cells but occurs in large quantities in bone marrow where it is required for the production of red blood cells. Until recently it was thought that cobalt in humans was found only as a constituent of vitamin B₁₂ (cobalamin), but it is now known to have a role in some enzymes. Sources of cobalt include liver, lean meat, poultry, fish and milk. Recommended intakes have not been established, but excessive intakes (29.5 mg per day), which were used to treat certain anaemias, have proved toxic. High doses of cobalt salts may also contribute to heart disease. This was a problem in the 1950s when cobalt salts were added to beer in Belgium and Canada to retain the head.

cocaine

An addictive drug that acts as a powerful stimulant on the central nervous system. Cocaine is an alkaloid derived from the leaves of the coca plant, *Erythroxylon coca*, which grows in the Andes. Because of the dangers inherent in administering the drug, there are no controlled experiments of cocaine's effects on athletic performance. Nevertheless, some athletes do take cocaine in the belief that it enhances performance. The drug makes them feel more euphoric, more alert, and physically less tired. Although speed of reflexes may be increased, cocaine abuse disturbs muscular coordination and distorts the athlete's perception of his or her ability. Other more serious side-effects include irregularities of heartbeat, high blood pressure, blockage of the coronary arteries, and mental seizures. Cocaine abuse is potentially fatal and is believed to have contributed to the deaths of several prominent American athletes, including the basketball star Len Bias and professional footballer Don Rogers in 1986, and the footballer Dave Waymer in 1993.

coeliac disease (gluten intolerance; sprue)

A digestive disorder caused by hypersensitivity to gluten, a mixture of two proteins found in wheat, barley, oats, and rye. The name 'coeliac' is derived from the Greek for 'suffering in the bowels'. The condition is characterized by swelling of the intestinal wall and disappearance of the microvilli (the very fragile, highly folded membrane of some intestinal cells) in the presence of gluten. This results in impaired absorption of all nutrients (general malabsorption). Coeliac disease can be controlled by eating a strict and lifelong, gluten-free diet (i.e. a diet excluding wheat, barley, and rye products). The structure and function of the intestine returns to normal if gluten is removed from the diet.

coenzyme Q

A chemical that occurs naturally in every cell in the body where it plays an important intermediary role in aerobic respiration. It also has some anti-oxidant properties and may help protect cells from damage by free radicals.

Coenzyme Q is now being manufactured and sold as a product which, it is claimed, encourages weight loss, boosts energy, combats fatigue, and delays ageing. The body makes its own coenzyme Q in the liver, but manufacturers of the enzyme claim that the ability to do so may decline with age. Supplements may be useful to those who cannot make sufficient quantities of their own coenzyme Q. There is no unequivocal evidence that coenzyme Q will accelerate weight loss nor that supplements have beneficial effects.

coffee: *See* caffeine.

cold

Medically termed a coryza or rhinitis, a cold in the head is caused by a viral infection. There is some concern that exercising during a viral infection can worsen the disease and may, albeit rarely, lead to myocarditis (inflammation of the heart muscle which can in some cases cause sudden death). Studies on the effects of exercising during a viral infection are inconclusive, but it is generally agreed that it is safe for a person with a mild cold to continue with light to moderate levels of physical activity, provided the cold is not accompanied by a fever. A person with a body temperature higher than 38°C should not exercise.

cold therapy

Indirect application of ice or a cold compress is often the first line of treatment for an acute sports injury. The low temperature decreases the metabolic rate of injured tissue and constricts blood vessels. Since most internal bleeding occurs a few minutes after an injury, immediate application of ice for about 10 minutes reduces bruising and swelling. The low temperature also stops muscle spasms and deadens pain receptors in the injured tissue. The painkilling effect of ice is sometimes too effective. A victim who feels no pain may return to activity prematurely and exacerbate the injury. *See also* **RICE**.

collagen

Collagen is the most abundant protein in the body comprising up to 6 per cent of our total weight. It is one of the main constituents of skin, bones, tendons, cartilage, and ligaments, forming fibres that bind together and strengthen these tissues. Collagen (from the Greek, meaning 'glue-maker') is a remarkably strong material, having a tensile strength equal to that of light steel wire, but it is relatively inelastic.

As a person ages, the three-dimensional shape of collagen fibres changes, resulting in the formation of wrinkles. Collagen treatment has been available in Britain since 1984 to counteract this ageing process. Approximately 4000 people each year ask cosmetic surgeons to inject preparations of bovine collagen into their skin to remove wrinkles, creases, and folds. About 3 per cent of the women cannot have the treatment because of an allergic reaction, but for the others the treatment may remove wrinkles. However, the effects are short-lived as the collagen is usually reabsorbed into the body within 6 to 18 months.

Collagen from animal bones is extracted by boiling them to form a sticky resin from which gelatin can be extracted.

Gelatin is, of course, edible and is used in jellies, some cheesecakes, and other foods as a gelling agent because it swells on contact with water.

collar bone (clavicle)

A slender, doubly-curved long bone extending horizontally across the upper part of the chest. Many muscles of the chest and shoulder attach onto the clavicle which forms the front part of the pectoral girdle. The clavicle is easily fractured when the arms are outstretched in a fall. Those who perform strengthening exercises of the shoulder and arm muscles develop larger, stronger clavicles, more resistant to fractures.

collateral circulation

Collateral circulation refers to the development of new branches of blood vessels. Regular, vigorous aerobic exercise may stimulate the formation of new branches of the coronary arteries. This may offset the effects of a thrombosis. If one of the coronary arteries becomes blocked, the new vessels can provide the blood with an alternative pathway to maintain the supply of oxygen and nutrients to the heart. Good collateral circulation may also accelerate recovery from a heart attack.

colonic fermentation

The breakdown of dietary fibre, resistant starch, and some other undigested foods by bacteria in the large intestine. The end products of fermentation include volatile fatty acids that may contribute up to 10 per cent of human energy requirements. One of the volatile fatty acids, propionic acid, is thought to lower blood cholesterol levels. Another, butyric acid, may have an anti-cancer effect by stimulating the growth of normal cells in the bowel wall rather than cancer cells. A less desirable result of colonic fermentation is that the bacteria cause flatulence containing gases that may include methane. *See also* **gut bacteria**.

Columbus Nutrition Plan

A reduced calorie diet high in carbohydrates, low in fats, and moderately high in fibre and protein. The plan was devised by Dr Janet McBarron-Liberatore and combines dieting with exercise. Dr McBarron-Liberatore advocates vigorous walking for at least 30–45 minutes per day, six days a week. Although the recipes do not give the values of carbohydrate, fat, and protein, the diet appears to be nutritionally sound and in line with most dietary recommendations.

combining diets: *See* **food combining diets**.

comfort eating

Some people eat to satisfy psychological needs, such as wanting to feel comfortable, happy, and relaxed. Comfort eating appears to be more prevalent among women than men. Many women eat to relax or relieve feelings of depression. Chocolate appears to be a favourite comfort food (*see* **chocoholic** and **carbohydrate addict's diet**). Comfort foods such as chocolate may contain chemicals that affect the brain, producing a calming effect and making a person feel happier. Comfort eating may also develop as a result of social conditioning. Confectionery, for example, is often given to children as a sign of social approval and adults may indulge in confectionery because of the pleasant feelings with which it is associated. *See also* **mood swings**.

comfort index

An arbitrary index that indicates the suitability of environmental conditions for physical activity. It is expressed as an equation:

comfort index = T+RH/4

where T is temperature in degrees Fahrenheit and RH is the relative humidity. When the comfort index is above 95 and the wind speed is low, it may be necessary to acclimatize to the conditions before attempting very strenuous activity; the presence of wind allows higher values to be tolerated.

comfort zone

The weather has marked effects on the ability of a person to exercise comfortably. The comfort zone is the range of temperatures and humidities within which people feel comfortable under calm wind conditions. In general, as temperature increases, tolerance to humidity decreases, and vice versa. For people adapted to most temperate regions, the comfort zone has air temperatures of 20–25°C and relative humidities between 25 and 75 per cent. In Britain, it is generally agreed that the optimum conditions for comfort are 15°C and 60 per cent relative humidity. Wind speed, however, has a great effect on the comfort zone. Increases in wind speed up to about 40 miles per hour lower the effective temperature, a phenomenon known as the wind-chill factor. When air temperature is 20°C and wind speed is 20 miles per hour, the effective temperature is −10°C, and −21°C when wind speed is 40 miles per hour.

compartment: *See* **compartment syndrome**.

compartment syndrome

A compartment is a section of the body containing a group of muscles and other tissue enclosed by tough connective tissue. A compartment syndrome develops when the space within a compartment is reduced. During exercise, the muscle swells, fluid accumulates and cannot escape immediately, pressing on structures which become tense and painful. *See also* **anterior compartment syndrome**.

complete protein

Animal protein or mixture of plant proteins which contain all of the essential amino acids in adequate amounts to meet human requirements.

complex carbohydrate

Complex carbohydrates are polysaccharides. They include starches and cellulose. The more complex a carbohydrate is, the longer it takes to digest and be absorbed; cellulose is not digested at all. Therefore foods containing complex digestible carbohydrates such as starches release their sugar constituents into the bloodstream over a long period. This makes them a good source of energy for endurance activities. Complex digestible carbohydrates are common in unrefined foods, such as wholemeal breads, potatoes, cereals, fruit, and vegetables, which are also rich in vitamins, minerals, and fibre. *Compare* **simple carbohydrate**; *see also* **carbohydrates** and **fibre**.

compression neuropathy

An inability to transmit nerve impulses because compression has damaged nerve fibres either directly, or indirectly by restricting their supply of oxygen. During cycling, the ulnar nerve in the palm of the hand is often compressed onto the handlebars leading to a loss of sensation and weakening of the hand, a condition known as ulnar compression syndrome. Compression neuropathy can lead to permanent paralysis of the hands. It is easily treated in its early stages by altering the hand position frequently and protecting the hands with tape or cycling gloves.

compulsive overeating

An addiction to eating large amounts of food even when not hungry. Compulsive eaters binge for pleasure rather than to satisfy nutritional needs. Such excessive eating usually leads to obesity. *See also* **bulimia nervosa** and **comfort eating**.

computerized tomography

An application of computer technology to radiography. It involves making X-ray images in layers or 'cuts' through the body. Computerized tomography provides excellent images of internal body structures. It is used as a diagnostic tool and also for research purposes (for example, to determine body composition). The technique is also called Computerized Axial Tomography (CAT scan).

concentration

The ability to sustain attention and to focus on particular target stimuli. Concentration is an important skill for most sports activities. It can be learned and improved by specific training. Footballers and hockey players, for instance, play distraction games in which one person has to try to concentrate on performing a skill while others try to distract him or her.

A wide range of factors can affect concentration. Eating a heavy meal, very high levels of noise, and anxiety can reduce concentration. The morning is the best time to concentrate on complex

tasks which rely on memory (*see* **circadian rhythm**). It is difficult to sustain concentration at any time on tasks that are too simple, too complicated, or too repetitive.

concentric contraction: *See* **muscle contraction**.

concussion (knockout)

A sudden, transient loss of consciousness due to a blow to the head. The blow produces mechanical acceleration and deceleration forces that act on the brain. This impairs mental function, and can cause confusion. Concussion may last a few minutes or a few hours and is often accompanied by pallor, slowness, feebleness of heartbeat, shallow breathing, and reduction in reflex responses.

Individuals suffering from concussion are usually advised to avoid body-contact activities for at least three weeks. In some sports, such as Rugby Union football, this lay-off period is mandatory. Boxers suffering from concussion after being knocked out in the ring may also be required to avoid boxing for a time. In Britain, amateur boxers are not allowed in the ring again until 28 days after the first knockout, 84 days after the second knockout, and 1 year after the third knockout. In the USA, many team physicians in contact sports follow the '1–2–3' rule: one concussion and the player is removed from the game; two concussions results in the player missing the rest of the season; and after three concussions the player is advised to stop completely.

conditioning

Activities that exercise the whole body to improve overall physical fitness, especially aerobic fitness, muscle strength, and flexibility. Conditioning is not primarily concerned with developing a skill. For athletes, it forms part of the preparation period of their training programme. Conditioning enables an athlete to become fit enough to cope with specific training which may be physically very demanding.

confidence

A belief and a self-assurance in one's own abilities. In competitive sport, confidence includes having an expectation of success.

Very often the most successful sports people have high levels of confidence, but it is situation-specific: e.g. a person who is highly confident when playing tennis may not be confident when swimming.

Lack of confidence is thought to be an important factor in the development of some eating disorders (*see* **anorexia nervosa** and **bulimia nervosa**). One of the main ways of treating such disorders is to boost self-confidence.

conjunctivitis

Inflammation of the conjunctiva, the thin protective membrane lining the eyelids and covering the front surface of the eye. Conjunctivitis may be due to a viral or bacterial infection, or chemical irritation. Bacterial infections can cause pus to form. Such purulent infections can be exacerbated by exercise. Chlorine in swimming pool water commonly acts as a chemical irritant resulting in conjunctivitis, similar to that caused by bacterial infections. Wearing goggles offers protection against this condition.

connective tissue

A tissue found in all parts of the body. Its functions include support, storage, and protection. All types of connective tissue have a good blood supply. Most types, especially bones, cartilage, tendons, and ligaments, are strengthened by collagen fibres. This enables the tissues to endure high levels of abuse from physical trauma and abrasions. Adipose tissue is a fairly loose connective tissue that is not very strong. Its main function is to store fat.

connective tissue massage: *See* massage.

constipation

Contrary to popular opinion, you are not constipated if you do not pass faeces once a day. Constipation exists only when bowel movements are difficult or accompanied by discomfort, and if there is failure to empty the bowels at least three days in succession. Many people who are not constipated, but who believe that daily bowel movements are important, resort to using laxatives to achieve their

objective. Laxatives, however, may disrupt normal bowel reflexes and cause true constipation. Fluid losses associated with laxatives may also contribute to dehydration and induce abdominal cramps which restrict physical activity.

Changes of environment and diet, or inactivity can lead to intermittent bouts of constipation. Chronic constipation is often linked to low dietary fibre. It can affect physical performance and make a person feel unwell. Risk of constipation can be reduced by:

- eating high fibre foods, such as fruits, vegetables (especially legumes), and unrefined cereals
- drinking plenty of fluids, at least eight glasses or cups a day
- exercising regularly.

Constipation lasting more than a week warrants seeking medical advice, because it can be a symptom of an underlying disorder.

constitutional theory: *See* somatotype.

contact sport

Any sport in which the impact of one person against another is an inherent part of the sport. Contact sports include boxing, football (especially American football and rugby), ice hockey, lacrosse, martial arts, and wrestling. Contact sports carry a high risk of injury and some people are advised not to take part in them: for example, those with a history of epileptic seizures triggered by a collision, and those suffering from certain contagious skin infections (e.g. impetigo, herpes, scabies, and boils). It is also unwise for any injured person to compete in a contact sport until completely recovered (*see* **concussion**).

continuous exercise

Aerobic exercise performed to completion at a steady pace without any periods of rest. It is also called continuous training or continuous work. The most popular forms of continuous exercise at low to moderate intensity are walking and jogging. They tend to have less drop out rates than more intensive, anaerobic forms of exercise. *Compare* **interval training**.

contraception

The contraceptive pill contains chemicals that prevent fertilization of the ovum by a sperm. Other options for preventing unwanted pregnancies include abstinence (not popular with many!); the rhythm method, which restricts sexual intercourse to periods when the chances of conception are low; barrier methods, such as condoms, a diaphragm or sponge; and intrauterine devices. Each has its own advantages and disadvantages so it is important to obtain comprehensive advice from a doctor when deciding which form of contraception to use.

Little is known about the effects of most contraceptives on athletic performance although some women endurance athletes found that their weight increased when they took steroid contraceptive pills. New low-dose oral contraceptives have much lower hormone concentrations than the older pills. Their side-effects (e.g. weight gain) have been greatly reduced. However, many athletes are still wary of using these pills because there have been reports that they reduce maximal oxygen consumption and aerobic power. Also, some athletes still believe that use of such pills may lead to weight increase and fluid retention.

Contraceptive pills containing steroids are sometimes taken by athletes to control the menstrual cycle so that blood flow does not coincide with important competitions. The onset of a period can be delayed for up to 10 days. The potential health risks of this practice are not known but women are advised not to engage in it repeatedly.

contraceptive pill: *See* contraception.

contraindicated

A contraindicated procedure, technique, or exercise is one that is inadvisable or undesirable. Contraindicated exercises include any which pull a body part out of alignment, or force the body beyond its normal limits. An exercise may also be contraindicated for an individual because of a medical condition; for example, strenuous exercise and isometric exercises are contraindicated for people with serious heart disease. Several ballistic stretch-

ing exercises that have been practised for years and advocated in popular magazines and books, are now known to be contraindicated for most people (figure 23). These include standing toe

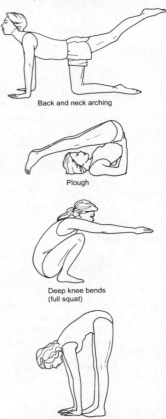

Figure 23 Contraindicated. Four exercises that may be harmful

Back and neck arching

Plough

Deep knee bends (full squat)

Standing toe touch with knees locked

touches and sit-ups performed with straight legs (an abdominal curl-up with legs bent is much safer and more effective at developing abdominal muscles). As a general rule:

● do not overstretch the upper back and neck (e.g. avoid the plough)
● do not hyperextend the lower back (e.g. avoid straight leg sit-ups)

- do not hyperextend the neck (e.g. avoid neck circling)
- do not flex the knee joint more than ninety degrees (e.g. avoid deep squatting)
- do not perform exercises that cause muscle imbalance (e.g. avoid strengthening pectorals at the front of the chest without also strengthening the rhomboids and trapezius muscles at the back).

contrast baths

A common treatment for sports injuries, such as a sprained ankle. Two baths or basins are used, one filled with hot water and the other filled with cold water. Plunging the injured part into the baths alternately stimulates blood supply to the immersed part, accelerates metabolic processes, decreases pain, and increases the elasticity of the ligaments. The ratio of heating time to cooling time is adjusted according to the likelihood of creating tissue swelling. Short periods in the hot water and longer periods in the cold water are used for acute injuries.

control group

When the safety and effectiveness of a diet or exercise are tested, it is important to ensure that the observations are due to the factors under consideration, and not to any other coincidental factor. It is necessary to compare the results of at least two groups of subjects: one (the experimental group) is subjected to the factor under consideration, while the other (the control group) matches the experimental group in all aspects except that the factor under investigation is kept at a constant level (often zero). Incorporating adequate controls is an essential part of the design of scientific investigations. It is also one of the most difficult aspects, and many studies of the effects of diet and exercise lack adequate controls, making their results suspect. *See also* **placebo**.

contusion: *See* bruise.

conversational index

The conversational index is reached when an exerciser can no longer hold a conversation because the supply of oxygen is only enough to meet the demands of the exercise. It is an approximate indicator of the upper limit of aerobic exercise (*see also* **anaerobic threshold**).

cool down (warm down)

Most people are aware of the importance of warming up before exercise. It is also important to cool down afterwards. When you stop exercising suddenly, blood vessels contract and the waste products of exercise become trapped in muscles. One function of the cool down is to help eliminate these products, such as lactic acid, and to reduce the risk of muscle stiffness. Another function is to allow body temperature to return to normal and lessen the risk of chills. Cool down procedures vary, but they usually involve a gradual reduction in activity which includes jogging (or slow swimming), and static or slow stretches to reduce muscle tension and maintain flexibility. Low intensity activities maintain the flow of blood through muscles so that the waste products can be carried away. They also enable the body to adjust gradually from exercise to rest. *See also* **pooling**.

Cooper points: *See* aerobic points.

Cooper twelve-minute test

A test of aerobic fitness in which the total distance a subject runs in twelve minutes is recorded. The Cooper twelve-minute test is a maximal test. The subject must run to exhaustion if the results are to be reliable. A variation of the test is based on the time taken for a subject to run 1.5 miles. Although the exact fitness rating will depend on age and sex, men covering 1.5 miles in 12–13 minutes and women doing the same distance in 14–15 minutes are generally regarded as having a good level of aerobic fitness.

coordination

Coordination is one of the main components of physical fitness. It is the ability to perform smooth and accurate movements involving different parts of the body. It requires good awareness of relative limb and body positions, and good integration between the senses and muscles involved in the movement. Ball juggling is regarded as a good way to develop eye to hand coordination.

copper

An essential element involved in many processes including red blood cell formation, respiration, and bone formation. Copper deficiencies are rare, mainly because most domestic water supplies are contaminated with copper from pipes, but low intakes can lead to anaemia. Oysters and liver are good sources of dietary copper. In the UK, the adult Reference Nutrient Intake for copper is 1.2 mg each day. In the USA, the estimated safe and adequate daily intake of copper is 1.5–3.0 mg. Blood levels of copper often decrease after exercise indicating that athletes may need higher than normal intakes. Copper and zinc appear to be antagonistic; high intakes of one tend to reduce the absorption of the other. Copper toxicity is rare, but intakes greater than 20 mg cause vomiting and nausea.

core temperature

Temperature in the part of the body containing the vital organs (the brain, heart, lungs, and kidneys). The core temperature is measured internally (e.g. in the rectum or oesophagus) and it usually remains within a narrow range, between 36.5 and 37.5°C. This is the temperature at which the majority of the chemical reactions in the body work most efficiently. During exercise, heat is generated and the muscle temperature may rise to 39 or even 40°C. Skeletal muscle functions best at 38.5°C. *See also* **hyperthermia** and **hypothermia**.

corn

A hard pad of skin that develops on or between the toes as a result of friction or pressure. It is often caused by shoes that do not fit properly. The corn has a small fluid sac below the hard pad that allows the pad to slide back and forth without damaging the underlying tissue. Pressure on top of the corn (e.g. from a shoe) pushes it downward causing pain. Corns can be treated with warm water or other softening agents. Also, the pressure on the corn can be relieved by using specially designed pads. Radical treatment by surgical resectioning of the bone underlying the corn, is generally reserved for very difficult cases that do not respond to other forms of treatment.

coronary heart disease

Malfunction of the heart caused by blockage of one of the arteries supplying the heart muscle. Coronary heart disease has been linked to unhealthy eating and lack of exercise. In the USA more than 500 000 people die from coronary heart disease each year. In Britain, it is responsible for one in four of all deaths. More than 800 people a day suffer heart attacks and it costs the National Health Service more than 700 million pounds a year to treat them.

The disease is not confined to the elderly. Children as young as seven years old can have abnormal electrocardiograms indicating the beginnings of heart disease. These abnormalities are thought to be linked to the children's lack of exercise: in the UK, about a third of 10-year-olds walk continuously for less than 10 minutes a week. Most are transported to school by car and spend a lot of their leisure time in front of a television or computer screen.

A new test has been devised to screen children's susceptibility to the disease. It involves tying a tight band round a child's arm or leg. When the band is removed, there is a sudden increase in pressure, causing the artery to expand. The degree of expansion is measured using ultrasound. Slow or restricted expansion is believed to be an early warning sign of artery disease that may develop into a fatal condition in later life.

The risk of succumbing to a coronary heart disease at any age is reduced by regular aerobic exercise and a healthy diet. Physically active people have a lower incidence of the disease. Health experts in the USA estimate that 30 000 deaths would not occur each year if more people engaged in regular exercise. As little as 5–10 miles (8–16 km) walking or jogging each week can offer some protection against heart disease.

coronary heart disease risk factor

A factor that increases the risk of suffering a coronary heart disease. The factors include:

- age
- family history of heart disease
- high blood pressure

- high blood cholesterol level
- high stress
- lack of exercise
- obesity
- tobacco smoking.

Males, particularly those who are bald-headed, are at greater risk than females. Of these factors, high blood pressure, high blood cholesterol, and smoking are the three major risk factors which operate independently of the others. This means they influence the risk of heart disease whatever other factors are involved. Age, sex, and family history (i.e. genetic factors, as yet ill-defined) have the greatest effect on coronary heart disease, but they are beyond an individual's control. The three independent factors are controllable. Smoking can be avoided. Blood pressure and cholesterol levels can be reduced by eating a well-balanced, healthy diet, and by taking exercise. Experts generally agree that the risk of heart disease can be reduced by eating less salt and fat (particularly saturated fat), and by eating more fibre. It may also be beneficial to eat less sugar. The exercise should be regular (at least three times a week), vigorous, (but not over-strenuous), and aerobic. Such exercise does not guarantee immunity, but exercisers are less likely to have a heart attack than those who are inactive.

coronary-prone personality
The personality of an individual whose patterns of behaviour are thought to increase the risk of suffering a coronary heart disease. Such an individual is usually highly aggressive and competitive, and always seems to be in a hurry to get things completed. This pattern of behaviour is sometimes called type A behaviour, but recent research suggests that only particular aspects of type A behaviour are related to coronary heart disease.

corticosteroids
Hormones released from the outer part of the adrenal gland (adrenal cortex). Drugs similar to corticosteroids are produced synthetically. There are two main groups of corticosteroids: glucocorticoids are essential for carbohydrate, fat, and protein metabolism; and mineralocorticoids

which are involved in salt and water balance. The glucocorticoids are also powerful anti-inflammatories and painkillers, normally involved in reactions to stress. Synthetic glucocorticoids are used to treat sports injuries. They are administered in and around damaged muscles, tendons, or joints. They are not given directly into damaged structures because of the risk of weakening them and hindering the healing process. Except under certain conditions, use of artificial corticosteroids is banned by the International Olympic Committee and many other sports federations.

cortisone
A corticosteroid sometimes used to treat sports injuries. If applied directly into an injured joint, it can have serious side-effects, including damage to bone and muscle.

coryza: *See* cold.

cosmetic surgery
Surgical techniques used to beautify the body. Sometimes cosmetic surgery is used to reduce psychological suffering, but often it is practised without good medical reason by people whose prime motive is profit.

counter-conditioning
A method of reducing stress. When a person is faced with a potentially stressful situation, counter-conditioning attempts to replace unpleasant feelings of anxiety with pleasant feelings. *See also* **desensitization**.

cramp
A sudden, uncoordinated, prolonged spasm in a muscle, causing it to become taut and excruciatingly painful. Cramps commonly occur in the calf, thigh, and hip muscles after strenuous exercise. As yet, there is no complete explanation for their development. Several causes have been suggested including muscle damage, dehydration, low blood glucose levels, and restriction of the blood supply to the muscles. Exercisers are more likely to suffer cramps if they are out of condition, wear low-heel shoes, or do not take enough fluids and electrolytes during

exercise (*see also* **heat cramps**). Cramps are often relieved by gentle static stretching, gentle massage, and rest. To reduce the risk of cramps:

- warm up properly; include static stretching
- increase exercise intensity gradually during a workout
- take it easy when performing a new type of workout
- drink plenty of fluids before and after exercise.

crash diet

A diet designed to produce a dramatic decrease in body weight in a short time. Losses may be as high as 3 kg (more than 6 lb) in the first 3 days, but much of this loss is water rather than fat. This is because water is associated with carbohydrate stored in the body as glycogen. Crash diets are usually high in protein and low in carbohydrate, resulting in a reduction of glycogen and its associated water. The weight lost due to water losses is regained when the dieter returns to a balanced diet with normal levels of carbohydrate.

Some crash diets do result in reduced body fat, but usually lean tissue is also lost. It can be dangerous to lose lean tissue from vital organs. When the dieter returns to a normal calorific intake, weight is more likely to be regained as fatty tissue than as lean tissue. Fatty tissue has a lower metabolic rate, consuming less calories, so that the dieter is likely to gain more weight than before the diet started. *See also* **Yo-Yo diet**.

creatine

A chemical made naturally in the body from amino acids readily obtained from meat and fish. Inside the body, creatine is involved in energy expenditure during exercise. Much of it is phosphorylated (i.e. a phosphate group is added to it) to form phosphocreatine, an energy-rich compound used by muscles during very short bursts of explosive activity (*see* **phosphagen system**).

The average person's body has about 120 grams of creatine; 98 per cent in the muscles, 1.5 per cent in nervous tissue, and 0.5 per cent in other organs. The recommended intake is about a gram a day.

Studies have shown that dosages of about 24–30 g of creatine per day for two days can raise the level of phosphocreatine stored in muscle, increasing the energy available for high intensity exercise where there is a short recovery between bouts of activity. When individuals performed multiple sprints of 10–15 seconds duration with less than 30 seconds recovery between each sprint, then after the 6th, 7th, or 8th sprint those who consumed creatine were not so fatigued as those who took a placebo. Creatine supplementation increased power output by as much as 7 per cent in high intensity exercise of an intermittent nature, but there is no evidence that it improves peak power output or sprint ability in a continuous sprint. A dosage of 24 to 30 g per day is equivalent to eating approximately 6 kg (13lb) of beef. Ingesting so much meat would create dietary problems, so a pure form of creatine has been produced as a supplement. Further research has shown that the greatest improvements in short-term performance occur if exercise is performed immediately after taking the supplement, and the improvements are retained longer if relatively small doses of creatine are ingested over a long period of time.

Creatine supplements have been used by a number of successful sports people, including the Cambridge University crew who won the 1993 boat race, and many competitors at the Barcelona Olympics. However, there is concern that the large amounts consumed by athletes may put their health at risk because kidney failure can occur if too much creatinine (the end product of creatine metabolism) is excreted after muscle damage.

creatine phosphate: *See* phosphagen system.

Creutzfeldt-Jakob disease

A fatal disease characterized by spongy degeneration of the brain and progressive dementia. It is thought to be caused by peculiar proteins called prions that can be transmitted in human growth hormone extracted from human pituitary glands. Creutzfeldt-Jakob disease may be related to BSE (*see* **bovine spongiform encephalopathy**).

cricket

A dynamic team sport characterized by short bursts of activity punctuated by irregular periods of inactivity. It is often assumed that you do not have to be very fit to play cricket. This is a misconception. Fast bowlers, batsmen running between the wickets, and fielders chasing a ball have to be able to move suddenly, extremely quickly, and powerfully for brief amounts of time. This pattern of inactivity followed by dynamic movement carries a high risk of injury. Fast bowlers are particularly vulnerable if they are unfit or if their running and bowling technique is poor. Injuries of the shoulders, back, knees, and ankles are common. The risk of injury can be reduced if players are in good physical condition; if they warm up and perform stretching exercises before playing; and if they keep mobile during periods of relative inactivity.

Crohn's disease

A disease that results in local inflammation of the gut wall, usually the ileum. Acute inflammations can mimic appendicitis. Chronic inflammation causes abdominal pain, diarrhoea, and malabsorption of nutrients. Treatment includes anti-inflammatories (commonly corticosteroids), or surgical removal of the offending portion of the gut. Sufferers of the disease usually perform badly in sports because of the nutritional deficiencies caused by malabsorption, but those who have been treated successfully can lead a fully active life.

cross-country skiing: See skiing.

cross-frictional massage: See massage.

cross-training

A training programme involving more than one type of aerobic activity; for example, one that combines running, swimming, and cycling. Cross-training is an integral part of the preparation for a triathlon. Many exercisers also use cross-training to develop all-round fitness. For example, swimming combined with running develops muscles of the upper and lower body respectively. Many people cross-train to improve their cardiovascular fitness needed for endurance activities. However, the effects gained from one activity are not readily transferred to another. For example, training on a stationary cycle for several weeks may improve your cycling by a significant amount, but it is unlikely to improve your running or swimming by the same amount. This demonstrates the importance of specific training; to improve endurance for running, for example, the best training is running. Nevertheless, many runners cross-train, exercising in water when they are recovering from muscle injuries that would be exacerbated by the high impact of running. Other elite, single-activity athletes cross-train to add variety to their training programmes and to improve fitness components not developed by their main activity.

cruciate ligaments

Ligaments that span the capsule of the knee, binding the femur to the tibia. The cruciate ligaments cross each other forming an X-shaped structure which helps to prevent displacement of the bones. *See also* **anterior cruciate ligaments**.

crunch programme

A programme of exercises designed to correct postural misalignments, particularly in the back, and to tone the abdominal or stomach muscles. The abdominals help to stabilize the torso and can be used to draw the ribcage and pelvis together in a 'crunching' movement. The exercises in a crunch programme specifically emphasize this action so that the abdominals are strengthened. It is claimed that properly performed crunches reduce lower back injuries because the abdominals work in opposition to the lower back muscles, helping to relieve them of excess stress and strain. There are several forms of crunching, but a typical crunch is described below.

■ Lie on your back on the floor. Your knees should be bent and the soles of your feet on the floor. Rest your hands on your abdomen so that you can feel the muscles contract as you perform the crunch. Exhale and pull your abdomen in and up as you slowly round your spine forward to lift your shoulders and ribcage off the floor and towards your pelvis (the 'crunch 'movement). Lift only as far as you are able without straining. At the top of the movement, contract your abdominals a little, hold the position for a few seconds, then relax, inhale and return to the start position. During the whole exercise, keep your middle and lower back in contact with the floor to stabilize the pelvis and protect the back.

cryotherapy

Treatment of an injury or disease with cold. Cryotherapy includes the use of ice packs, cold baths, and coolant sprays. It reduces pain and swelling, decreases muscle spasms, and lowers the metabolic and oxygen needs of damaged tissue. It is particularly useful in the treatment of acute muscle and soft-tissue injuries. *See also* **cold therapy** and **RICE**.

cult of slenderness

An intense interest in, and devotion to, the development of a body that is shapely and slender. The cult of slenderness has been propagated by a range of groups with a vested interest in promoting the concept that the ideal shape for women is slim, and for men is muscular. Advertisers of fashion products and weight-loss diets portray slim people as healthy and attractive; those who are not slender are portrayed as unhealthy and unattractive.

curl-up

An abdominal exercise similar to a sit-up, but which involves curling the chin onto the chest. The exercise is performed slowly with the lower back held flat on the ground, to reduce the mechanical stress on the backbone in the lumbar region (figure 24).

Figure 24

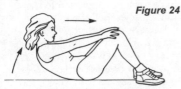

■ Lie on your back with your knees bent and your hands resting on your thighs. Slowly and gently, roll your head and neck forwards, then your shoulders. Roll forwards, sliding your hands onto your knees without

lifting your lower back off the floor. Hold, then return slowly to the starting position.

cut: *See* **laceration**.

cyanocobalamin: *See* **vitamin B$_{12}$**.

cyclamate

An artificial sweetener, thirty times sweeter than sucrose, discovered in 1937. It quickly became the world's most popular artificial sweetener until the 1960s when a few experiments using very high doses suggested it might cause bladder cancers in rats. Cyclamate was banned in the USA and Britain, although subsequent research has indicated that it is not carcinogenic unless taken in abnormally high amounts. Its use is now permitted in the European Union, and always has been permitted in Canada, Switzerland, and Norway.

cycle training

A planned training programme in which the year is divided into cycles, often of different duration. Each cycle has a different purpose. The training programme usually starts with a cycle devoted to general conditioning, then it gradually progresses through cycles of increasing intensity in which training becomes more specifically directed towards the targeted activity. Macrocycles are the main periods of training, e.g. off-season, pre-season, competition, and recovery (transition) cycles. Mesocycles are phases of training within macrocycles. There might be a mesocycle for general conditioning, another for strength training, and a third for speed work. Microcycles refer to daily and weekly training sessions and are described in terms of the type of exercise, its intensity and duration. Cycle training is the US equivalent of periodization.

cycling

Cycling has always been a popular activity in northern Europe and it has recently been taken up by an increasing number of people in North America. It is estimated that more than 85 million people in the United States ride bicycles. One of the main attractions of cycling is that the bicycle keeps the body weight off load-bearing joints, so that cyclists are less prone to ankle and knee injuries than joggers or runners. A number of studies have shown that cycling is as effective as running for developing aerobic fitness. Although cycling uses mainly the large lower body muscles, the upper body is also used to steady the cyclist in the saddle and transmit extra drive to the legs. This may explain why echocardiographs (images of the heart produced from ultrasound waves) indicate that trained cyclists have a significantly greater heart-muscle mass than trained runners.

The major disadvantage of outdoor cycling is the danger of being in collision with other road users. In the United States, cycling injuries accounted for over 500 000 hospital emergency visits and 1300 deaths in 1985. The most common cause of serious disability was head injury. The use of cycle helmets significantly reduces the severity of head injuries but unfortunately many people, especially children, are reluctant to wear them. Unless you can cycle in an area where the air is relatively clean, another disadvantage of outdoor cycling is the risk of breathing in noxious chemicals, especially from vehicle exhaust fumes. So, as well as a helmet, you might want to wear an anti-pollution mask which prevents air pollutants from getting deep into your lungs.

The dangers of cycling outside can be avoided by using a stationary indoor machine but, much of the appeal of outdoor cycling, the scenery and the sense of speed, will be lost. Before buying a home exercise bike, be sure that you really want it. Less than one quarter of long-term owners use their bikes three or more times a week. Many regular users make indoor cycling more enjoyable by watching television or listening to the radio while they pedal. If you do decide to buy an indoor bike it should have the following features:

- VARIABLE RESISTANCE. You should be able to change easily from a low level of exercise for warming up and cooling down, to a higher level during a workout. You should also be able to increase the level of the workout progressively as you become fitter
- STURDINESS. The bike should be strong and well constructed so that it is stable when you sit on it and when you are pedalling fast. It should stand up to the wear and tear of regular use over a long time
- ADJUSTABILITY. You should be able to adjust the seat and handle-bar height to suit your own individual requirement.

Whether cycling indoors or outdoors, you should always stretch before you start and finish a cycle ride. You should also cycle gently for about 5 minutes at the beginning and end of each ride to ensure that your muscles are adequately warmed up before you cycle hard and to cool them down afterwards.

cyproheptadine hydrochloride

A drug taken to increase appetite and weight. It may work by stimulating the appetite centre in the brain. It is a also a potent antihistamine administered to treat allergies and itching skin conditions. Drowsiness is a common side-effect of the drug.

cytotoxic testing

A technique used to identify and treat nutritional disorders by testing an individual's blood for food allergies. The tests are often conducted by non-medical people and the results are sometimes incomplete or misleading. Most dietitians believe that the best way to evaluate an individual's nutritional status is by a medical examination to determine the overall level of health, and a complete inventory of dietary intake.

D

"I am resolved to grow fat and look young till forty, and then slip out of the world with the first wrinkle and the reputation of five-and-twenty."
John Dryden, *(1631–1700), The Maiden Queen IIIi.*

Daily Values

Daily Values are used on food labels; they are a legal requirement of food labelling in the USA. A Daily Value for a particular nutrient is the percentage of the amount of the nutrient recommended for a person consuming 2000 Calories daily. So if a label states that the food contains 6 g of total fat, that represents 10 per cent of the total amount of fat the person should have in one day. Daily Values are based on Daily Reference Values. These form a set of nutritional standards for consumption of total fat, saturated fat, cholesterol, sodium, potassium, and fibre, based on the levels people should consume if they are on a 2000 Calorie diet.

dance

There are many types of dance ranging in intensity from the slow waltz to energetic jazz dancing and ballet. Elite dancers require total body fitness, including cardiorespiratory and muscular endurance, agility, balance, and coordination. Most people, no matter what their age or level of fitness, can find a form of dance that suits them. Dance is a beneficial form of exercise but it is difficult to be specific about the exact contribution it will make to each fitness component because it comes in so many varieties. Generally, however, the more energetic the dance, the more it will help you build stamina and protect bones. Many leisure centres offer sessions in dancercise or dance aerobics (dance movements specially designed to develop aerobic fitness). In addition to benefiting general fitness, dance also helps to strengthen leg muscles, improve flexibility, and develop balance and coordination.

dart thrower's elbow

A tender swelling around the tip of an elbow owing to inflammation of a bursa (*see* **bursa**). It is caused by repeated physical flexing of the elbow, or by rubbing the elbow.

dead-lift

A weight-training exercise in which a barbell is picked up from a rack or the floor and slowly brought up to thigh height. It is a simple exercise that increases mobility of the thighs, hips, and lower back muscles, and increases the strength of the back and abdominal areas.

■ Stand upright, feet a shoulder's width apart. Bend your legs in order to pick up the barbell and then straighten them to lift it; keep your back and arms straight during the lift; make your legs do most of the hard work.

deep friction massage: *See* **massage**.

deep stroking: *See* **massage**.

dehydration

Dehydration (loss of fluids from the body) is a hazard in many sports and can be a serious medical problem. It is also a problem associated with some weight loss techniques, such as steam baths, plastic sweat suits, and diuretic pills (water tablets). Dehydration can result in overheating, a potentially dangerous lowering of blood pressure, and a reduction in the rate at which blood is pumped out of the heart. These effects can lead to illness, heat stroke, and even death. Dehydration can occur during exercise when the amount of fluid lost through sweating is greater than fluid replacement through drinking. It can cause poor performances even in temperate climates. A 2 per cent loss of body weight due to water loss, can lead to a 20 per cent drop in the working capacity of muscles. Dehydration reduces both the speed and strength of muscular contractions. To minimize the risk, water should be freely available during exercise and competitive sports. *See also* **heat stroke** and **water replacement**.

deinhibition training
A potentially dangerous form of training performed by some weight-lifters and body-builders. Usually, when the mechanical strain on muscles exceeds a threshold level, stretch receptors are stimulated and the central nervous system (brain and spinal cord) inhibits further muscle activity. This is an important safety mechanism designed to prevent muscles from being overstretched, but it tends to stop them from working to their full capacity.

Deinhibition training aims to remove the inhibition, enabling muscles to work with greater loads, thus accelerating strength development. It requires high amplitude or explosive movements that stretch muscles and tendons fully. However, with the natural safety mechanism removed, the risk of overstretching and damaging nerves, muscles, and tendons is high. This form of training is definitely not suitable for a beginner.

delayed onset muscle soreness: *See* muscle soreness.

deltoid muscle
A thick, flat triangular muscle responsible for the round shape of the shoulder. One end is attached to the collar bone and shoulder blade, and the other to the humerus bone in the arm. The deltoids (delts) take part in all movements of the upper arm, but their main action is to abduct the shoulder, lifting the arm sideways away from the midline of the body. They also rotate the arm: the anterior fibres rotating the arm inwards and the posterior fibres rotating it outwards. The deltoids are particularly active during rhythmic swinging movements of the arms during walking, and during the propulsive phase of the front crawl. Weight training exercises for strengthening the delts include dumbbell curls,

the dumbbell punch, and the military press.

delts: *See* **deltoid muscle**.

dementia pugilistica: *See* **punch-drunk syndrome**.

dental caries: *See* **tooth decay**.

depression
A melancholy mood; a feeling of hopelessness or an attitude of dejection. Depression varies from mild forms, which most people experience, to very severe clinical forms that require expert medical treatment. Although depression can affect the motivation to exercise, it is generally agreed that aerobic activity can protect against and relieve depression. Aerobic exercise sustained for at least 30 minutes, five times a week, can have remarkable anti-depressant effects. The reason is unclear, but may be linked to the production of endorphins during exercise, or increased self-esteem and control.

descending sets (multi-weight sets)
A weight-training method in which a particular resistance is lifted the maximum number of times. The resistance is reduced and the trainee continues the exercise with the lighter weight, again until failure. Again, the resistance is reduced and the procedure repeated. As many as 10 sets can be completed using this method, but usually three to five sets is as much as most people can tolerate. This is not a routine for the novice; it can be quite painful.

desensitization
A stress-management technique, more accurately called systematic desensitization, which induces relaxation. Desensitization is a form of counter-conditioning in which feelings of anxiety are replaced by feelings of pleasure. The subject compiles an ordered list of anxiety-inducing situations (such as those associated with performing physical activities in public), placing the one causing the most anxiety at the top. Then, the subject completes a progressive muscle relaxation routine. Once relaxation is

achieved, each anxiety-inducing situation is visualized, starting with the one causing least anxiety. At the same time, the subject visualizes that he or she is performing well in public.

designer foods

A new category of foods that are genetically engineered to contain higher than normal amounts of health-promoting nutrients.

It is theoretically possible to transfer the nutritional attributes of one plant to another and to design a plant genetically that combines the attributes of a number of different plants. For example, potatoes, renowned for their high starch content, could be engineered to have additional chemicals, such as the beta-carotene of green vegetables and the flavanoids of citrus fruits. One day it might be possible to order food on a computer by choosing characteristics from a palette of tastes, colours, textures, and nutrients.

detached retina

Separation of the whole or part of the retina from the main wall of the eye, causing loss of vision in the region of separation. The actual separation may be due to increased pressures in the eye following extreme physical exertion, such as lifting a heavy weight or bungee jumping, but the underlying cause of the detachment may be a hole or tear in the retina associated with degenerative changes. Treatment involves re-attaching the retina. People who are susceptible to detached retinas, such as those with degenerative eye conditions, are advised to avoid contact sports (e.g. boxing) and sports that may induce high pressures in the eye (e.g. bungee jumping and skydiving).

detox diets: See detoxication.

detoxication (detoxification)

Detoxication and detoxification are used synonymously when referring to the process whereby toxins (poisons) are removed or toxic effects neutralized. Detoxification also refers to the withdrawal process for those who are addicted to alcohol and drugs such as opiates.

Natural foods often contain toxins. Wild potatoes, for example, contain glycoalkaloids that cause vomiting, diarrhoea, and nervous disorders (see **solanine**). Over thousands of years, we have evolved biological and cultural methods of avoiding toxicity, and metabolic reactions that reduce the toxicity of ingested compounds. We grow less toxic varieties of food and prepare them in ways that reduce their toxicity. We have learnt to avoid foods that make us ill, and to be attracted by those that do not. We also share with other primates the habit of nibbling at strange food and leaving it a while to see if there are any ill-effects. If these cultural and behavioural adaptations fail us and food toxins enter the bloodstream, our livers provide another line of defence. The liver produces a wide range of detoxication enzymes, the best known of which is alcohol dehydrogenase. The toxins are often converted to substances that can be eliminated in the bile or urine. This elimination is helped if the toxin makes us feel thirsty so that we drink plenty of water.

If, despite all our efforts, toxins accumulate in our bodies, we are likely to suffer from toxicity and feel ill. Some people believe that the risk of toxicity has increased because our food is becoming overloaded with artificial chemicals. Some of these chemicals may be fat-soluble toxins which are stored in adipose (fatty) tissue. They do not harm vital organs until they are released when the fat is broken down.

Several diets are designed to promote detoxication. Many claims made for 'detox diets', however, are exaggerated. They are based on the unfounded assumption that most normal foods are toxic in some way. There is little scientific support for such diets. Some of these diets are based on the belief that fruit, vegetables, and yoghurt are virtually free of toxins, while meat and fish are high in them. Although this may be the case for artificial toxins (it will depend on the source of the food and how it has been treated), there tends to be higher levels of natural toxins in plant products than in meat and fish. Some detox diets claim that they contain enzymes or other chemicals that act as detoxication agents. Again, there is little scientific support for these claims.

Most doctors believe that our bodies are usually quite capable of eliminating toxins from a normal, balanced diet without the need for extreme measures. Sensible eating of a variety of foods helps you avoid toxicity. A diet with sufficient vitamins and minerals enables your liver to function efficiently, and certain components in a well-balanced diet, such as water-soluble fibre found in oat bran, bind to some toxins helping the body to eliminate them.

detoxification: See detoxication.

detraining effects
The loss of the beneficial effects of training after regular, vigorous physical activity has ceased. If a person stops exercising completely, most training effects are lost within eight weeks. However, if a person continues exercising at a moderate level, many of the beneficial effects are retained: for example, endurance levels can be maintained for several months by continuing a light exercise programme for one or two days a week. In addition, detraining is affected by the way people have acquired their training benefits. Those who have trained at gradually increased intensities over a number of years, tend to lose the training effects much more slowly than those who have trained intensively for only short periods.

development: See growth.

dextrin (starch gum; starch sugar)
A carbohydrate formed as an intermediate breakdown product in the digestion of starch by the enzyme, amylase. Dextrin is also formed by the application of dry heat on starch (e.g. toasting bread). Dextrin added to water forms a sticky gum used as a food thickener.

dextrose
An alternative name for glucose.

diabetes
Diabetes is the commonly used abbreviation for the medical condition diabetes mellitus, a disorder characterized by an increased blood sugar level. This may be due to the body's inability to produce enough insulin (called Type I diabetes,

insulin-dependent diabetes, or juvenile-onset diabetes), or an inability to use insulin properly (called Type II diabetes, adult-onset diabetes, insulin-independent diabetes, or non-insulin-dependent diabetes). In addition to high blood glucose levels, diabetes results in a depression of carbohydrate utilization. This causes the formation of ketones in the liver, toxic chemicals which damage the nervous system and may lead to convulsions and a diabetic coma.

Type I diabetes develops primarily in young people under 30 years and accounts for about 10 per cent of diabetics. Signs and symptoms include weakness and fatigue, irritability, nausea, thirst, and frequent passing of urine. Type I diabetics frequently suffer extreme hunger and weight loss. Consequently, they are typically lean or have a normal body weight. If left untreated, they often have abnormally high levels of potentially toxic ketones in their blood. To counter the pancreas's lack of insulin production, Type I diabetics take artificial insulin to maintain blood glucose concentrations within the normal range. Regular physical activity has been shown to help Type I diabetics control their blood glucose levels. It also reduces the risk of cardiovascular diseases.

Type II diabetes results from a resistance to insulin. It usually develops gradually in people over 40. Its development is sometimes linked to obesity. One of the highest incidence of Type II diabetes in the world is among a group of people in a district of Port Moresby, the capital of Papua New Guinea. In the past, fat was usually in short supply, so it is believed that the people evolved a genetic ability to store fat in times of plenty. This may have predisposed them to diabetes when they adopted a Western, high fat diet. In type II diabetes, the production of insulin by the pancreas may be normal or even greater than normal, but the liver and muscle cells become relatively insensitive to the hormone. Primary treatment of Type II diabetics includes diet and exercise to achieve a desirable body weight, and to control blood glucose. Development of Type II diabetes is less likely in those who lead physically active lives, and physical activity is generally recommended as an effective means of managing the disease. The risk of Type II diabetes falls by about 6 per cent for every 500 Calories of energy expended per week (approximately equivalent to jogging or swimming for an hour). Regular aerobic exercise reduces the concentration of insulin in blood serum, and increases the sensitivity of the cells to insulin. This increased sensitivity applies to diabetics as well as non-diabetics: sedentary diabetics require about 0.5–1.0 insulin units per kilogram; exercising diabetics require 0.5–0.6 units. Exercise may also reduce the risk of cardiovascular complications. The protection provided by exercise is greatest among obese and elderly people, and those with a family history of diabetes.

Although exercise may benefit diabetics, it also presents some dangers. Overexertion may cause hypoglycaemia (low blood glucose) and, paradoxically, in Type II (non-insulin-dependent) diabetics, it can result in hyperglycaemia (high blood glucose) because the exercise reduces insulin production. Clearly, vigorous exercise may not be safe unless blood glucose levels are well controlled. Certain types of high impact exercise, such as road running, may also harm diabetics who have a decrease in the sensory nerve function of their feet. Diabetics who suffer from some degeneration of the retina should avoid exercises, such as weight lifting, that raise the pressure in the eye, increasing the risk of further damage to the retina.

Treatment of diabetes includes a diet, carefully controlled so that it provides just the right amount of carbohydrate for the body's needs. If adhered to, the diet can prevent some long-term complications of diabetes. Oral hypoglycaemic agents or administration of insulin may be needed to lower blood glucose levels.

diabetes insipidus

A rare metabolic disorder caused by an inadequate release of anti-diuretic hormone (ADH). This hormone helps the body to reabsorb water from the kidneys. Without it a person produces excessively large volumes of watery urine. Diabetes insipidus is accompanied by intense thirst and may result in dehydration. It is treated by the administration of ADH.

diabetes mellitus: *See* diabetes.

diarrhoea

A digestive disorder that occurs when too much water is passed along with a stool. It can result from bacterial or viral infection, from eating contaminated food and drink, from high intake of sugar alcohols such as sorbitol, or from extreme physical exertion and exhaustion. Water in the digestive tract is usually reabsorbed through the intestinal walls, but during a bout of diarrhoea this process is disturbed. Diarrhoea usually resolves itself in one or two days, but it can cause dehydration which limits physical activity. The dehydration can be especially severe and dangerous in the very young and elderly. The most important treatment is to drink plenty of fluid to restore the water balance. Salt and water may need to be added to water to make rehydration effective and to replace losses of mineral salts, especially in young children. Diarrhoea which lasts more than 48 hours, or which recurs, requires medical attention. *See also* **traveller's diarrhoea**.

diastase

A plant enzyme that accelerates the breakdown of starch to maltose. Some sufferers of digestive disorders take it as a supplement to aid digestion of starch. Diastase is common in barley seeds.

diastolic blood pressure: *See* blood pressure.

diathermy (short wave diathermy; SWD)

A form of heat treatment using high frequency electromagnetic currents. These cause molecules in deep tissue to vibrate, heating the tissues and increasing blood flow to them. Diathermy is used to accelerate recovery and reduce pain in sports injuries such as bursitis, strains, and sprains. It is not used on acute injuries where there has been recent bleeding.

diet

The word diet comes from the Greek word 'diaita', used in the past to refer to a person's whole mode of life. Today, the term diet is usually restricted to people's eating and drinking habits: their daily pattern of eating, the quality and quantity of their food, and the frequency of eating. To many people the word means a prescribed allowance or selection of food for some specific purpose. In this sense, a diet may be used to control weight or for health reasons. Weight control diets may be used to maintain a constant weight, to gain weight, or to lose weight. Most people, however, think of diets as restrictive and aimed at weight loss. Around 15 million people in the UK are on some kind of weight-loss diet. These diets are rarely successful. One sports nutritionist estimated that 95 per cent of those who go on a strict diet to lose weight quickly not only regain the weight within a year, but also regain proportionately more fat than muscle. *See also* **weight-loss maintenance**.

dietary exchange lists
(food exchange system)
A dietary management system first developed in the USA for diabetics. The lists consist of six types of food that have been grouped together because they have a similar calorific content and similar composition of carbohydrates, fats, and proteins. The groups are:

- milk and milk products (skimmed milk recommended)
- vegetables
- fruit
- bread (starchy foods)
- meat (lean, low fat products recommended)
- fat.

Each group contains lists of foods and the amounts which provide equivalent energy and macronutrients. For example, one teaspoon of oil is equivalent in fat and energy content to one rasher of bacon; and half a banana has a similar content of energy, carbohydrate, protein, and fat, to one small apple. Nutritionally balanced, calorie-controlled diets can be constructed on the basis of the dietary exchange system. Consequently, the lists are used by a wide range of people to plan a structured diet for weight control. In the UK, special carbohydrate exchange lists are used by some people with diabetes, and protein exchange lists by people who need to restrict their protein intake (e.g. those people with kidney disease need to keep their protein intake as low as possible but still obtain adequate amounts of all the essential amino acids).

dietary fibre
Part of food that cannot be digested and absorbed. The term is sometimes used to distinguish fibre in the diet from crude fibre, a chemical analytical form of fibre. *See also* **fibre**.

Dietary Reference Values
Dietary Reference Values (DRVs) are standards set in the UK by the Committee on Medical Aspects of Food Policy (COMA). The Values are established specifically for population groups and not for individuals. The Reference Nutrient Intake (RNI), for example, is a level of intake greater than required by 97.5 per cent of the population, and therefore more than adequate to meet the needs of most people. However, if an individual's intake is below the RNI, this does not mean that the individual will suffer a deficiency because his or her specific requirements are not known. DRVs give the daily requirements for energy and 33 nutrients. The standards were presented in a comprehensive report entitled *Dietary Reference Values for food energy and nutrients for the United Kingdom*, available from HMSO. The DRVs are provided as four values:

- ESTIMATED AVERAGE REQUIREMENT (EAR): The average requirement for a particular nutrient or for energy
- REFERENCE NUTRIENT INTAKE (RNI): The amount of a nutrient which is sufficient for almost all individuals (97.5 per cent of the population). The RNI is equivalent to the previous Recommended Daily Amount (RDA)
- LOWER REFERENCE INTAKE (LRNI): The amount of a nutrient which is sufficient for only a few individuals (2.5 per cent of the population); therefore most people need more than this
- SAFE INTAKE: A range of intakes sufficient for almost all individuals' needs but not so high as to cause harmful effects. This level is given for nutrients for which there is insufficient information to set more precise levels.

In addition, the DRVs include High Intakes indicating the upper levels of intake for a nutrient above which there is no further benefit and effects may be harmful.

Desirable intakes of total fat, saturated fats, sugars, and starches are expressed as a percentage of the EAR for energy. The estimates are based on the calories expended during sleep or rest, plus the energy expended in physical activity. COMA concluded that, as a population, we have become less active and require less calories than previously recommended. Of course, if you are very active, you would expend more energy and require a higher calorie intake.

ESTIMATED AVERAGE KILOCALORIE
REQUIREMENTS PER DAY

AGE	MALE	FEMALE
0–3 mths	545	515
4–6 mths	690	645
7–9 mths	825	765
10–12 mths	920	865
1–3 yrs	1230	1165
4–6 yrs	1715	1545
7–10 yrs	1970	1740
11–14 yrs	2220	1845
15–18 yrs	2755	2110
19–49 yrs	2550	1940
50–59 yrs	2550	1900
60–64 yrs	2380	1900
65–74 yrs	2330	1900
75+ yrs	2100	1810

Separate energy requirements for pregnant and lactating mothers are also given in the report.

RNIs have been set for vitamins A, B_1 (thiamin), B_2 (riboflavin), B_3 (niacin), C, D, and folate. The RNI for vitamin C is 40 mg compared with the 1979 Recommended Daily Amount of 30 mg. RNIs are also given for calcium, iron, phosphorus, magnesium, potassium, and zinc. Calcium requirements, especially in premenopausal women, are now thought to be higher than in previous recommendations.

Dietitians have considered the information in the report and, in a briefing paper by the Health Education Authority, say that the DRVs provide the scientific basis for the following advice to the average person:

- reduce energy intake slightly to match physical activity
- reduce energy from total fat intake from 40 per cent to 35 per cent
- reduce energy intake from saturated fats from 17 per cent to 11 per cent
- increase consumption of non-starch polysaccharides (a more precise term which replaces fibre) from 12 g to 18 g per day
- reduce average sugar consumption by about a quarter
- reduce salt intake from about 10 g (sodium 3.2 g) per day to about 4 g (sodium 1.6 g)
- eat a varied diet to ensure adequate mineral and vitamin intake
- increase consumption of fruit and vegetables
- increase intake of fibre-rich foods such as pasta, rice, and bread.

diet induced thermogenesis
(thermic effect of food)

When we have a meal, our body temperature tends to rise. This is because we need to expend energy to digest food, and to absorb and assimilate nutrients. Consequently, the calories available to you from food may not correspond exactly to the calorific content described on a food label. It is estimated that diet induced thermogenesis uses between 5 and 10 per cent of a meal's total energy, but the exact amount varies with the type of food. Our bodies seem to be relatively inefficient at utilizing carbohydrate, and less energy is available from it for storage and growth. Diet induced thermogenesis accounts for up to 23 out of every 100 calories when we eat complex carbohydrates, but only 3 out of every 100 calories when we eat pure fats. This is one reason fatty meals are so fattening!

diet pill: *See* **slimming pills**.

digestion

The process by which complex food is broken down into simple compounds by chemical processes. Fats are broken down into glycerol and fatty acids, proteins into amino acids, and starch into glucose. Chemical digestion depends on enzymes secreted by cells lining the alimentary canal or by cells in the pancreas. Chemical digestion is aided by chewing which physically breaks down large chunks of food into smaller pieces; this is sometimes called mechanical digestion. Fat digestion is accelerated by bile secreted by the liver. Bile is stored in the gall bladder until needed in the small intestine where it emulsifies fat, increasing the surface area on which enzymes can act.

digestive disorders

The digestive system consists of a complex tube which extends from the mouth to anus and is linked to several specialized glands and organs. Digestive disorders afflict nearly everyone at some time. The most common include constipation, diarrhoea, diverticulosis, food poisoning, haemorrhoids, heartburn, and irritable bowel syndrome (*see* separate entries).

digestive juices

Juices secreted into the alimentary canal. Digestive juices contain enzymes that help to break down food into its components (mainly amino acids, monosaccharides, and fatty acids) so that they can be absorbed and assimilated by the body.

dilutional hyponatremia: *See* water intoxication.

dimethylglycine: *See* methyl donors.

dimethylnitrosamine: *See* nitrosamine.

dimethyl sulphoxide (DMSO)

A drug used to treat sports injuries. It is rubbed into the skin to reduce swelling and inflammation.

dips

An exercise for strengthening the arms and shoulders (figure 25). It is best performed on parallel bars, but many exercisers improvise by using benches, chairs, or other furniture. However, you must make sure the 'equipment' is anchored securely before you start the exercise.

Figure 25

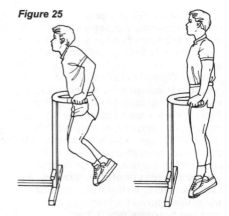

■ Grasp the two bars so that your upper arms are flexed. Lift your feet off the ground and cross your legs at your ankles. Lift your body by straightening your arms. Make the movement in a strict vertical line. Slowly return to the starting position and repeat the exercise.

There are a number of variations of this exercise, including adding weights to a special harness, and reversing the grip so that the knuckles are pointing inwards.

DIRT

A mnemonic used for the components of interval training in running. 'D' represents the distance to be covered; 'I' is the interval of rest between each run; 'R' is the number of repetitions in each set of runs; and 'T' is the target time for each run.

disaccharide (double sugar)

A carbohydrate resulting from the combination of two monosaccharides (single sugars). For example, when glucose and fructose combine, they form the disaccharide sucrose; glucose and galactose form lactose; and two glucose molecules form maltose. During digestion, disaccharides are broken down into monosaccharides which are absorbed into the bloodstream and carried to the liver for processing, after which their main use is as a source of energy.

disc (intervertebral disc)

Discs are flexible, cushion-like pads between two adjacent vertebrae. They enable the backbone to move, and act as shock absorbers during movements. Each disc is composed of an inner semifluid material (nucleus pulposus) and a strong outer ring of fibrous cartilage (annulus fibrosis). The discs are thickest in the neck and lower back, increasing their flexibility. Discs have to be able to bear very high loads, particularly during high-impact exercises such as jumping. In very fit people, a single disc in the lower back can withstand loads in excess of 1000 kg without being damaged. Regular exercise aids the flow of nutrients into intervertebral discs and is essential for maintaining back strength and flexibility. See **prolapsed intervertebral disc**.

dislocation (luxation)

Complete separation (displacement) of the bones forming a joint when the joint is forced beyond its maximum range of movement. A joint becomes immobile or unstable when dislocated, but there is little pain unless the bones press against a nerve. The most common dislocations involve shoulder joints. Dislocations of the knee are rare but when they do occur they are true emergencies requiring expert medical treatment.

Partial dislocations (subluxations) are more common. They result when a joint moves beyonds its maximum range, distorting the alignment of joint surfaces. Unlike complete dislocations, the articulating bones retain partial contact with each other. Partial dislocations are often temporary and the bones usually go back to their normal position without any special treatment.

When a bone has to be put back in place, care needs to be taken even if the dislocation is partial. If an unskilled person uses an inappropriate technique, a great deal of damage can be done to surrounding blood vessels and nerves. It is usually relatively easy for a skilled person to replace dislocated bone (it may even realign automatically) within a few hours of injury. If treatment is delayed, however, the condition may be as difficult to correct as a fracture because the ligaments damaged during the dislocation tend to stick together.

distance running: See **jogging**.

distraction strain: See **muscle strain**.

distraction rupture: See **muscle strain**.

diuresis

The excretion of large volumes of urine. An increase in urine output may be caused by exercise, disease, or drugs (see **diuretic**).

diuretic

A diuretic is any substance (including alcohol and caffeine) that increases the elimination of fluid from the body through urination. It is also the name of a pharmacological class of drugs banned by the International Olympic Committee and many other sports federations.

Diuretic drugs form an important part of the treatment for certain disorders such as oedema (a process which results in accumulation of fluid and swollen tissues). Diuretics have also been used by sports people and slimmers to lose weight quickly. Weight-lifters, jockeys, wrestlers, and boxers use diuretics so they can meet strict weight controls. Diuretics are included in diet pills (sometimes called water tablets) to accelerate weight loss, but their effects are temporary.

Chronic use of diuretics can be dangerous. The elimination of large volumes of water may result in a loss of mineral salts and increase the risk of dehydration, hypertension, and cardiovascular disorders.

diverticulitis

Inflammation of one or more of the pouches or sacs that sometimes form in the wall of the large intestine (see **diverticulosis**). In extreme cases, the diverticulitis obstructs the bowel and is very painful. The disease is linked to poor dietary habits (especially a reliance on highly refined foods) and is made worse by inactivity. A well-balanced diet with plenty of fibre combined with regular exercise, can alleviate uncomplicated diverticulitis by improving mobility of the gut and easing the passage of stools.

diverticulosis

The formation of a small pouch (called a diverticulum) in the wall of the colon. It is a type of hernia that seems to be related to ageing. There is also evidence that a diverticulosis can result from high pressure in the gut lumen, associated with a low fibre diet. Diverticulosis is not usually serious, but the pouch can become infected with bacteria which cause diverticulitis.

DLPA: *See* DL-phenylalanine.

DL-phenylalanine (DLPA)

A special, synthetic form of phenylalanine taken by injured athletes in the belief that it prolongs the painkilling effects of endorphins (natural chemicals secreted by the brain in response to injury). DLPA is thought to inhibit the enzymes that normally break down endorphins.

Some people are sensitive to phenylalanine and related chemicals. DLPA should on no account be used during pregnancy or by those who suffer from phenylketonuria. *See also* **phenylalanine**.

DMG: *See* methyl donors.

DMSO: *See* dimethyl sulphoxide.

Doctor's Quick Weight Loss Diet: *See* high protein diet.

doping

A term derived from the African Kaffirs who used a local liquor called 'dop' as a stimulant. In sport, doping is generally regarded as trying to gain an unfair advantage over other competitors by the use of:

● substances which are alien to the body (e.g. cocaine)

● normal body substances in abnormal amounts (e.g. blood doping)

● abnormal procedures (e.g. altering the integrity of urine samples to mask drugs).

Defining which drugs and methods constitute doping is a major problem. There is no universally agreed definition for all sports.

dose regime

The amount of drug or chemical taken, expressed in terms of the quantity of a drug and the frequency at which it is taken.

double-jointed: *See* hypermobility.

double progressive system

A system of weight training in which both the resistance (load) and the number of repetitions are increased as the trainee becomes stronger.

double sugar: *See* disaccharide.

drive

A psychological force thought to energize behaviour. Some early psychologists postulated that specific drives (e.g. hunger drive, sex drive, and thirst drive) were responsible for energizing each type of behaviour. They distinguished between primary, innate drives associated with satisfying biological needs (hunger), and secondary drives associated with satisfying social needs (e.g. status). Other early psychologists claimed that a single general drive was responsible for energizing all behaviour.

The term drive is still used descriptively to convey the idea of a psychological force, but it is not generally used by modern psychologists because of confusion with the scientific concepts of force and energy. *See also* **motivation**.

dropout

An individual who has stopped participating in an exercise programme. Lack of time, loss of interest, and, especially, failure to achieve goals seem to be critical factors. The vast majority of exercisers who do not achieve their pre-set goals drop out, while most exercisers who attain their goals continue exercising. This emphasizes the need to set personal goals which are reasonably easy to achieve before embarking on an exercise programme. *See also* **exercise adherence**.

drugs

Drugs are substances that alter the body's actions and natural chemical environment. They include medications and narcotics. In sport, drugs are used to enhance physical or mental abilities (*see* **stimulants**); to gain weight (*see* **anabolic steroids**); to lose weight (*see* **amphetamines** and **diuretics**); or to reduce pain (*see* **narcotic**). They are often taken by sports people to gain an unfair advantage over competitors. Drugs taken to prevent or cure a disease, or to alleviate a body disorder are referred to as medicines.

Most drugs are potentially harmful. For example, anabolic steroids can cause aggressive behaviour; amphetamines may induce depression; diuretics may increase the risk of cardiovascular disorders; and narcotic analgesics such as morphine can cause loss of appetite, constipation, and nausea. Chronic use of certain drugs can lead to physiological and psychological dependence. Withdrawal from drug use may then induce unpleasant symptoms which act as a disincentive to give up the drug. In addition, drug tolerance increases with repeated use, so larger doses are needed to maintain the same effects. See also **banned substances**.

dumbbell

A hand weight consisting of a short bar with weights, sometimes adjustable, at each end. They are usually used in pairs during weight training, one for each hand. Some weight-trainers prefer dumbbells to barbells when performing exercises such as bench presses, because dumbbells allow them to stretch their muscles further.

dumbbell curls

A strength-training exercise in which two dumbbells, one held in each hand, are alternately raised and lowered between the chest and the thighs. It is quite a difficult exercise because each arm has to work independently. You cannot do more work with the stronger arm to compensate for a weakness in the other arm.

dumbbell punch

An exercise for strengthening the deltoid, pectoral, and triceps muscles in the upper body.

■ Stand upright, feet slightly astride and hold a dumbbell at shoulder height in each hand. Punch the dumbbell in your left hand upwards by fully extending your arm. Lower it to shoulder height and punch the other dumbbell upwards. Try to maintain a smooth rhythm, remembering to breathe in as each dumbbell is punched upwards, and to breathe out when it is lowered.

duodenal ulcer

An ulcer located in the first part of the duodenum. See also **peptic ulcer**.

duodenum

The first part of the small intestine connecting the stomach to the ileum. The walls of the duodenum are highly folded to increase the surface area for the absorption of nutrients. These are also lined with cells that secrete an alkaline fluid and enzymes, which helps to digest food. The duodenum also receives digestive juices from the pancreas and the gall bladder.

duration of exercise: See **training duration**.

dynamic strength: See **strength**.

dynamogeny

A phenomenon thought to occur when someone moves alongside or just ahead of another moving person. It is suggested that the movement stimulates the production of nervous energy that enables the person being passed to move faster. Dynamogeny may explain why athletes perform better in competition or when using a pacemaker than when training alone.

dynamometer

A device which measures forces. In sport, dynamometers have been designed to measure the forces exerted by specific groups of muscles.

dysentery

A very infectious disease of the gut causing severe diarrhoea accompanied by loss of blood and mucus. In amoebic dysentery the gut is infected with a protozoan, *Entamoeba histolytica*, which is spread by food or water contaminated by faeces. The infection sometimes results in intestinal ulcers and abscesses. Treatment is with specific antibiotics. In bacillary dysentery, the gut is infected by a bacterium, *Shigella*. Transmission is by contact with an infected person, a carrier, or with water contaminated by their faeces. In addition to diarrhoea, symptoms include nausea, cramp, and fever.

Again, treatment is with antibiotics. Patients should not handle food for other people until they are completely free of the disease.

dysmenorrhoea
Pain during menstruation. There are many possible causes including reduced blood supply to the uterus and psychological factors. Dysmenorrhoea is less common in physically active women. *See also* **amenorrhoea** and **menstruation**.

dyspepsia: *See* indigestion.

dyspnoea
Laboured breathing that usually causes some distress because it seems out of proportion with the demands being placed on the body. Shortness of breath at the end of a vigorous exercise session is not dyspnoea, because the effort of breathing is appropriate, passes quite quickly, and causes no real distress. Dyspnoea occurs when the airways are restricted, as in bronchitis and asthma; when circulation to the lungs is impaired, as in heart failure; or if the blood cannot carry enough oxygen, as in anaemia.

E

"Of all the countless evils known through Greece, none is worse than the race of athletes, slaves of their belly."

Eurypides, Greek playwright. Quoted in Green, J. and Atyeo, D. (1979)
The book of sports quotes. Omnibus Press.

....

Eastern prayer
An exercise often used in cool-down routines.

■ Lie face down on the floor with your legs and feet extended. Bend your arms and place the palms of your hands on the floor at the side of your hips. Keeping your palms fixed on the floor, slowly and smoothly push upwards and backwards, first to a high kneeling position and then to a low kneeling position resembling that adopted by people praying towards Mecca. Your head should be tucked well into your body and your buttocks should be touching your heels. Hold for a few seconds and then slowly return in the opposite direction to the start position. Repeat three to five times.

eating diary (food diary)
A daily record of all food eaten. An eating diary usually includes the time of day that eating or drinking took place, rough estimates of the amounts ingested, and the diarist's feelings. For example:

DATE:
Time
Food and drinks consumed
Location
Feelings/mood

The eating or food diary is used by nutritionists, dietitians, and food researchers to study what people eat and the relationship between diet, health, and well being. The diary should record everything you consume (even the 'naughty-but-nice' treats you would rather keep secret), not just what you think you should consume. If compiled honestly, the record can be used to analyse the nutritional content of the diet, and identify ways in which it could be improved. It can also be used to identify the foods responsible for a food intolerance. A person showing symptoms of intolerance records everything eaten in a meal and any symptoms that develop. Foods associated with unpleasant symptoms, such as headaches, dizziness, irritability, nausea, and sneezing, are avoided and replaced by a nutritionally equivalent substitute (e.g. dairy products may be replaced by soya milk products).

eating disorder
A potentially dangerous disturbance in the pattern of eating. It usually has an underlying psychological basis, but is sometimes caused by a malfunction of the appetite centre in the hypothalamus at the base of the brain. Eating disorders are usually classified into two main groups: anorexia nervosa and bulimia nervosa. In reality there is a spectrum of disorders and it is not always easy to assign a particular disorder neatly into either of the two main groups. Patients who do not meet all the criteria for either anorexia nervosa or bulimia nervosa are said to suffer an 'eating disorder not otherwise specified' (NOS).

Eating disorders of any type are more prevalent among females than males. More than 90 per cent of those with eating disorders are women, mostly adolescents. Many sociologists and psychiatrists blame the disorders on the preoccupation of Western culture with slimness and the negative stereotyping of women who are plump. Women are continually bombarded with images from the media reinforcing the notion that they have to be slim to be beautiful, successful, healthy, and happy.

There now appears to be a significant

change in cultural expectations for men, with a greater emphasis on good looks and a muscular physique. This has resulted in many young men becoming compulsive exercisers and resorting to the use of anabolic steroids and special bodybuilding diets. The obsession of men with physical appearance may parallel that of women; both can result in psychological disorders, but of different types. *See also* **anorexia nervosa**; **bulimia nervosa**; and **eating disorder not otherwise specified**.

eating disorder not otherwise specified (NOS)

An eating disorder which cannot be classified as either anorexia nervosa or bulimia nervosa. A person suffering from NOS may exhibit behaviour characteristic of both specific eating disorders, or may alternate between the two disorders. NOS may also occur in a person who has not yet developed the full clinical disorder of anorexia nervosa or bulimia nervosa. This form of eating disorder is relatively easy to treat compared with the full clinical disorders.

eccentric contraction: *See* **muscle contraction**.

eccrine glands: *See* **sweating**.

ECG: *See* **electrocardiogram**.

ectomorph: *See* **somatotype**.

ectopic heartbeat

A heartbeat which momentarily loses its rhythm. The heart may miss a beat which is then followed by a heavy jolt. It is not a cause for concern as long as a person with ectopic beats has an otherwise normal heart, and as long as the ectopics occur during rest. If they occur during exercise and increase in frequency with the intensity of exercise, or if the ectopics combine with other abnormalities, the sufferer should seek medical advice.

Well-trained athletes have a relatively high incidence of abnormal heart rhythms but, in the absence of other symptoms, these variations are normal and do not indicate heart disease. Ectopics can be caused by drugs such as caffeine.

eczema

A non-infectious skin disorder characterized by itching and often accompanied by small blisters. One form may be induced by cold, windy conditions, or chemical irritants dissolved in water. Another form is caused by an allergy to one of a wide range of substances. Flexural or atopic eczema affects mainly children at sites frequently involved in flexion, such as the back of the knees. Atopic eczema is partly inherited, but is also believed to be related to the mother's diet during pregnancy, the child's diet after birth, and other factors. Certain foods, such as cow's milk, chocolates, tomatoes, and nuts, may increase the risk of eczema in infants who are genetically predisposed to the condition. Breast-fed infants are less likely to have eczema, especially if the mother avoids eating foods suspected of triggering eczema. Eczema often worsens under conditions of stress.

Irritant eczema has little effect on participation in sport and exercise, with the exception of swimming, which is not generally suitable for eczema sufferers. Contact sports carry the risk of bacterial infection of eczematous blisters for sufferers of flexural eczema.

EEG: *See* **electroencephalogram**.

effleurage: *See* **massage**.

effluage: *See* **massage**.

eicosapentaenoic acid (EPA)

A long chain polyunsaturated fatty acid used in the formation of anti-clotting agents. EPA is an omega-3 fatty acid. It is one of the active components in fatty fish diets, such as those of the Inuit of the Arctic regions, that appear to provide some protection against coronary heart disease. *See also* **Eskimo diet**.

elastic belt

A belt claimed to increase the temperature round the waist and melt away fat. The same claim is made for inflatable belts. These claims are false: the belts may increase temperature and water loss, but they do not burn off fat. A temporary reduction in waist size may result from the water loss and compression of tissues, but this will be regained quickly. The belts often come with instructions for abdominal strengthening exercises. These exercises may account for reports of more permanent loss in waist size.

elastic strength: *See* strength.

elbow joint

The elbow is a very complex structure. It is the meeting point of many nerves and blood vessels as they pass from the upper to the lower arm. It actually consists of three joints enclosed in a common joint capsule: the humeroulnar joint, between the humerus and ulna; the humeroradial joint, between the humerus and radius; and the radioulnar joint, between the radius and ulna. The elbow functions mainly as a hinge joint, allowing bending and straightening of the arm, but the radioulnar joint also allows the forearm to rotate.

Elbow injuries are quite common in sports, especially those which use hand-held equipment. Hitting a ball with a racket, for example, imposes great stress on the shoulder, elbow, and wrist. Repeated movements can damage tendons attached at the elbow. Over a dozen muscles cross the elbow and the tendon attachment sites are very small. The cumulative microtrauma associated with repeatedly hitting a ball can cause the tendons to fray, much like a nylon rope would if repeatedly stretched. They may even become detached. Elbow injuries require skilled treatment, particularly in children, because damage to the complex internal structures can be permanently disabling. Many of the injuries are named after the sport in which they most often occur (*see* **boxer's arm; dart-thrower's elbow; golfer's elbow; judo elbow; tennis elbow**; and **thrower's elbow**).

electric muscle stimulator

A device for stimulating a muscle by passing a current of electricity through the skin. Electric muscle stimulation (EMS) is used to treat muscle injuries and muscle atrophy when a limb has been immobilized. It is claimed that regular EMS passively exercises muscles, reducing fat levels, but it has been shown that 30 minutes of EMS results in less than 10 extra calories being used.

Charlie Francis, the Canadian athletics coach, believes that EMS can accelerate muscle growth. He used the technique to train his squad of elite athletes, which included Ben Johnson. The general opinion of exercise scientists, based on existing scientific literature, is that EMS appears to be a valuable aid to rehabilitation, but that its use for muscle building is unproven. Improper use of EMS or poorly designed devices can be dangerous. In 1970, a home EMS device was banned by the Food and Drug Administration after users testified that they suffered varying degrees of injury, including severe burns.

electrocardiogram

A tracing on a graph of the electrical changes occurring during a heartbeat. It is one of the most useful records of heart function. It can reveal irregular heartbeats and damage to heart muscle. Specific irregularities in the trace may indicate enlargement of the heart chambers, mineral imbalances in the blood, or whether someone has had, or is having, a heart attack. ECGs are usually recorded while the subject is at rest. An exercise ECG, sometimes called a stress test, provides information about the heart's response to physical exertion.

electroencephalogram (EEG)

A graphical record of the electrical activity of the brain. Three types of brainwaves are associated with different levels of arousal: theta waves occur during sleep, alpha waves are associated with wakefulness, and beta waves with excitement. EEGs can be used to monitor the effects of exercise since there is a close correlation between certain EEG wave patterns and fatigue or overtraining. They are also used to determine the extent of injuries inflicted to the head (for example, after a knockout in boxing).

electrogoniometer: *See* goniometer.

electrolyte drink

A drink that contains mineral salts, such as sodium. It is taken during or after exercise to replace mineral salts lost by sweating and to avoid heat cramps.

There are three main types of electrolyte drink:

- HYPOTONIC DRINKS are watery and have a lower mineral salt concentration than body fluids; they provide the fastest possible rehydration. The mineral content of these drinks is present simply to ensure rapid uptake of fluid across the small intestine
- ISOTONIC DRINKS have a mineral salt concentration the same as normal body fluids; they are designed to rehydrate and deliver energy to working muscles
- HYPERTONIC DRINKS have a mineral salt concentration greater than that of body fluids; they have a high carbohydrate content and are designed to boost energy during endurance activities.

Fluid uptake from the small intestine is greater if the drink has a lower salt concentration than body fluids. Hypotonic electrolyte drinks, therefore, are the most effective at preventing dehycration. During exercise, the salt content of sweat decreases while the salt concentration of the body fluids increases. Therefore, replacing salts without also replacing enough water will increase the state of dehydration and may adversely affect performance. Any individual can restore their electrolytes (salts) by eating a well-balanced diet. There are no conditions encountered by normal athletes or recreationally active individuals when salt tablets are required. *See also* **water replacement**.

electrotherapy

Forms of physiotherapy that use electrical devices to treat injuries. In most cases, their effects include warming deep tissue. They are potentially hazardous and need expert knowledge for their safe application. *See also* **electric muscle stimulator**; **diathermy**; and **ultrasound**.

elevation

1 The type of movement that occurs when a body part is lifted, such as when the shoulder blades are elevated during a shoulder shrug.

2 The process of keeping a limb raised after injury. Many sports injuries reduce the ability of peripheral muscles to pump blood back to the heart. This results in pooling of blood. Elevation allows gravity to return the blood to the heart, and reduces the risk of swelling.

elimination diet

A procedure used to identify foods responsible for food intolerance. First, all suspected foods are excluded from the diet. After several days, the foods are reintroduced one at a time at intervals. An eating diary is kept which logs the foods eaten and any unpleasant symptoms associated with them (e.g. nausea, headaches, insomnia). The aim is to eliminate from the final diet all foods that cause an intolerance reaction, and to substitute them with foods of equivalent nutritional value. Dairy products, for example, that induce lactose intolerance can be replaced by fortified soya milk products.

Individuals who suspect they are suffering from food intolerance are advised to consult a physician and dietitian to confirm the condition. The experts will also be able to help plan and monitor an effective elimination diet. Self-diagnosis and self-treatment are rarely successful.

emergency muscle

A muscle brought into action to assist other muscles only when an exceptional amount of total force is needed. For example, the biceps is an emergency muscle for some movements of the shoulders.

emotions

Psychologists tend to get entangled in a web of words when they are asked to define emotions; some prominent scholars even deny the existence of the concept. However, most people associate emotions with feelings that are either pleasant, like joy and excitement, or unpleasant, like fear or humiliation. Regular, strenuous aerobic exercise commonly induces pleasant emotions (*see* **runner's high**). An exercise programme that evokes feelings of joy and satisfaction is often more effective than a utilitarian programme aimed only at improving health or athletic performance. The message conveyed by most exercise psychologists is that, for long-term involvement, exercise should be fun. An exercise programme based on coercion and fear is rarely adhered to for very long.

emphysema

A degenerative disease associated with chronic coughing. It is fairly common in the elderly. The tissue in their airways loses its elasticity, trapping air in the lungs. This effectively reduces breathing capacity and causes breathlessness. Emphysema is exacerbated by smoking but is sometimes alleviated by taking sensibly graded exercise. However, exercise will not cure the condition.

empty calories: *See* sugar.

emulsification

A process that forms a liquid, known as an emulsion, containing very small droplets of fat or oil suspended in a fluid, usually water. Fats and oils are made into an emulsion in the small intestine by the action of bile salts. Emulsification increases the surface area of these lipids making them much easier to digest. Unemulsified fat usually passes through the intestines and is eliminated in faeces.

emulsifiers (mixers)

Substances added to foods, such as puddings and frozen desserts, to keep oil or fat particles evenly suspended in the water or fluid mixture; they also help disperse oils and flavours within the food. Most emulsifiers, such as lecithin, come from natural sources.

encephalins: *See* endorphins.

encephalopathy: *See* punch-drunk syndrome.

endometriosis

The presence of uterine tissue at sites in the pelvis other than the uterus. The tissue undergoes similar monthly changes to that in the uterus and can cause severe pain during menstruation. Endometrial tissue may adhere to other pelvic tissue. Endometriosis is often treated with hormones, but sometimes surgical removal

of the uterus, Fallopian tubes, and ovaries may be necessary to relieve symptoms. Moderate, regular exercise may reduce the risk of endometriosis.

endorphins

A group of painkilling chemicals secreted by the brain. Endorphins, like encephalins, are produced naturally and have effects similar to those of artificial narcotics such as morphine and heroin. The release of endorphins is believed to increase during prolonged exercise. This may explain the development of conditions such as runner's high in which exercisers experience a sense of elation during prolonged, vigorous activity. There is also a theory that the pain relief induced by acupuncture and transcutaneous nerve stimulation is due to the release of endorphins.

endotoxin

A poison produced within bacterial cells, such as those that cause salmonella poisoning. The toxin is released only when the bacteria die. Our immune systems are unable to produce an antitoxin, so they attack the bacteria directly. Heat, if sufficient, destroys salmonellae and the toxin in food.

end point: *See* range of movement.

endurance (stamina)

The maximum duration an individual can maintain a specific activity; it is commonly called staying power. Sports scientists sometimes distinguish between activities which demand short-term endurance (between 35 seconds and 2 minutes), medium-term endurance (2–10 minutes), and long-term endurance (longer than 10 minutes). Short-term endurance activities are associated with high levels of arousal and use special white muscle fibres that can contract very quickly. The energy release for these activities (e.g. an 800 metre run) depends mainly on anaerobic respiration. Medium term endurance (e.g. 1500 metre run) uses a combination of muscle fibre types, some of which can contract slowly and others quickly. The energy for these contractions comes from both anaerobic respiration and aerobic respiration.

Long-term endurance activities (e.g. the marathon) mainly use red muscle fibres that contract slowly and aerobic respiration.

Slimmers are believed to benefit most from vigorous long-term endurance exercises because the body tends to respire more fat as exercise duration increases and exercise intensity decreases.

energy balance

The relationship between energy intake (food and fluid consumption) and energy output (energy expenditure for body maintenance and activity). A balance occurs when energy input equals energy expenditure. If you ignore weight changes due to water retention and loss, you lose weight only if you have a negative energy balance (i.e. your energy expenditure exceeds energy intake) and you gain weight only if you have a positive energy balance (i.e. energy consumption exceeds expenditure). As a general rule of thumb, most women go into a negative energy balance when they consume less than 1200 calories each day, and men when they consume less than 1500 calories each day.

energy continuum

A concept used to describe the type of respiration demanded by different physical activities. Those activities demanding 100 per cent anaerobic respiration (e.g. 100 metre sprint) are at one end of the continuum; those requiring almost 100 per cent aerobic respiration (e.g. the marathon) are at the other end. In between these two extremes are activities requiring different combinations of aerobic and anaerobic respiration.

energy drink

A drink, usually containing glucose, especially designed to replace or supplement energy expended during exercise. Consumption of low concentrations of liquid glucose (less than 2.5 g per 100 ml) may help to maintain blood sugar levels, delay fatigue, and prevent dehydration. However, many energy drinks are more concentrated; some common sports drinks contain the equivalent of twelve or more teaspoons of sugar per can. These hypertonic drinks are absorbed in the small intestine slowly. They actually accelerate dehydration and, paradoxically, lower blood sugar levels for a short time (see **insulin rebound**). Several drinks are marketed as complete replacement drinks; the manufacturers claim that these not only replace water and energy used during exercise, but also that the amino acids and creatine they contain contribute to muscle growth and repair. There is little scientific support for this last claim. See also **electrolyte drink**.

energy expenditure

The energy expended during exercise is commonly expressed in calories, although scientists tend to use the joule. Energy can be measured either directly from heat production, or indirectly from oxygen consumption (see **calorimetry**).

Daily energy expenditure is dependent on a person's sex, basal metabolic rate, body-mass composition, the thermic effects of food (see **diet induced thermogenesis**), and activity level. The approximate energy expenditure of a man lying in bed is 1.0 kcal/kg/h; for slow walking (just over two miles per hour), 3.0 kcal/kg/h; and for fast steady running (about 10 miles per hour), 16.3 kcal/kg/h. Females expend about 10 per cent less energy than males of the same size doing a comparable activity. For people weighing the same, individuals with a high percentage of body fat usually expend less energy than lean people, because fat is not as metabolically active as muscle.

energy nutrient

A food which is a major source of energy. Carbohydrates and fats are the main energy nutrients, but dietary protein is also used as a metabolic fuel (protein can supply 5–10 per cent of the energy needed to sustain prolonged exercise). In extreme conditions (e.g. during starvation) protein within body tissue is broken down as fuel. Alcohol can also provide considerable amounts of energy.

ENERGY NUTRIENT	ENERGY (KILO-CALORIES PER GRAM)
fat	9
alcohol	7
protein	4
carbohydrate	4

enriched foods

Processed foods to which vitamins and minerals are added. This may be done to replace nutrients lost during processing; to make them more comparable to other foods (e.g. vitamins A and D are added to margarines to make them comparable to butter); or simply to increase people's intake of a nutrient. Enrichment can be statutory or voluntary. Enriched foods do not always have higher vitamin and mineral levels than unprocessed foods; on the contrary, many more nutrients are usually lost than have been replaced. For example, some bread made from white flour is enriched with vitamins B_1, B_2, and niacin, and with minerals such as iron, but may still contain less fibre and other nutrients than bread made with unprocessed, brown flour.

enteric bacteria: *See* gut bacteria.

entramine: *See* serotonin.

E-numbers: *See* food additives.

enzyme

Enzymes are proteins which act as biological catalysts accelerating specific chemical reactions, such as the digestion of food. Without enzymes, these reactions often require very high temperatures and pressures. Although enzymes take part in the reactions, they are not chemically altered by them. Consequently they are not used up and are required in relatively small concentrations. The body varies the concentration of a particular enzyme to regulate a specific activity; generally, the higher the enzyme concentration, the greater the rate of reaction.

Enzymes sometimes require additional, non-protein components to function properly; these are called cofactors. Many minerals and vitamins function as cofactors or coenzymes; deficiencies result in inefficient enzyme activity and ill health.

Enzymes work most effectively within narrow ranges of temperature and pH. Deviations cause the enzyme to change shape (denaturation) and to become less effective; this happens if the body overheats as a result of physical exertion or when lactic acid produced by anaerobic respiration lowers the pH of body fluids.

EPA: *See* eicosapentaenoic acid.

ephedrine

A stimulant drug sometimes used to treat asthma and respiratory complaints. It acts on the sympathetic nervous system to increase blood flow to muscles and promote a feeling of well being. Some people take ephedrine and ephedrine-related drugs as ergogenic aids to improve their physical performance. It is also included in some weight-reducing medications because of its stimulant effects; it may also act as an appetite suppressant. Side effects of ephedrine include heart irregularities and high blood pressure. Ephedrine is banned by most sports organizations including the International Olympic Committee and FIFA.

In 1994, Diego Maradonna managed to reduce his weight by more than 11 kg (25 lb) in the three months leading up to the World Cup. After Argentina's second game of the World Cup, against Nigeria, he was chosen at random for a drug test. Significant amounts of ephedrine-related drugs were found in his sample, described as 'a cocktail of banned substances'. Maradonna was banned from participating any further in the competition because of alleged drug abuse.

epilepsy

An established tendency to recurrent fits which may vary in seriousness; they are brought about by sudden abnormal discharges from brain cells.

Epileptics can participate in many sports. Exercise does not increase the risk of having a seizure. On the contrary, there is strong evidence to suggest that a regular physical exercise programme may be helpful in seizure control. The British Epilepsy Association advises only against sports in which a blow to the head is likely, and underwater sports, motor racing, or climbing, when an epileptic fit could be fatal. About 2 per cent of the population suffer from epilepsy. In most cases, it is adequately controlled by medication.

epiphyseal avulsion

A dramatic injury resulting in partial or complete detachment of a bone along one of its growth lines (the epiphyseal plates), between the head (epiphysis) and the shaft (diaphysis) of the bone. A complete avulsion is most common in preadolescent boys (12–14 years old). It may occur during rapid deceleration, such as when a basketball player comes to a sudden stop or when a long-jumper lands, causing the epiphysis to be pulled upward by the contracting quadriceps. The resulting fracture may extend all the way through the knee joint. Such injuries are a good reason to discourage adolescents from participating in excessively strenuous, high-impact exercises.

EPO: *See* **erythropoietin**.

ergocalciferol: *See* **vitamin D**.

ergogenic aid
An erogenic aid is anything that improves performance of physical activities beyond normally achievable levels. Chemical substances that act as performance boosters are called ergogens. They include drugs taken to improve performance during competition or to increase recovery during precontest training (this enables athletes to endure higher training loads). Ergogenic aids are frequently thought of as drugs only, but they may also be mechanical (e.g. equipment); psychological (e.g. hypnosis and mental practice), physiological (e.g. oxygen therapy); or nutritional (e.g. carbohydrate loading and vitamin supplementation).

ergogens: *See* **ergogenic aid**.

ergometer
An apparatus used to measure energy expenditure at different activity levels. A bicycle ergometer is a static bicycle which has had the drive wheel removed. The workload is adjusted by altering the weight attached to a flywheel. Modern ergometers are computerized to give continuous, direct readouts of workloads, heart rates, and speed. A well-designed bicycle ergometer will have a heavy flywheel to provide a smooth ride, a comfortable seat, and straps on the pedals. The handlebars and seat should be easy to adjust to individual requirements.

erythropoietin (EPO)
A hormone produced by the kidneys. It stimulates the production of red blood cells. Recently a genetically engineered form of the hormone, called recombinant erythropoietin (rEPO), has been made. It has been used successfully to treat anaemia.

Some athletes take rEPO to boost their red cell content in order to improve their endurance capacity. The beneficial effects of rEPO on athletic performance are unproven, but the possibility of gaining an advantage over competitors is too strong a temptation for some athletes to resist. There is great concern about the possible harmful effects of rEPO. High doses are associated with potentially dangerous increases in blood pressure which may lead to strokes and heart attacks. Some doctors suspect that the increase in the number of deaths among competitive cyclists in Europe may be attributed to rEPO abuse. Erythropoietin and related products are banned by most sports federations. However, detection is not easy because EPO is a naturally occurring substance.

Eskimo diet
Eskimos (more properly referred to as the Inuit) eat large quantities of fish rich in oils. Eskimos often appear to be relatively fat, yet suffer low levels of cardiovascular disease. This unexpected combination of a fatty diet and low heart disease is thought to be due to the special nature of the fish oils consumed. The blood of Eskimos takes significantly longer to clot than the blood of those on a Western diet. This longer clotting time is believed to reduce the risk of heart disease. The particular fatty acids thought to be responsible for this beneficial effect include omega-3 fatty acids (e.g. arachidonic acid and eicosapentaenoic acid) and other polyunsaturated fatty acids.

essential amino acid
An amino acid that must be obtained from the diet so that the body can synthesize vital proteins. The nine essential amino acids are isoleucine, leucine, lysine, methionine, phenylalanine, threonine, tryptophan, valine, and histidine. The essential amino acids must be

available in the body simultaneously and in the correct proportions for protein synthesis to occur. One of the problems with some crash diets is that they do not provide enough essential amino acids and, in some extreme cases, have resulted in death.

essential fat

A component of body fat that is essential for health and normal activity. It occurs in bone marrow, lungs, liver, spleen, kidney, muscles, the central nervous system (brain and spinal cord), and, in women, the organ fat within breasts.

essential fatty acid

An unsaturated fatty acid, such as linoleic acid, that is required for normal, healthy functioning of the body. Essential fatty acids cannot be made in the body; they must be obtained from foods such as nuts, oilseeds and their products (e.g. sunflower oil and other vegetable oils), and oil-rich fish. They are used as the raw material for several compounds, such as prostaglandins and leukotrienes, which help to control blood pressure and other vital bodily activities. Lack of essential fatty acid may result in hyperactivity, reduced growth, and even death.

Estimated Average Requirement: *See* Dietary Reference Values.

excess postexercise oxygen consumption: *See* oxygen debt.

exercise

An exercise may be any movement designed to improve a skill, but it generally refers to physical activities that involve large muscle groups. Exercise includes dance, callisthenics, games, and more formal activities such as jogging, swimming, and running. It may be of low-, moderate-, or high-intensity. The precise definitions of these vary, but as a general guide, low-intensity exercise requires 50 per cent aerobic capacity, little increase in respiration and no breathlessness; moderate-intensity exercise (also called vigorous exercise) requires between 60 per cent to 85 per cent aerobic capacity and causes mild breathlessness and some sweating; and high intensity exercise requires between 80

per cent to 120 per cent aerobic capacity. Exercise above 100 per cent aerobic capacity depends on anaerobic respiration and causes considerable breathlessness, sweating, and acute discomfort. Most people, unless they are ill or physically impaired, can perform low-intensity exercise which helps to expend calories (important in weight control) and reduce the risk of some diseases (e.g. diabetes and heart disease). Moderate exercise can cause some discomfort and may be unwise for those who are unfit. People with a body mass index of more than 30 should seek their doctor's advice before starting a vigorous exercise programme. But for healthy individuals this level is usually recommended as optimal for development of cardiorespiratory fitness. High-intensity exercise is suited only to individuals who are medically fit and interested in reaching a high level of physical performance.

exercise addiction (exercise dependence)

Do you:

- feel guilty when you miss an exercise session
- miss important social or business appointments to exercise
- exercise despite being injured?

If you answered 'yes' to these questions, you may be suffering from exercise addiction, a physiological or psychological dependence on regular exercise. A high dependence which produces unpleasant withdrawal symptoms when a person stops exercising is probably rare, but some sports psychologists believe that lower levels of addiction are quite common. The term exercise addiction is often used in a pejorative sense to imply that an individual has an uncontrollable craving for exercise. The cravings may be linked to the production of endorphins, brain chemicals that have narcotic effects similar to those of morphine. A person may be addicted to any exercise, but addiction is usually associated with distance running and weight training.

Most exercise addicts exhibit few harmful symptoms, but studies cited in the *International Journal of Eating Disorders* (January 1994) suggest that exercise addiction can lead to eating disorders, such as anorexia nervosa. The studies found that many anorexics started to exercise in order to become fit, not, as previously thought, to become slim. Apparently, their obsession with slimness developed only *after* they became addicted to exercise.

exercise adherence

Exercise adherence refers to the strength of an individual's commitment to performing physical exercise. People with strong exercise adherence continue physical activity despite opportunities and pressures to withdraw. However, many recreational exercisers quit within 6 to 8 weeks of starting. Adherence improves significantly when exercisers have good family support. Far fewer spouses who exercise together drop out compared with married people who exercise on their own. Exercise adherence is also higher among those who set themselves achievable but challenging goals; whose exercise is supervised or monitored by a coach or trainer; and whose exercise is not intensive to start with, but which becomes gradually harder.

exercise band: *See* **resistance exercise**.

exercise diary: *See* **training diary**.

exercise duration: *See* **training duration**.

exercise frequency: *See* **training frequency**.

exercise-induced asthma (EIA)

A form of asthma induced by physical activity. The bronchioles (air tubes leading to the lungs) are usually dilated during exercise, but in sufferers of EIA they constrict either during exercise or a few minutes after the exercise stops, making breathing difficult. The same intensity of exercise may provoke different degrees of asthmatic attack depending on the nature of the activity. Running provokes worse attacks than cycling, and both running and cycling provoke worse attacks than swimming which is generally considered to be one of the best activities for asthmatics. Asthmatic attacks are most likely if the exercise is of high intensity, continuous, and performed in cold, dry weather, or in a smoky or polluted environment. Attacks are also more likely in those who have poor levels of physical fitness and who have recently suffered a respiratory infection. Attacks are less likely if exercise is intermittent, of low intensity, and performed in a warm, moist environment free from air pollutants or pollen. In most cases, EIA can be prevented by using an inhaler before exercising.

About 80 per cent of asthmatics experience EIA compared to only 3–4 per cent of non-asthmatics. Interestingly, in 1984 the US Olympic team had 67 members who suffered EIA, 41 of whom won Olympic medals. This shows that the condition can be controlled and need not be a deterrent to sports participation at the highest level.

exercise-induced headache: *See* **headache**.

exercise intensity: *See* **training intensity**.

exercise machine

A machine used for strength training and general fitness. There are many kinds of exercise machines, designed either to develop different components of physical fitness, or designed to work different parts of the body. They include exercise bikes (*see* **cycling** and **ergometer**), rowing machines, and cross-country skiing simulators. *See also* **weight-training machine**.

exercise modification

Adjustment of an exercise programme to suit the physical condition, fitness, and health of the exerciser. Exercise components to consider include type of exercise, intensity, frequency, and duration.

exercise prescription

An exercise programme designed specifically for an individual. It is based on the individual's level of health and fitness, and his or her aims. It is very important to get the exercise prescription right: if it is too demanding it will result in overtraining and the risk of overuse injuries; if it is too easy, the exerciser will not acquire the full benefits of training. People often adopt an exercise prescription designed for someone else (usually a famous athlete); this is usually a mistake unless the prescription is modified to fit the abilities and needs of the person adopting it.

An exercise prescription should include mode, intensity, frequency, duration, and progression. The following prescription applies to healthy adults who wish to improve their aerobic fitness:

- **MODE**: rhythmical exercises using large muscle groups (e.g. aerobics; cross-country skiing; cycling; hiking; jogging; rope-skipping; rowing; running; skating; swimming; walking)
- **INTENSITY**: between 60 and 80 per cent maximal heart rate
- **FREQUENCY**: at least 3 days per week
- **DURATION**: 15 to 60 minutes of continuous or discontinuous activity, depending on the intensity
- **PROGRESSION**: increase the duration or intensity as fitness improves. (Duration should be increased before intensity.)

Nonathletic adults are advised to do low-impact exercises (e.g. swimming), at low to moderate intensity, and to progress very gradually.

exercise risks

All exercise carries some risk of injury, cardiovascular problems, and even death, but low-intensity exercise has a very low risk. In the USA, there is approximately one exercise-related death for every 15 000 to 20 000 people. Many more die from diseases caused by inactivity than from overactivity. However, risks increase with the intensity of exercise, and some forms of exercise are unsuitable for certain groups of people. Those with doubts about their health status should consult a medical practitioner before starting an exercise programme. *See also* **contraindicated** and **sudden death**.

exercise therapy

The use of exercise as a form of therapy for promoting psychological or physical well being. Running, cycling, and swimming are often used as psychotherapeutic tools. During rehabilitation from illness or injury, controlled exercise is often a key factor in returning a person to normal activity.

exhaustion: *See* **general adaptation syndrome**.

exotoxin

A poison released by live bacteria into food before it is eaten. The bacterium *Clostridium botulinum*, for example, causes botulism. Heat sufficient to kill the bacteria may not destroy the toxins. Exotoxins stimulate the immune system to produce specific antitoxins, but not before at least some of the toxin has had a harmful effect.

expedition-type endurance

A special type of endurance required for a physically challenging expedition. In addition to aerobic fitness, training may include acclimatization to the environment in which the expedition is to take place. Expeditions often occur in extreme environments, at high altitude, in hot, dry deserts, or in the extreme cold of the polar regions.

Expedition-type endurance requires psychological as well as physical fitness. The leader of an expedition must be able to sustain and motivate team members, and judge their levels of exhaustion. Every member must have tremendous reserves of will-power so that the team can marshall all its physical and mental resources for the supreme effort required for the successful completion of a challenging expedition.

extension: *See* **body movement**.

extensor

A muscle which straightens a joint.

extrinsic motivation: *See* **motivation**.

eye injury

The eye is surprisingly tough, but any injury should be regarded as potentially dangerous and requiring expert medical attention. Direct blows are very serious because the retina can become detached. This may lead to blindness. The sports with the highest risk of eye injuries are boxing and martial arts. Other high-risk sports include basketball, waterpolo, and soccer, with the eye injuries usually caused by fingers and elbows. Racket sports also carry a high risk, especially squash, because the ball can be forced inside the eye socket.

F

fad diet

The word fad, according to *The shorter Oxford English dictionary*, is derived from fiddle-faddle, an adjective meaning 'trifling' or 'fussy'. When used as an expletive, fiddle-faddle means 'Nonsense!' or 'Bosh!'. This is an apt description of many of the fad diets on the market.

Fad diets are those which tend to promote only one type of food. They are usually heavily marketed by people with a vested interest in the food. Exorbitant claims are often linked to the diet about its life-enhancing powers, or its weight-reducing properties. Some fad diets do result in weight loss. This can usually be attributed to a reduced energy intake due to boredom with eating one type of food, rather than to any special properties of the diet. A classic example is the man who lost a great deal of weight on a 'potato diet'. He could eat as much potato, jacketed, boiled, even roasted, as he liked. Unfortunately for him, he did not like potatoes, and his limited intake accounted for a large weight loss.

faeces

Body waste containing undigested food (mainly dietary fibre), bile pigments, bacteria, mucus, and water. Faeces are formed in the colon, stored in the rectum, and eliminated through the anus. Nearly 450 grams (1 lb) of faeces can be produced per day on a high fibre diet, but this is greatly reduced in low fibre diets. Very small amounts of faeces continue to be produced during starvation.

The appearance of the faeces is sometimes used as an indicator of health. Very watery faeces may indicate diarrhoea and a disruption of the normal water reab-

sorption which takes place in the colon. Small, bullet-shaped faeces usually signify lack of fibre in the diet which may lead to constipation. Such small, hard faeces often have to be forced out under pressure; this can contribute to the development of haemorrhoids (piles), diverticulitis, hiatus hernia, and varicose veins. Oily, smelly faeces are usually the result of poor fat digestion. The ideal faecal shape is that of a snake and has a firm, semi-solid consistency

fainting (syncope)

Loss of consciousness because of an insufficient blood supply to the brain. Fainting may occur in an otherwise healthy person because of emotional shock, overheating, or because of a sudden reduction in blood pressure on standing up quickly (postural hypotension). It may also result from severe injury or loss of blood.

Fainting during exercise is a classic warning of heart disease. It may indicate that the heart is not pumping enough oxygen-rich blood to meet the demands of active muscles. Fainting can occur in healthy, fit people when they are relaxing after strenuous exercise. This is due to pooling of blood in the legs.

fallen arches (flat feet)

A flattening of the arched shape of the foot between the heelbone and toes. Fallen arches usually result from excessive strain and weakening of the tendons and ligaments supporting the arches. The condition may develop after standing still for extended periods, or after running on hard surfaces with insufficient arch supports. Fallen arches are treated with appropriate foot supports (orthotics) and special foot exercises.

fanning: *See* massage.

fartlek training

Fartlek is a Swedish word meaning' speed play'. It is applied to a relatively unstructured form of training over natural terrain. It originated in Scandinavia where structured training during the snowy months of winter is difficult. Typically, the route is predetermined, but the pace is varied spontaneously according to the terrain and the disposition of the runner. A typical session includes short bursts of running at full speed, longer periods of sustained effort, easy running, jogging, and walking. Fartlek training is often used as an alternative to highly structured interval training to provide variety. If performed properly and energetically, fartlek improves both aerobic fitness and anaerobic capacity.

fascia

Tough connective tissue which may be superficial or deep. Superficial fascia is fatty and lies under the skin. It forms a lining separating the skin from the deep fascia. Deep fascia usually ensheathes muscles, blood vessels, nerves, and organs; it contains dense elastic tissue to give it flexibility.

fascial hernia (muscle hernia; muscle poops)

Protrusion of a muscle through the superficial fascia beneath the skin when the muscle is under pressure. It is sometimes accompanied by pain. If a person has a fascial hernia, a definite bulge can be felt where the hernia occurs during or immediately after exercise, and it is often possible to feel the hole in the fascia when the muscle is relaxed. The most common site for a fascial hernia is the anterior tibialis muscle at the front of the lower leg.

fashion

Fashion has a very strong influence on the attitudes and actions of people. This is particularly so with regard to diet and exercise. The predominant fashion in Western cultures is for women to have slim, almost boyish looks. Being slim has not always been fashionable. One has only to look at a Rubens painting to realize that his feminine ideal was a plump, curvaceous woman. It is unclear whether the fashion industry originally created the trend for slimness or merely followed it. Nevertheless, since the 1960s fashion designers have been accused of creating the cult of the super-thin model, reinforcing the desire for thinness. In order to follow the fashions worn by models, many women have needlessly subjected themselves to weight-loss diets and exercise regimes, not to keep fit and healthy, but to look acceptable. Not surprisingly, this has led to many impressionable young women going to extreme lengths to achieve their goal. An increase in the incidence of the eating disorders, anorexia and bulimia, have followed this fashion for thinness.

Until recently, apart from a few advertisements for body building, men were not under the same pressure as women to achieve a particular body shape. However, this has changed with the advent of mass parties where it is fashionable for young men to display their naked upper torsos. Consequently, there is an increasing trend for men to use artificial aids, especially anabolic steroids, to build bodies with well-defined muscles.

Regular exercise and a balanced diet are conducive to good health; an obsessive concern about diet and exercises which develop a certain fashionable body shape is potentially harmful, both physically and psychologically.

fast foods

Fast foods are convenience foods that can be prepared and served very quickly. On average, one-fifth of the population of the USA (45 million people) eat in a fast-food restaurant each day. Although it is possible to eat nutritious fast foods, menus tend to be stacked with items high on most dietitians' 'Avoid!' lists.

Fast foods include salty french fries, beefburgers, fried chicken, and pizzas with a thick cheese covering. These appeal to the Western palate by being fatty, low in fibre and nutrients, but high in salt (one beefburger can contain more than 1000 milligrams of sodium). To make matters worse, they are often served with sugar-laden soft drinks or creamy milkshakes full of empty calories or fat.

Those who regularly eat fast foods should be particularly selective, moderating the intake of unhealthy options and choosing healthy options, such as salads with low-fat dressings, wholegrain buns, and skimmed milk. *See also* **junk food**.

fasting

People may go without food for religious reasons, to lose weight, or in the belief that it is good for health, although there is no evidence of health benefits. Religious fasting usually involves going without food at certain times (e.g. between sunrise and sunset). It is rarely harmful to health and may be spiritually and psychologically beneficial. On the other hand, indiscriminate prolonged or repetitive fasting (i.e. going without food for more than 12 hours) to lose weight is generally regarded as unwise. Although a severe restriction of food intake has been used successfully to treat extreme obesity, this type of fasting should be used only under medical supervision. Weight loss during fasting is often in the form of water, and is quickly regained. If fasting is prolonged, muscle, vitamins, and minerals can be lost. Many people who fast say they experience a sense of heightened mental awareness. This may be related to the fact that the brain switches from using glucose as a fuel to ketones (chemicals that result from the breakdown of fat). The American College of Sports Medicine states, however, that prolonged fasting is scientifically undesirable and can be medically dangerous. It may cause loss of hair, dizziness, fainting, muscle cramps, and more serious problems that lead to permanent injury, such as kidney malfunction, and heart irregularities that can cause heart failure.

As well as being potentially harmful, prolonged fasting may also be ineffective as a means of losing weight. The body responds to prolonged fasting in the same way as to starvation. It adopts a kind of 'siege economy'; basal metabolic rate is lowered, the ability to store fat improved, and protein within muscles is broken down to yield energy. All these processes mean that when a person resumes a normal diet, body weight is likely to increase beyond the pre-fasting level.

fat (neutral fat; triglyceride)

True fats, neutral fats, or triglycerides (also called triacylglycerols) are lipids formed by the combination of glycerol and three fatty acids. Triglycerides are sometimes distinguished by their physical state: those which are liquid at room temperature (20°C) are called oils; those which are solid at room temperature are called fats. Often, however, fats and oils are both referred to as fats.

Fats contain carbon, hydrogen, and oxygen. They have a high proportion of hydrogen which makes them a more concentrated form of energy than either carbohydrates or protein. Each gram of fat or oil produces about 9 Calories of energy. Fats are the primary source of energy during prolonged aerobic exercise. The release of energy from fat requires more oxygen than the release of the same amount of energy from carbohydrates. Fat metabolism therefore puts a greater strain on the oxygen transport system.

Excess dietary fat is stored as body fat in adipose tissue. Excess dietary carbohydrates and proteins may also be converted into fat and stored in adipose tissue to provide energy (e.g. during the fasting state between meals), heat insulation, cushioning, and buoyancy.

There is a lot of confusion over the part dietary fat plays in causing disease. The confusion stems from the bewildering number of types of fat, and there is disagreement about how harmful or beneficial each type is (*see* **saturated fat** and **unsaturated fat**). Nevertheless, it is beyond dispute that high intakes of dietary fat are linked to obesity and coronary heart disease. Doctors speak with one voice when they say that we need to restrict our total fat so that it contributes no more than 35 per cent of the total calorific intake in the diet. Only 10 per cent of calorific intake should be saturated fat, the form of fat most clearly linked to disease. The average person in North America and the UK derives 40–45 per cent of his or her calories from fat.

Apart from the health risks, high fat diets may also impair physical performance. Athletes are usually advised to avoid fatty foods before competition because they can take 3–4 hours to digest. It seems that a high fat meal may also cause early fatigue by increasing the level of fatty acids in the blood.

It is wrong to try to eliminate fat from the diet completely. It is needed to absorb vitamins A, D, E, and K, and a little fat in the digestive system helps to delay hunger pangs. Some fatty acids are essential for the manufacture of other lipids, such as steroids. Other fatty acids appear to actually reduce the risk of coronary heart disease (*see* **omega-3 fatty acids**). Also, a modest intake of fat helps to maintain optimum levels of triglycerides in the muscles. These act as energy stores for aerobic activities.

fat blockers

Synthetic chemicals designed to stop the fat in food from being absorbed. Manufacturers claim that fat blockers provide an easy and quick slimming aid, and that users can eat fatty foods without putting on weight. Unfortunately, fat that is not absorbed may accumulate in the lower bowel where it can cause incontinence by reducing anal sphincter control. In addition, the stools will be smelly, fatty, and foamy. Fat blockers are being used experimentally in the USA but have not yet received approval for general use in Britain. Before approval, the authorities must be certain that fat blockers do not interfere with the absorption of fat-soluble vitamins and essential fatty acids.

fat cells: *See* **adipocyte**.

fatfold test: *See* **skinfold measurements**.

fat-free body mass: *See* **lean body mass**.

fat-free body weight

The weight of the body excluding storage fat and essential fat.

fatigue

Exercise fatigue is characterized by an overwhelming need to reduce the intensity of activity. When you become physiologically fatigued, no matter how hard you try, you are incapable of maintaining maximum power output from muscles. Fatigue is a safety device that conserves energy for vital activities and prevents irreversible damage to body tissues. It is caused by factors that act directly on muscles. These include depletion of energy stores (especially muscle glycogen, the main carbohydrate energy store in muscles), accumulation of waste proucts, and tissue damage caused by overuse of specific muscle groups. Fatigue may also be caused by chemicals which affect the brain. Some researchers suggest that concentrations of serotonin (a neurotransmitter) increase in the brain during exercise and cause fatigue. The increase may be associated with depletion of muscle glycogen and increases in fatty acids circulating in the blood. Serotonin levels in the brain may also increase when amino acids, called branched chain amino acids (BCAAs), are used as fuel, lowering the amount of BCAAs in the blood. Sports drinks containing BCAAs are now available. Manufacturers claim that they reduce fatigue by reducing serotonin levels in the brain, but the amount of BCAAs in the drinks is very low (less than 1 g per serving) and probably has a negligible effect. Exercise physiologists have warned that higher supplementations of BCAAs may lead to dehydration, toxic levels of ammonia in the body, and other dangerous effects. They suggest that until we know more about the relationship between BCAAs and fatigue, we should avoid taking supplements containing these amino acids.

Success in endurance activities often goes to the person who is best able to delay the onset of fatigue. There is a great temptation to take a short cut to success by using drugs (e.g. caffeine) that delay fatigue. This is contrary to the laws of most sports federations and can be dangerous. The following tips, suggested by exercise physiologists and sports scientists, may help you fight fatigue legally and safely:

● saturate your muscle glycogen stores by eating high-carbohydrate foods (*see also* **carbohydrate loading**)

- avoid high-fat foods, such as dairy products and doughnuts, which can increase the level of fatty acids in the blood (but *see* **fat loading**)
- be sure to reduce training before an endurance event (*see* **tapering down**).

Less reliable ways of delaying fatigue are increasing the alkali reserve (*see* **sodium bicarbonate**) and phosphocreatine levels in the muscles (*see* **creatine**). For exercise lasting more than 3 hours unique fats, called medium chain triglycerides (MCTs), may improve performance. MCTs are absorbed from the gut quickly. Tests on long-distance cyclists in South Africa showed that drinks containing 4.3 per cent MCTs and 10 per cent carbohydrate may delay fatigue by sparing muscle glycogen.

As well as physiological fatigue, exercisers commonly experience psychological fatigue due to the boredom of repeating the same exercise again and again. Although the muscles are physiologically capable of working harder, the exerciser can no longer be bothered to make the effort. Boredom can be avoided by making exercise varied and interesting. *See also* **overtraining**.

fatigue index

A concept used in the study of the development of fatigue during anaerobic activities. The fatigue index is expressed as the power decline (i.e. peak power minus minimum power) divided by the time interval in seconds between peak power and minimum power.

fat loading

Some sports nutritionists believe that fat loading (increasing the consumption of fat to fill fat stores within muscle cells) can delay fatigue. They suggest that the extra fat enables muscles to metabolize fat more efficiently during exercise, conserving muscle glycogen. Support for this belief comes from a study of a group of runners who increased their fat consumption by about 60 per cent for a week and improved their running performance by more than 30 per cent. They were able to continue running on a treadmill at 85–92 per cent maximal heart rate for significantly longer than those who had a normal diet or a high carbohydrate diet. However, the results have limited application because of the peculiar conditions of the experiment. Before the test, the runners fasted for 14–16 hours and had to complete a maximum treadmill test at 85 per cent effort, which probably depleted the muscles of glycogen. The results therefore apply only to moderate exercise intensities that do not require glycogen. At high exercise intensities, glycogen is the main energy source.

Because of the uncertainty about the advantages of fat loading and the potentially harmful effects of fat on health, most experts agree that athletes should avoid fat loading and eat foods with only a moderate fat content (10–25 per cent of the total calories). Dietary manipulations involving the high intake of fats must be proved safe and effective before they are recommended for general use. It is well established, however, that high fat diets are beneficial for activities which demand extremely prolonged endurance in very cold conditions. Polar explorers have been known to chew their way through one-pound slabs of butter so that they could obtain the calories needed to maintain body temperatures and sustain them on their arduously long treks.

fat malabsorption

A reduction in the ability to absorb fat from food in the gut, usually due to a deficiency of bile salts or coeliac disease. Fat malabsorption results in the body becoming deprived of fat soluble vitamins, the stools become fatty, and the gut becomes bulky.

fat mobilization

The breakdown of fat into glycerol and fatty acids so that it can be transported and used as an energy source by active muscle. Fat stored in fat cells (adipocytes) cannot be used until it is broken down. An enzyme, lipase, exists in the membranes of these cells and accelerates the breakdown. The performance of marathon runners improves significantly if fats can be mobilized and used as fuel early in a race so that glycogen stores can be conserved for later use.

fat pad

A pad of fatty tissue occurring in and around bony joints. Fat pads act as a cushion helping to protect the joints from mechanical damage.

fat-soluble vitamins

Vitamins A, D, E, and K dissolve in fats. They dissolve in dietary fats and are absorbed along with digested products. Anything interfering with fat absorption, such as a deficiency of bile, will interfere with the uptake of fat-soluble vitamins. All, except vitamin K, are stored in adipose tissue. An excessive intake of vitamins A and D can cause toxicity called hypervitaminosis.

fatty acids

Components of neutral fats or triglycerides. Chemically, they are long linear chains of carbon, hydrogen, and with an organic group (-COOH) at one end. They have the general formula R-$(CH_2)_n$-$COOH$, where R represents a hydrocarbon group, e.g. $-CH_3$ or $-C_2H_5$.

Fatty acids are classified as either saturated or unsaturated (*see* **saturated fat** and **unsaturated fat**). Those which attach loosely onto proteins in blood are called free fatty acids. They are an important source of energy for exercises of long duration. Persistently high levels of free fatty acids in the bloodstream are considered by some to indicate high reserves of energy and high levels of fitness. On the other hand, increases in circulating fatty acids have been linked with the onset of fatigue.

FDA

Food and Drug Administration; a federal government agency in the USA that regulates and monitors food and drug safety. Initially it was concerned only with food additives and drugs already in use and proven harmful. Subsequently its jurisdiction has widened. The Delaney clause, introduced in 1958, empowers the FDA to prohibit any substances in foods that cause cancer in laboratory animals. Since 1962, it has enforced regulations to ensure that new drugs are effective as well as safe.

feedback

Information provided either during or after an activity and which enables a performer to assess how well an activity has been done. Feedback is regarded by many sports coaches as the single most important factor in training; without it, a person does not know how well he or she is progressing. Some feedback is a natural consequence of performing an activity; athletes see and feel how well the activity is being accomplished. However, the most effective feedback is often provided by an external observer (e.g. coach) or from some other objective source (e.g. a video camera). A good coach or exercise trainer should always ensure that those being trained are getting high quality feedback.

Feedback is also important for those who are trying to maintain or achieve a certain body weight. It is obtained by keeping an eating diary and regularly weighing oneself. *See also* **biofeedback training**.

Feingold diet

A diet that excludes colourings, flavourings, and naturally occurring aspirin-like compounds (salicylates). The Feingold diet was devised for hyperactive children and those suffering from attention deficit disorder in the belief that the excluded substances contribute to the development of the conditions. The diet can be difficult to manage. To ensure it remains 'well balanced' and nutritionally sound, it is best to obtain the advice of a fully qualified dietitian. There is no clear evidence that the additives cause the problems or that the Feingold diet is beneficial.

fencing

The art of fighting with swords. Today, it is practised as a sport using three weapons: the foil, epee, and the sabre. Fencing demands quick reflexes, poise, balance, and good muscular coordination combined with mental discipline. Although competitions usually consist of short bursts of anaerobic activity, practice sessions can be long and require stamina as mind and body are trained to carry out the complex fencing movements.

fenfluramine

An appetite suppressant, chemically related to amphetamine, but without its addictive properties. Fenfluramine is used in the treatment of obesity. Adverse side-effects include depression and irregular heart beats.

fermentation

The breakdown of organic substances by organisms to release energy in the absence of oxygen. It is especially applied to the anaerobic breakdown of carbohydrates by yeasts to produce alcohol and carbon dioxide, and the bacterial breakdown of milk sugar to give lactic acid (as in the production of cheese and yoghurt). See also **colonic fermentation.**

fermented foods

Foods such as cheese and yoghurt are made by bacterial or yeast fermentation. In Asia and Africa cooked soya beans and cereals are fermented to make a number of important foods, including koji, miso, sufu, and tofu. Fermented foods contain the bacteria or moulds which helped to produce them. These can improve the taste of bland foods and may provide valuable nutrients that are especially difficult for vegans to obtain. In addition, some bacteria (e.g. *Lactobacillus* in natural yoghurt) can take up residence in the intestine where they may produce enzymes, vitamins, and other chemicals beneficial to the health of their host (*see also* **gut bacteria**). Fermented milk products (e.g. yoghurt) are tolerated by people lacking the enzyme lactase who cannot tolerate fresh milk (*see* **lactose**), but fermented milk products are no use for people who cannot tolerate milk because of an allergy to milk proteins.

ferritin

A protein containing iron. It occurs mainly in the liver, kidney, and spleen where it acts as an iron store.

fertility vitamin: *See* vitamin E.

fever (pyrexia)

A condition in which the body core temperature is higher than normal (oral temperature more than 37°C). Fever is usually caused by an infection that disturbs the temperature control centre in the brain, but it is sometimes linked to an emotional disturbance. It is often accompanied by headaches, shivering, and nausea. It can result in dehydration if sufficient liquids are not taken.

One golden rule of exercise is that you should avoid physical exertion during a fever which raises the core temperature above 38°C. The fever not only diminishes muscle strength and endurance, but it also increases the risk of heat exhaustion during exercise. More seriously, exercising during fevers may lead to inflammation of the heart (myocarditis). Although this may be very rare, myocarditis is a potentially fatal condition.

fibre

Fibre is the indigestible part of plants. It includes cellulose, hemi-cellulose, lignin, pectin, and gums. It is sometimes called bulk or roughage. Fibres are grouped into two basic types: insoluble fibre and soluble fibre.

Insoluble fibre absorbs many times its own weight in water and swells up in the alimentary canal. People on high fibre diets tend not to suffer from obesity because they feel full and so consume less food. By increasing the bulk of faeces, fibre promotes efficient waste elimination from the colon and may help to prevent colon cancer. The bulk also provides a resistance against which the gut muscles can work. These muscles produce the peristaltic waves of contraction that push food along the gut. Efficient peristalsis reduces the risk of intestinal disorders such as constipation. Insoluble fibre is found in wholegrains and vegetables; it includes cellulose and lignin. Much of it is resistant to human digestive enzymes and therefore passes through the alimentary canal virtually unaltered.

Soluble fibre is found in many plant foods, but is especially rich in oat bran. Some types are broken down by microorganisms in the large intestine into substances that can be absorbed through the gut wall and into the bloodstream. Fibre regulates the transit time of faeces and reduces the risk of constipation. It may prevent or reduce the absorption of cholesterol (high cholesterol levels are a risk factor of coronary heart disease). It may also delay the entry of glucose into the blood. This means that blood glucose levels do not fluctuate widely, reducing the risk of glucose overload or deficiency, and diabetes.

Most nutritional experts agree that Western diets are deficient in fibre. The National Institute of Cancer in the United States, recommends that 25–50 grams of fibre should be eaten per day. Although wholegrain cereals are an excellent source, the fibre should be provided from a variety of sources (for example, fruits, vegetables, beans, and whole baked potatoes). In addition to providing fibre, these foods provide valuable minerals and vitamins.

People on high fibre diets should drink plenty of water or the fibre may partially block the gut, inhibit digestion, and cause intestinal problems. They should also be aware that fibre can reduce protein absorption. This problem can be reduced by eating plenty of protein and by getting fibre from a variety of foods. Some types of dietary fibre, such as unprocessed bran, are not recommended as sources of fibre because they contain high levels of phytic acid which may interfere with the absorption of minerals. *See also* **fibre supplements**; **F-plan diet**; and **non-starch polysaccharide**.

fibre splitting: *See* **muscle growth**.

fibre supplements

Manufacturers produce pills that contain fibre. They claim that the pills provide the same benefits as dietary fibre. However, natural fibre is a complex of a whole variety of substances. No one knows the combinations that are the most beneficial, so the supplements may be unbalanced or incomplete. Fibre tends to reduce the absorption of some minerals (e.g. iron). Most sources of dietary fibre are rich in minerals and vitamins, which compensates for this reduction. Fibre supplements are usually lacking in nutrients. Some of the early fibre supplements available in the UK contained high concentrations of guar gum. This swells in the stomach, reducing feelings of hunger, but it may also swell and block the intestine or even air passages in the throat. The British government has now

banned the sale in the UK of all fibre supplements with more than 15 per cent guar gum.

fibrin

A fibrous, insoluble protein formed during blood clotting. Molecules of fibrin form a network trapping cells and debris that seal off a damaged vessel. Unwanted fibrin formation can occur inside undamaged vessels, causing thromboses. One theory (the fibrin deposit theory) suggests that regular aerobic exercise reduces fibrin deposits in the blood, lowering the risk of thromboses and some other cardiovascular disorders.

fibrositis

A term often applied rather loosely to any condition in the shoulder or upper back characterized by a dull ache. True fibrositis is an inflammation of the fibrous connective tissue of muscles and tendon sheaths. The affected area is painful and tender when touched. Although fibrositis is exacerbated by exercise, range of movement is not usually affected. Fibrositis may result from chills, toxins, chronic strain, or physical fatigue. It often responds well to heat therapy and massage.

fish-oil supplements

Fish oil supplements are usually taken in the form of pills or capsules. They contain oils from fish, such as mackerel and herring, which are rich in monounsaturated and polyunsaturated fats. These fats are believed to protect the heart against disease by lowering blood cholesterol levels and triglyceride concentrations, and reducing the tendency of blood to clot. Chemicals, such as prostaglandins, derived from some of the fish-oil fats (e.g. arachidonic acid, an omega-3 fatty acid), help to regulate blood pressure, and play an important role in the inflammatory and immune responses. Although it is generally agreed that fish oils are beneficial, many dietitians advise that the oils should be obtained directly from fish and not from supplements because the effectiveness of supplementation is unproven. There is also doubt about the optimum dietary levels of the oils and it is easy to overdose on supplements. An excessive intake may prolong clotting time to a dangerous extent, increasing the risk of bleeding after accidents or during surgery. Also, pills containing cod liver oil are rich in vitamins A and D, which can be toxic in large amounts.

fitness

Fitness is generally defined as the ability of a person to live a happy, well-balanced life. It embraces the physical, intellectual, social, and spiritual aspects of a person's life. It is a relative term, depending on individual circumstances and for what a person needs to be fit. Fitness has health-related components and skill-related components. Health-related components include aerobic fitness, muscular strength, muscular endurance, flexibility, and body composition. Skill-related components include agility, balance, coordination, speed, power, and reaction time. Both sets of components interact and are interdependent. A deficiency in any component reduces overall fitness. *Compare* **unfitness**; *see also* **physical fitness**.

fixed-weight machine

A solid weight-training machine that usually uses a weighted pulley system to vary resistance. Some fixed-weight machines are designed for a wide range of muscle-strengthening exercises (*see* **multi-gym**); others are used for exercises on specific muscle groups. The butterfly machine, for example, has pads which are moved by the arm and chest muscles in a manner reminiscent of butterfly wings. The lateral pull-down machine has a bar which is grasped above the head. The exerciser pulls down on the bar, working the muscles in the arms and back, particularly the latissimus dorsi muscles. The total hip machine has padded rollers that can be pushed back and forth by the leg muscles, enabling an exerciser to tone the hips and thighs. The total calf machine has a fixed seat and a back plate against which the feet are pushed to strengthen the calf muscles. The recumbent leg press helps to work buttock and thigh muscles when a foot pad is pushed in an effort to make the seat slide backwards and forwards.

Although variable in design, all fixed-weight machines tend to be easier and safer to use than free weights, because if any weights are dropped they merely fall back into the machine.

flat feet: *See* fallen arches.

flatulence

The expulsion of gas from the alimentary canal. Most belching is due to swallowing air. Rectal flatulence is usually caused by excessive gas produced by bacteria in the alimentary canal. The bacteria fermentation results in the breakdown of indigestible complex carbohydrates, such as those in beans and lentils. The fermentation results in the production of gases including hydrogen, methane, and carbon dioxide. Flatulence may be reduced by chewing food thoroughly, drinking plenty of fluid, and avoiding too much food that causes the flatulence. Although flatulence is associated with high fibre diets, the problem tends to decrease as a person becomes accustomed to the diet. Intestinal gas is also common in those who cannot digest lactose (*see* **lactose**).

flavour enhancers

Substances added to food to exaggerate its taste or aroma. Flavour enhancers include monosodium glutamate, hydrolyzed vegetable protein, and maltol (a substance that occurs naturally in malt and tree bark). They are commonly added to gravies, oriental foods, and soups. *See also* **food additives**.

flexibility

Flexibility is the ability to move a joint smoothly through its complete range of motion. There are two main types: static flexibility is the ability to move slowly into a stretched position and to hold the body still (e.g. the ability to sit in a splits position); dynamic flexibility is the ability to move quickly or at normal speed into a stretched position (e.g. a gymnast performing a split leap).

Flexibility is one of the main components of physical fitness and is believed to be important for optimum health. Flexibility exercises have been prescribed for the relief of menstrual disorders, general neuromuscular tension, and low back pain. A certain amount of flexibility is needed for body movement; conversely, lack of flexibility restricts movement.

Flexibility of a particular joint is limited by factors such as the bony structures of joints, and the size, strength and extensibility of the muscles, ligaments, and tissues associated with the joint. Most flexibility exercises focus on improving the extensibility of muscles and associated tissues, usually by static or very slow stretching. To be effective, flexibility training must incorporate an element of overload. This can be achieved by

- stretching the muscle more than is normal (but within tolerance limits)
- holding a stretched position for longer than is normal
- increasing the number of stretches.

It takes several weeks of regular training to produce improvements; for maximum benefit flexibility exercises should be performed on a daily basis. Many adequate routines take only a few minutes each day to complete, but warm-ups and cooldowns must also be included in good flexibility programmes.

Flexibility tends to be specific for each part of the body and type of movement. Training must take this into account. To develop overall flexibility, different stretching exercises using each of the major muscle groups must be performed at different speeds. The composition of the training will depend on the requirements of individual sports and activities. The needs of a gymnast are quite different from those of a footballer. In addition, a person should not concentrate on flexibility exercises at the expense of strength training as this may reduce joint stability, and increase the risk of sprains and dislocations. *See also* **stretching**.

flexion: *See* **body movements**.

flexor
A muscle that causes a joint to bend.

flotation therapy
A form of relaxation therapy that involves floating on very salty water in a light-proof and sound-insulated room. To many people who have not experienced flotation therapy, it appears to be a form of self-inflicted sensory deprivation. If imposed by an outside agency, such as army interrogation officers, it would be banned under the Geneva Convention of Human Rights. However, regular practitioners (called floaters) claim that they experience feelings of great relaxation and euphoria during a float. Some use the float as part of their weight-loss activities and state that it gives them the opportunity to focus their thoughts on positive images about themselves, their diet, and their exercise regime.

flow
A psychological state of extreme well being sometimes felt when exercising. A person experiencing flow has feelings of great pleasure, satisfaction, and enjoyment. To many competitive sports people, this subjective experience is often more important than the actual outcome of the activity. Flow tends to occur when there is a perfect match between the challenge of an exercise and the capability of a performer to complete it successfully. Some sport psychologists believe that flow may be related to the secretion of endorphins in the brain, although others think that this is unlikely.

fluid retention (water retention)
The human body is about 60 per cent water. Everybody's fluid content is kept relatively constant at this level; excess fluid is eliminated by the kidneys. However, fluid retention increases significantly with high carbohydrate diets. When carbohydrate is stored as glycogen in muscles, extra water becomes bound to the glycogen (*see* **carbohydrate loading**).

Excessive fluid retention is linked to some diseases (e.g. heart failure or kidney disease) and fluid may accumulate in tissues where it causes swelling (oedema) in places such as the ankles. Diuretics (water tablets) help to remove this excess fluid.

In women, fluid retention also varies during the menstrual cycle, tending to increase just before menstruation. These variations in fluid retention can often mask changes in real body weight. Furthermore, in the first stages of many weight-loss programmes, much of the loss is attributable to water loss.

Sometimes, when fat is lost from tissue, fluid retention increases to fill the spaces left by the fat. Most dietitians advise people to monitor their weight over a long period and not to be unduly influenced by daily variations, which are probably due to differences in fluid retention.

fluoride: *See* fluorine.

fluorine

A highly toxic gas that usually occurs in combination with other elements, forming fluorides. Fluorine is an essential trace element needed for the healthy development of teeth and bones. A low fluorine intake increases susceptibility to dental caries. Fluorides are present naturally in hard water, but they are also added to drinking water in some areas, and to most toothpastes to harden teeth. A concentration of 1 part per million (1 ppm) in tap water retards tooth decay by more than 50 per cent. Too much fluoride (above 10 ppm) can damage enamel, causing discolouration of the teeth. Higher concentrations of fluoride may also increase the risk of developing brittle bones (osteoporosis). It is generally accepted that the average daily intake of fluorine should be between 1 and 3 mg. The best sources are tea and seaweeds.

fluoxetine: *See* prozac.

flushing methods

A method used by body-builders to improve the appearance of muscles. A single muscle group performs several different exercises, one after the other to fill the muscles with blood. Flushing tends to be avoided by competitive weight-lifters and those weight training for sport because it does not usually improve muscle strength.

foetal stretch

An exercise that prevents lordosis (an accentuated inward curvature of the lower part of the spine) and relieves backache. It also stretches the lumbar muscles and gluteals (figure 26).

■ Lie on your back. Grasp the back of your thighs and slowly bring both knees to your chest, curling your pelvis and upper body off the floor. Hold for 30–60 seconds.

Figure 26 (a) Foetal stretch; (b) Modified stretch.

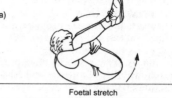

(a)

Foetal stretch

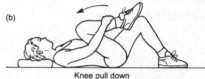

(b)

Knee pull down
(potentially harmful)

A modified foetal stretch is sometimes performed by grasping the shin and drawing one leg at a time up to the chest. This form of the exercise can be harmful and is generally not recommended.

folacin: *See* folic acid.

folic acid (folacin; pteroyl-l-glutamic acid)

A member of the B complex of vitamins. Folic acid is a bright yellow, crystalline, water soluble substance that is stable to heat but easily oxidized. It acts as a co-enzyme in the synthesis of a number of important chemicals in the body, including some amino acids and DNA. Because of its involvement in DNA synthesis, it is also essential for the formation of cells, especially red blood cells and embryonic cells. Just before and during the early stages of pregnancy, greater amounts are required for the growth of embryonic and maternal tissues. The Medical Research Council Vitamin Study at St. Bartholomew's hospital in London demonstrated a direct link between taking folic acid before pregnancy and avoiding neural tube defects (NTDs) in the embryo. The defects occur when the embryonic neural tube that forms the brain and spinal cord fails to close properly. NTDs are the most common birth defects in the Western world and cause babies to be born with spina bifida or, worse still, without a brain. In the UK, the Department of Health recommend that all women eat foods rich in folates and take 400 micrograms of folic acid each day if they are planning a pregnancy and for the first 12 weeks of pregnancy. Research undertaken in Northern Ireland, suggests that synthetic forms of the vitamin are better assimilated by the body than folate from foods such as broccoli. Supplementation must begin before conception because the neural tube closes about day 21 of pregnancy, usually before the woman knows that she is pregnant. Women at greater risk of folic acid deficiency (e.g. those who are anaemic, have had multiple pregnancies, or have used oral contraceptives for a long period) are often prescribed greater amounts.

Folic acid deficiency causes anaemia, diarrhoea, gastrointestinal disturbances, and other disorders. The risk of cervical dysplasia increases as levels of folic acid in the blood or cervix decrease. Cervical dysplasia is an abnormal growth of tissue in the cervix, linked to a viral infection. It is thought that folic acid may increase resistance to the virus.

Little is known of the effects of folic acid on physical performance, but a deficiency is likely to affect endurance athletes adversely owing to anaemia.

Folic acid is supplied in the diet from foods such as leafy green vegetables, liver, pulses, eggs, and wholemeal cereal products. The richest source is dried brewer's yeast (2400 micrograms of folic acid per 100 grams of yeast). It is also made in the body by intestinal bacteria, but this folate is probably not absorbed. In the UK, the adult daily Reference Nutrient Intake is 200 micrograms; in the USA, Recommended Dietary Allowance (1989) is 180 micrograms for females and 200 micrograms for males.

food additives

Food additives may be natural or artificial. Common natural additives include sugar, salt, corn syrup, baking soda, and pepper. Many modern additives, such as vitamins and some flavours, are made in a laboratory but most of them are exact replicas of naturally occurring substances and the body is unable to distinguish between the natural and artificial forms. The most controversial additives are those which are completely synthetic and have no natural counterpart.

In the European Union, food additives are often given 'E' numbers: a set of standard codes which have been approved by the European Union. The main categories of additives are colours (e.g. E100, curcumin), preservatives (e.g. E200, sorbic acid); antioxidants (e.g. E300, L-ascorbic acid); emuslifiers and stabilizers (e.g. E322, lecithins); and sweeteners (e.g. E421, mannitol). Other food additives include:

- acids (e.g. citric acid, give a sour taste)
- anti-caking agents (e.g. some phosphates, to help food flow easily)
- antifoaming agents (e.g. oxystearin, to prevent excessive frothing)
- bases (e.g. bicarbonate, as a raising agent and acid neutralizer)
- bulking agents (e.g. guar gum, adds bulk without adding any calories)
- firming agents (e.g aluminium salts, to retain crispness)
- flavour modifiers (reduces flavour)
- flour improvers (e.g. cysteine)
- glazing agents (e.g. waxes, to give polished appearance)
- humectants (e.g. glycerol, to prevent foods, such as marshmallow, drying out)
- liquid freezants (e.g. liquid nitrogen, to freeze food quickly)
- packaging gases (e.g. nitrogen, to control the atmosphere within a package)
- propellants (e.g. carbon dioxide, to form an aerosol, forcing food out of containers)
- release agents (e.g. silicates, to prevent food sticking to pans)
- sequestrants (e.g. sodium hydrogen diacetate, to help remove heavy metals from food
- solvents (e.g. glycerol, to dissolve solids in food).

food allergy: *See* allergy.

Food and Drug Administration: *See* FDA.

food aversion

A psychological repugnance to some foods provoked by emotions associated with the food rather than by any chemical properties within the food. Unlike a food allergy or food intolerance, there is no adverse reaction if the food causing the aversion is given in an unrecognizable form. Anorexia nervosa is regarded by some as an extreme form of food aversion.

food combining diets

Food combining diets were first introduced by Dr William Hay in the 1930s. He believed that everything we eat is either acid- or alkaline-forming, and that the intake of acid-forming foods (e.g. meat and cereals) should be reduced and alkaline-forming ones (fruits and vegetables) increased. He also believed that it was best to eat only one type of food at a meal, otherwise the body could become overwhelmed with toxins, which could lead to acidosis and fat formation. You should never, for example, eat carbohydrate (e.g. potatoes) and protein (e.g. meat) at the same meal.

Since the 1930s, other food combining diets have been devised, but they all share this idea that food should be eaten in specified combinations only. They promote the idea that certain combinations are incompatible, harmful, and 'putrefy' the body, while other combinations are conducive to good health and weight loss. Many accounts which support these diets neglect to point out that all foods (including potato and meat) contain a combination of protein and carbohydrate. There is no scientific evidence to support the use of particular combinations of food, except that a diet should be balanced and contain adequate amounts of all the nutrients.

food diary: *See* eating diary.

food exchange system: *See* dietary exchange lists.

food group

A group of foods that have similar nutritional properties. There are various classifications, but one commonly used in the USA and UK divides foods into four groups:

- milk group
- meat or protein group
- fruit and vegetable group
- cereal group.

The milk group includes milk itself, cheese, and yoghurt. These are rich sources of calcium, riboflavin, and protein.

The meat group includes all types of meat (lean meat is the highest in nutrient density) and fish, and also nuts and pulses. They are good sources of protein, phosphorus, vitamin B_6, vitamin B_{12}, zinc, magnesium, iron, niacin, and thiamin.

The fruit and vegetable group is the main source of minerals and vitamins. Those which have the highest density and which are especially important sources of vitamin A, vitamin C, riboflavin, folate, iron, and magnesium include apricots, bean sprouts, broccoli, Brussel sprouts, cabbage, cantaloupe, carrots, cauliflower, cucumbers, grapefruit, green beans, green peas, leafy greens (e.g. spinach), lettuce, mushrooms (though not strictly a fruit or vegetable), oranges, peaches, strawberries, and tomatoes.

The cereal group includes all grains, such as wheat and rice, and their products. They are rich sources of carbohydrate, riboflavin, thiamin, niacin, iron, protein, and magnesium. The best sources are wholegrains (wheat, oats, barley, millet, rice, and rye). These unrefined foods are good sources of dietary fibre.

The food groups can be used as a guide when devising balanced diets. They are sometimes called food exchange groups, because one food can be freely exchanged with any other food belonging to same group. Quantities eaten also need to be comparable. For example, most health experts advise us to eat at least five servings of fruit and vegetables each day. A serving is half a cup or a typical portion (one medium orange, half a grapefruit, or a wedge of lettuce).

food guide pyramid

A diagrammatic guide to daily eating (figure 27a). The food guide pyramid has been adopted by the US Department of Agriculture and the Department of

Figure 27 (a) Food guide pyramid; (b) Plate model

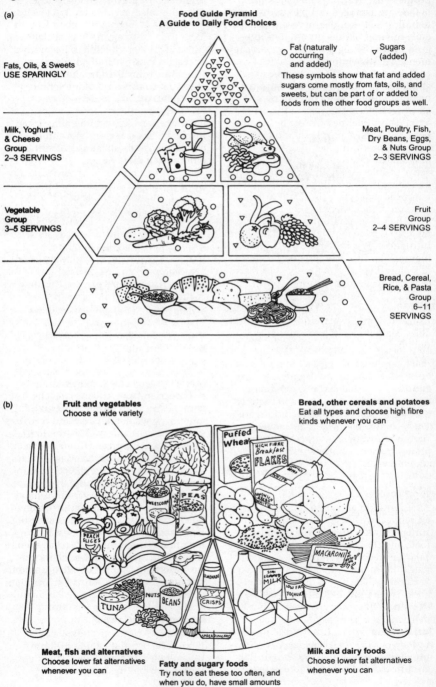

(a)

**Food Guide Pyramid
A Guide to Daily Food Choices**

○ Fat (naturally occurring and added) ▽ Sugars (added)

These symbols show that fat and added sugars come mostly from fats, oils, and sweets, but can be part of or added to foods from the other food groups as well.

Fats, Oils, & Sweets
USE SPARINGLY

Milk, Yoghurt,
& Cheese
Group
2–3 SERVINGS

Meat, Poultry, Fish,
Dry Beans, Eggs,
& Nuts Group
2–3 SERVINGS

Vegetable
Group
3–5 SERVINGS

Fruit
Group
2–4 SERVINGS

Bread, Cereal,
Rice, & Pasta
Group
6–11
SERVINGS

(b)

Fruit and vegetables
Choose a wide variety

Bread, other cereals and potatoes
Eat all types and choose high fibre kinds whenever you can

Meat, fish and alternatives
Choose lower fat alternatives whenever you can

Fatty and sugary foods
Try not to eat these too often, and when you do, have small amounts

Milk and dairy foods
Choose lower fat alternatives whenever you can

Health and Human Services to encourage people to eat healthily. Six major groups of food are arranged in a pyramid shape to indicate the number of recommended daily servings of each group: the food group with the highest number of recommended daily servings (bread, cereal, and pasta group) form the base of the pyramid; the group with the lowest recommended number of servings (fats, oils, and sweets) form the apex of the pyramid. The guidelines are for the average person. All active people should have at least the lowest number of servings recommended for each food group. Very active people, especially serious athletes and those in physically demanding jobs, may need more than the larger number of recommended servings.

In the UK an alternative diagrammatic guide to the food guide pyramid has been introduced. It is called the 'plate model' (figure 27b). This diagram takes the form of a plate divided into five sections representing the main food groups: bread, other cereals, and potatoes; milk and dairy foods; fatty and sugary foods; meat, fish, and alternatives; and fruit and vegetables. Market research found that the public preferred this approach to the pyramid.

foodie

A person who takes pleasure in the preparation, presentation, and eating of food. The term is sometimes used in a pejorative sense to describe someone who is always searching for new, exotic taste sensations.

food intolerance

An unpleasant and abnormal reaction to a chemical within a food. Sometimes the sufferer cannot identify the offending food, and the condition is not psychological (*compare* **food aversion**), nor is it a true immunological reaction to the food (*see* **allergy**). The mechanism of intolerances is not fully understood. Most are unexplained, but some are due to inherited deficiencies of the enzymes needed for the efficient metabolism of specific chemicals. For example, lactose (milk sugar) intolerance is due to a deficiency of the enzyme lactase, needed to break the

double sugar (lactose) down into the single sugars, glucose and galactose.

Food intolerance can develop towards a wide range of foods. Some chemicals in foods (such as tyramine in chocolate) can stimulate the production of histamines in certain sensitive individuals. Histamine is involved in immunological reactions, so this form of intolerance is sometimes called a pseudo-allergy because it simulates a food allergy. Identification of food intolerance often involves a blood test or a slow process of elimination to establish the culprit (*see* **elimination diet**).

food labelling

Food labelling differs from one country to the next, but most pre-packaged foods have the following labels:

- name or description of food
- net quantity (weight, volume, or number of items in packet)
- ingredients (arranged in descending order of weight)
- date mark (indicating by when it should be consumed)
- instructions for use
- name and address of supplier
- place of origin.

In the UK, food labelling regulations require prepacked foods to bear the name; list of ingredients (in descending order by weight); the name and address of manufacturer, or packer, or seller established within the European Union; and the appropriate indication of durability (a 'use by' or 'best before' date mark). The regulations also set conditions for claiming foods have certain properties (e.g. that it is an aid to slimming). Rules are also set for nutrition labelling. Such labelling is compulsory when a nutrition claim is made (e.g. that a food is 'low fat'), and the label must include the minimum amount of energy, protein, carbohydrate, and fat provided by 100 ml or 100 g of the food. Many labels provide additional information voluntarily about the nutritional value of the food (e.g. vitamin content and types of fat). In the USA, it is a legal requirement to give nutritional information on food labels (*see* **Daily Values**).

food poisoning

A disorder of the digestive system caused by eating food contaminated with bacteria, fungi (such as moulds), viruses, their products, or a non-biological poison. Symptoms vary depending on the type of food poisoning, but usually include nausea, abdominal pain, diarrhoea, and a headache. Some types of bacterial and viral infections can be fatal to the elderly, the young, and those with poor immune systems. Most food poisoning is caused by bacteria, such as the well-known *Salmonella* and *Listeria*. Less well known is a group of bacteria called *Campylobacter* which are transmitted in untreated water, unpasteurized or poorly pasteurized milk, and insufficiently cooked meats. Apparently, in the UK the disease may also be spread by birds pecking at milk bottle tops. Symptoms of food poisoning by *Campylobacter* range from mild diarrhoea to death. Food poisoning associated with the bacterium *Bacillus cereus* is also a major problem. The bacterium thrives in cooked rice kept warm but not hot in some take-away restaurants.

Nearly all food contains bacteria, but most are harmless unless they are allowed to multiply quickly. Cooking at high temperature kills most bacteria, and refrigeration retards their growth. However, food left at room temperature for long periods may enable certain bacteria (e.g. *Clostridium perfringens*) to multiply and produce high levels of toxin which is still effective after heating or freezing. The risk of food poisoning is greatly reduced by proper hygienic handling and preparation of the food. *See also* **botulism**; **campylobacteriosis**; **cholera**; **listeria**; **parahaemolyticus food poisoning**; **salmonellosis**; **shigellosis**; **staphylococcal food poisoning**.

food transit time

The time it takes for food to pass through the gut. This is not only of academic interest as it can have important consequences for health and comfort. If food passes too quickly through the gut, there is little time for it to be digested and nutrients will be lost in the faeces. If food is retained for a long time, constipation may result and faeces become hard and bullet-like. In addition, the longer food remains in the gut, the more calories can be absorbed: efficient in biological terms, but not what someone on a weight-loss diet wants.

Food rich in fibre tends to normalize the food transit time of those whose food either passes through the gut too quickly or too slowly. High fat levels in the diet tend to delay the passage of food and may contribute to constipation. Exercise stimulates peristalsis (the movements of the muscular wall which pushes food along the gut). This is a possible cause of 'jogger's trots', the urgent need for early-morning joggers to find a lavatory or some other place to relieve themselves. The quicker passage of food through the gut associated with regular physical activity may also offer some protection against cancers of the colon and rectum.

football: *See* **American football** and **soccer**.

footballer's ankle (impingement exostosis)

An ankle joint in which spiky outgrowths (osteophytes) of bone develop. Footballers commonly suffer from this complaint because they are prone to overstretching the soft tissue in the ankle as they make lunging tackles. The overstretching causes the edges of bones that make up the ankle to rub against each other, stimulating the growth of the spikes. This happens particularly at the front of the shin bone (tibia), which knocks against the main ankle bone (the talus). Although the spikes are not malignant, they may break off, damaging soft tissues, causing pain, and reducing flexibility of the joint. When this happens, surgery may be required to remove them from the joint.

footballer's migraine: *See* **headache**.

forced expiratory volume (FEV)

The volume of air that a person with fully inflated lungs can breathe out in one second. The forced expiratory volume (FEV) is used in the diagnosis of respiratory conditions such as asthma. A low FEV indicates difficulty in breathing, which usually restricts the ability to exercise. People who can expel less than 75 per cent of their vital capacity (the maximum volume which can be breathed out from fully inflated lungs) are generally advised to consult a doctor. *See also* **exercise-induced asthma**.

forced repetitions: *See* forced reps.

forced reps (forced repetitions)
A method of weight training in which a partner helps a lifter to continue training beyond their normal limit of fatigue. When the lifter has completed the number of repetitions that causes fatigue, the partner physically assists the lifter to perform more repetitions (usually three to five more). This is believed to stimulate the growth of muscles and improve strength.

form
Gymnasts, dancers, ice-skaters, and other sports people who perform in front of judges, have to develop good body form to be successful. Their movements have to be graceful, controlled, and precise if they are to be awarded high marks. Good form usually results from efficient movements. Different muscles share the strain so that energy is not wasted and mechanical stress is distributed as evenly as possible.

Cyclists, runners, and other athletes whose performance is measured by the stopwatch and by their position in a race, are often concerned only about how fast they can go and give little thought to how they look. However, all exercisers can benefit from improving their form so that they move more efficiently and with less risk of injury.

If you wish to improve your form during exercise you should pay attention to the following general points, unless instructed otherwise:

- keep your body straight
- avoid hunching your shoulders
- keep relaxed, do not strain, and do not tense your muscles unnecessarily
- keep your buttocks tucked in and avoid an arched back
- keep your elbows and knees unlocked. This allows movement to flow freely from the limbs to the torso and vice versa
- move your upper and lower body in opposing directions to maintain balance. For example, as you move forwards with one leg, move the arm on your opposite side backwards
- move slowly and gently, focusing on the muscles you wish to use
- do not perform movements that are painful or very uncomfortable
- breathe comfortably at all times; never hold your breath during an exercise.

formula diet
An artificial diet usually in the form of powders or drink supplements. Formula diets are designed to provide complete balanced meals and are usually intended to be used for a short time by people who are ill or recuperating from illness. They may used as complete meal replacements, or supplements after meals to increase energy and nutrient intake. They are also often used by dieters to lose weight because they make it easy to keep track of the calories consumed. Although these diets provide all the nutrients needed to survive and help people to recover from malnutrition and infection, laboratory experiments indicate that they are not optimal for growth and health. People using formula diets over a long period often develop nutrient deficiencies. The deficiencies are easily identified and corrected, but they show that many diets are not perfect. Another disadvantage of formula diets is that they are rather bland and boring. They are rarely a long-term solution to weight control. *See also* **meal replacement diet**.

fortified foods
Foods containing added vitamins and minerals which were originally not present or were present in smaller amounts. Many breakfast cereals are fortified.

F-plan diet
A very popular low fat, high fibre diet developed in 1982 by Audrey Eyton, co-founder of *Slimming Magazine*. The F-plan diet was based on the recommendation of the Royal College of Physicians, that a fibre-rich diet can help weight control by making the dieter feel full on relatively few calories. Fibre absorbs water, providing bulk which fills the gut and contributes to the feeling of being full.

Audrey Eyton also believes that the prolonged chewing associated with eating high fibre foods reduces feelings of hunger. She claimed that followers of the diet should find it easier to slim and lose weight quickly, and would gain health advantages from eating high fibre meals. Critics of the diet suggest that the feelings of satiation associated with high fibre diets are gradually lost as the stomach adapts by stretching. Some users complain of high levels of flatulence in the first few weeks of the diet. Nevertheless, in addition to a number of health benefits (*see* **fibre**), high fibre diets are usually effective for losing weight because they tend to decrease calorific intake.

fracture

A break in a bone, usually the result of an instantaneous application of excessive force, relatively common in contact sports. There are several different types of fracture but they fall into two main categories: simple fractures, in which the bone breaks cleanly but does not penetrate the skin; and compound fractures, in which the bone does not break cleanly, often shattering with the broken ends protruding through the skin. The latter type of fracture is the more serious because it may result in severe bone infections. The gruesomely named green stick fracture occurs when a bone breaks incompletely, in much the same way as a green twig breaks. It is common in children whose bones are more flexible than those of adults. Green stick fractures are more difficult to treat than simple fractures. Suspected fractures require expert medical treatment. This usually includes taking an X-ray.

framing: *See* **segmenting**.

free fatty acid: *See* **fatty acids**.

free radicals

Free radicals are unstable, chemically incomplete substances that 'steal' electrons from other molecules. They are highly reactive, damaging chemicals in the body such as enzymes, making them less effective. Free radicals occur naturally as products of oxidation and are formed in the body during respiration

and other chemical processes. Exposure to pollution, cigarette smoke, and strong sunlight can increase the formation of free radicals. Once in the body, free radicals can damage tissues and delicate cell membranes. They can also damage DNA, disrupting our store of inherited information; this may lead to the initiation of certain cancers. Medical scientists believe that free radicals also contribute to at least fifty other major diseases including atherosclerosis, heart disease, rheumatoid arthritis, and lung disease. They may even accelerate the ageing process. Fortunately, our bodies have a good defence system to deal with free radicals. The system is based on chemicals, such as the enzyme sodium dismutase, which can donate electrons to the free radicals, quelling their hyper-reactivity. Chemicals in food, called antioxidants, also disarm free radicals. These antioxidants include beta-carotene, and vitamins A, C, and E.

We use much more oxygen during intense physical activity than when we are inactive. Consequently, we are likely to produce many more free radicals that could harm us. It is thought, however, that regular aerobic exercise may stimulate the formation of more chemicals with antioxidant properties to protect our bodies from free radical damage.

free weight

A weight, such as a barbell or dumbbell, not attached to a specialized weight machine or exercise device. Free weights allow movement in any direction and so lend themselves to a wide variety of exercise routines for weight training. However, they do not isolate muscle action as precisely as weight-training machines. Homemade weights can be constructed from pieces of pipe and plastic bottles filled with water.

frequency of exercise: *See* **training frequency**.

friction burn

A burn that occurs when the skin rubs against another surface. Friction burns range from a superficial redness where two areas of skin rub together, to deep burns (for example, on the thigh and buttocks of a footballer who makes a sliding tackle on a dry pitch). Burns, called mat burns, often occur on wrestlers when the skin over bony joints rubs against the unyielding surface of a mat. Mat burns are notorious for becoming infected with bacteria. Friction burns should be treated in the same way as any other type of burn: if minor, the injured part should be placed under slowly running water and then covered with a clean, sterile, non-fluffy dressing. Medical advice should be sought if there is any doubt about the seriousness of the burn. *See also* **blister**.

frostbite

Tissue destruction resulting from exposure to very low temperatures. Usually associated with polar regions and high altitudes, frostbite can even occur in subtropical deserts at night. The extent of the frostbite depends on the temperature, the length of exposure time, and the wind-chill factor. In very serious cases, the damaged tissue can decay and gangrene could occur. Frostbite is treated by gently warming the frozen tissue in tepid water; the affected parts should not be rubbed because this is likely to damage the tissues even more. No thawing should be attempted if there is a risk of the damaged part being refrozen: the alternation of freezing and thawing is more harmful than continuous freezing. Frostbite can develop during any activity performed in freezing temperatures. The late David Niven relates in his autobiography, *The moon's a balloon*, an account of a rather nasty case of frostnip (a mild, though still painful, case of frostbite in which the tissues become numbed but remain pliable). While skiing, he caught frostnip in a very sensitive and precious part of his anatomy. His treatment, not to be found in medical textbooks, was to immerse the damaged appendage in a glass of brandy. This peculiar therapy revived the organ successfully, but David Niven promised himself that he would never go again into cold climes inadequately clad.

frostnip: *See* frostbite.

frozen shoulder

Chronic pain, inflammation, and restricted movement in the shoulder. It is a common overuse injury in the 50+ age group. During exercise it may be caused by wrenching the shoulder, and inducing a protective spasm in a shoulder muscle. However, it may also be linked to a cardiovascular disorder, or it may develop for no apparent reason. Treatment is by gentle massage and special exercises, sometimes combined with the application of steroids.

fructose

A simple sugar, found naturally in honey and most fruits. Fructose combines with glucose to make sucrose (table sugar). It is often added to drinks in preference to glucose because, weight for weight, it is about twice as sweet. Fructose also has the nutritional advantage that it is absorbed more slowly than glucose and is converted in the liver to glycogen. Consequently, it tends not to cause a rapid rise in blood glucose levels, a feature which makes it suitable for some diabetic diets. However, excessive intake of fructose should be avoided; because of its slow absorption it can cause diarrhoea. There has also been a suggestion that very high levels of fructose intake may damage the liver.

fruitarian

A vegetarian who only eats raw or dried fruit, nuts, seeds, honey, and vegetable oil. *See also* **vegetarian**.

fulminant exertional rhabdomyolosis: *See* sickle cell disease.

functional short leg: *See* short leg.

fungal infections

Diseases caused by fungi which either digest dead tissue such as skin (e.g. athlete's foot) or parasitically feed on living tissue in the body (e.g. thrush). Fungal infections of the skin are usually characterized by itchy, red patches that may develop into pus-filled blisters. They tend to be very contagious and occur in warm, dark, moist regions of the body (e.g. in the groin). Primary treatment usually consists of washing with soap and water, drying thoroughly, and applying an antifungal agent. You are advised to consult a doctor if you suffer repeated or persistent fungal infections.

G

". . . the aims of sport embody the same principles for the disabled as they do for the able-bodied; in addition, however, sport is of immense therapeutic value and plays an essential part in the physical, psychological, and social rehabilitation of the disabled."

Sir Ludwig Guttmann, a famous neurosurgeon. Quoted in Guttmann, L. (1976), *Textbook of sport for the disabled*. HM & M Publishers, Aylesbury, Bucks.

GABA: *See* gamma-aminobutyric acid.

galactose
A simple sugar found in milk, yeast, and liver. It is absorbed into the bloodstream and transported to the liver where it is converted to glucose. Galactose combines with glucose to form lactose (milk sugar).

gall-bladder
A small sac lying beneath the right lobe of the liver. It stores bile.

gallstones
It is estimated that, in the USA, more than 5 million men and 15 million women have gallstones. More than 75 per cent of the gallstones are formed in the gall-bladder from cholesterol, sometimes in association with bile pigments and calcium salts. The high incidence is thought to be related to fatty diets which slow down food transit times (the length of time food is in the gut) and increase the likelihood of constipation. Pregnant women may be more susceptible because of their tendency to suffer from constipation. Other factors that increase the risk of gallstone development include obesity, high blood cholesterol levels, and diabetes. A high fibre diet is thought to stimulate bile flow from the liver and prevent bile reabsorption. This may reduce the risk of gallstone formation. A high fibre diet also accelerates movement of food in the gut.

Gallstones may exist for many years without causing symptoms. However, they can produce severe pain if they enter and obstruct the bile duct. Blockage of the duct may lead to jaundice or an acute inflammation of the gall-bladder or pancreas. If gallstones are causing severe problems, the stones or the entire gall-bladder are usually removed by surgery.

gamekeeper's thumb: *See* skier's thumb.

gamesmanship
The art of winning competitions or defeating opponents by cunning practices that do not break any rule. In these days of sexual equality, it is wrong to assume that only men can stoop to such devious practices and perhaps the term 'gamespersonship' should be adopted.

gamma-aminobutyric acid (GABA)
A chemical released by nerves in the brain. Some anti-anxiety drugs are thought to stimulate the release of GABA which tends to have an inhibitory effect on brain activity. It also acts as a muscle relaxant. It is suspected that GABA has been used by some sports people to reduce muscle tension so that they can make smooth movements more easily (e.g. in archery and pistol shooting).

gamma-linolenic acid (GLA)
A constituent of evening primrose oil, starflower oil, and human milk. GLA is a source of linolenic acid, one of the essential fatty acids. Linolenic acid is used in the body to form hormone-like substances called prostaglandins that play an important role in a number of metabolic processes.

GLA is used as a treatment for an

impressive list of disorders. It is reputed to have an almost magical effect on chronic skin itching. It might also help to reduce some symptoms of premenstrual stress, such as irritability and breast tenderness. Additional reports suggest that GLA is beneficial in treating alcoholism, multiple sclerosis, hyperactivity in children, arthritis, and disorders of the immune system.

The optimum daily dose of GLA has not been established, but usual intakes are 40 mg per day, taken as oil of evening primrose. It is probably unwise to take excessive amounts because high levels of fatty acids may depress the immune system.

gamma-oryzanol (GO)

A white powder extracted from rice bran oil. Some body-builders who consume it in food supplements claim that it increases lean body mass, decreases fatty tissue, and relieves stress. These claims have not yet been fully tested scientifically.

garlic

A hardy, widely cultivated herbal plant, *Allium sativum*, belonging to the onion family. When crushed, the bulb of this plant releases a pungent odour. Since Hippocrates first recommended garlic for the treatment of battle wounds, it has had a reputation for potent medicinal properties. It is highly regarded as a cure for colds, coughs, and other viral infections, including verrucas, but there is little scientific evidence of its efficacy. It may also offer some protection against stomach ulcers (one theory suggests that it eradicates *Helicobacter pylori*, bacteria that are implicated in the development of some ulcers). Several clinical trials have shown garlic to reduce blood cholesterol levels and the risk of blood clots. Those with low to moderate cholesterol levels (average 220 mg/dl) have been able to reduce their cholesterol levels by as much as 10 per cent after taking a daily dose of 900 mg of garlic for 12 weeks. Since reports of garlic's anti-cholesterol properties gained publicity in the mass media, a multi-million pound garlic-based industry has developed. However, some pills and oils sold in shops have been processed in such a way as to remove the active ingredients. Also, garlic may upset the digestive systems of young children.

gaseous exchange

The exchange of gases between air in the lungs and blood, and between respiring tissue and blood. The essential feature of gaseous exchange is that oxygen is absorbed into the body and carbon dioxide, the waste gas of respiration, is eliminated. Efficient gaseous exchange is essential for health and fitness. If it is impaired in any way, for example because the lungs are clogged with soot from tobacco smoking or diesel exhaust particulates, then the ability to exercise is greatly reduced.

gastric balloons

A balloon inserted into the stomach and inflated to restrict food consumption. Many experts question its effectiveness and safety.

gastritis

A blanket term covering any inflammatory irritation of the stomach lining not due to an identifiable gastrointestinal disorder, such as a stomach ulcer. Gastritis is characterized by pain in the pit of the stomach, nausea, and sometimes vomiting. The layer of mucin protecting the stomach lining from acids may have become damaged, for example by bile salts which have entered into the stomach from the duodenum. As a result, the acidic gastric juice irritates and burns the lining, causing gastritis. Factors that might provoke or aggravate the disorder are alcohol, coffee, indigestible foods, and stress. Antacids are effective in relieving the symptoms, but the condition often resolves itself if the provoking factors are eliminated. If gastritis is not treated properly, there is a risk that it will develop into a peptic ulcer. There is a growing body of evidence to suggest that, as with some types of peptic ulcer, gastritis may be associated with an infection of bacteria (*Helicobacter pylori*), in which case treatment with appropriate antibiotics may be effective.

gastroenteritis

Inflammation of the stomach and intestines. It is usually caused by a bacterial or viral infection associated with food poisoning. Symptoms include nausea, vomiting, and diarrhoea. Gastroenteritis may cause dehydration, which precludes vigorous physical activity. Victims of gastroenteritis should drink plenty of fluids and maintain a good salt balance. Infants are at particular risk of dehydration and may require intravenous fluid replacement.

gastroplasty: *See* **banded gastroplasty**.

gastroporn

A term used to describe the colourful photographs in magazines that entice people to indulge in food fantasies. The term is usually used by those who believe that food should only be consumed for sustenance.

gelatin: *See* **collagen**.

gender

A social classification of people, attributes, and activities into categories such as male, female, and neuter. Gender is frequently based on anatomical differences between men and women, but does not necessarily coincide with them. Gender is socially and culturally determined; it is not biologically determined.

There is a strong tendency in Western cultures to indulge in gender role stereotyping, labelling certain activities and forms of behaviour as being appropriate to one sex but not the other. This stereotyping is still rife in sport and exercise; some people still regard activities such as rugby and boxing as being unladylike, while others think that activities such as dance and synchronized swimming are unmanly. Gender stereotyping has resulted in a psychological conflict among some males taking part in activities ascribed as feminine, and among females taking part in activities ascribed as masculine. However, the boundaries of cultural acceptance are continually being extended. It is now more commonplace to find female boxers, rugby players, and body-builders, and some professional soccer clubs, such as Birmingham, are employing female managers.

gender role stereotyping: *See* **gender**.

gene: *See* **genetic endowment**.

general adaptation syndrome

A set of characteristics manifested in the body as a response to stress. The syndrome typically has three stages. The first stage (alarm reaction) occurs when there is an increase in heart rate and mobilization of glucose as an energy source. This stage often happens when somebody starts exercising or increases exercise intensity. It is usually associated with a lowering of tolerance to disease and injury. During this stage, the body's defence systems become more active. During the second stage (resistance stage) the body develops maximum adaptation to stress, including an increase in heart rate and muscle tone. There is also an increase in the production of stress hormones, which help the body to cope with the increased stress. If the stress persists, a third stage (exhaustion) results in the defence mechanisms of the body beginning to breakdown. Overstress may have a wide range of harmful effects, including development of ulcers, heart disorders, and a predisposition to musculoskeletal injuries. The key to successful exercising is to impose sufficient stress for the body to enter the resistance stage, but to avoid exercising so much that the body enters the stage of exhaustion.

genetic endowment

A person's characteristics are determined by an interplay between genes (the carriers of inherited information) and environment. Genetic endowment predisposes a person to exhibit certain behaviours, inclines a person to put on or lose weight, and sets the ultimate limit to physical and intellectual potential. Genetic endowment is believed to be the most important single factor in determining fitness potential: the type of muscle fibre, capacity to respond to training; and physical traits, such as heart size, are all largely determined by inheritance. However, this is not a recipe for complacency if you are genetically well endowed, or despondency if you have a poor inheritance. Very few individuals achieve their full physical potential; realization of that potential depends on what each individual does during his or her life. People with a low genetic potential for fitness may become fitter than those who are well endowed, by training harder; people with a genetic predisposition to obesity may still maintain a healthy body weight by sensible eating, but they may have to work harder to achieve their goals. *See also* **obesity gene**.

ginseng
A herbal root obtained from the plant *Panax ginseng* (Siberian ginseng is obtained from a different species, *Eleutherococcus senticosus*). It is one of the best known of the traditional Chinese medicines and is said to bestow a long and happy life. The active ingredients within ginseng are thought to be soapy chemicals called saponins or ginsenosides. Ginseng is sold whole or as an extract in capsules, powders, or tea, and marketed as an 'energizer'. However, although taken by athletes as an ergogenic aid, there is no concrete, irrefutable evidence that ginseng improves physical performance. One of the problems with its use by sports people is that unrefined products sometimes include traces of other drugs, such as ephedrine, which are banned by many sports federations. Ginseng may also be harmful in doses as low as 3 g per day, causing high blood pressure, insomnia, and depression. *See also* **adaptogen**.

GLA: *See* **gamma-linolenic acid**.

glass jaw
A jaw vulnerable to a blow, such as an uppercut from a boxer. Glass jaw is a phenomenon recognized not only by screenwriters of films such as 'Rocky', but also by boxing trainers and other sports coaches. A person with a glass jaw is relatively easy to knock out and is more likely to sustain a fracture from a blow to the jaw.

gliadins: *See* **gluten**.

gloves: *See* **clothing**.

glucagon
A protein hormone secreted by the pancreas. It has the opposite action to insulin, causing blood glucose levels to rise. Glucagon is secreted in the fasting state to maintain blood glucose levels and mobilize fatty acids. Secretion usually increases during exercise because of the increased need for fuel mobilization, but the response is lower in people who are physically fit. Consequently, blood glucose levels tend to fluctuate less in those who exercise regularly.

glucose
A simple sugar belonging to the group of carbohydrates called monosaccharides. It is the main form of carbohydrate used by the body.
   Glucose is the primary fuel for the brain and muscles. Because the brain is very sensitive to shortages, there are a number of control mechanisms in the body which tend to keep blood glucose level constant. Excess glucose is either converted by the liver and muscle cells into glycogen, or turned into body fat. The glycogen store is readily converted back to glucose when blood glucose levels fall (for example, during exercise and between meals). In some circumstances, glucose can also be derived from glycerol and proteins stored in the body. Complex carbohydrates, such as starches, are the best source of glucose in the diet, because they release their glucose molecules gradually. *See also* **carbohydrate loading** and **sugar fix**.

glucose polymers
Short chains of glucose molecules sometimes added to sports drinks to provide more energy with less sweetness than normal glucose. They are popular with endurance athletes because they leave the stomach quickly and do not upset it as much as other sugars.

glucose tolerance test
A test of the ability of the body to cope with sudden, high intakes of sugar. A person takes a sugary drink (most commonly containing 50 g of glucose) after overnight fasting. At half-hourly intervals, blood sugar levels are measured. After 4 or 6 hours, most people's blood sugar returns to normal, but it rises higher and remains elevated for longer in diabetics. The test is used in the diagnosis of diabetes mellitus.

glutamate: *See* **glutamic acid**.

glutamic acid
An amino acid, the salt (glutamate) of which functions as a transmitter of nerve impulses in many parts of the brain and some areas of the spinal cord. It is used as a flavour enhancer in various processed foods and, like its salt monosodium glutamate, it can provoke allergic reactions in some people. *See also* **Chinese restaurant syndrome**.

glutathione
A substance produced in the body, and consumed in foods such as spinach and parsley. It is a tripeptide formed by the combination of three amino acids: cysteine, glutamic acid, and glycine. It is used in the body to make glutathione peroxidases, chemicals that act as antioxidants, protecting red blood cells from damage and destruction by mopping up toxic free radicals. It is also needed for the action of insulin.

glutathione peroxidase: *See* glutathione.

gluteal lift
An exercise that helps prevent an exaggerated curvature of the lower spine and strengthens the gluteal muscles (figure 28).

Figure 28

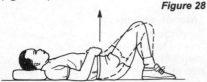

■ Lie on your back with knees bent and feet close to your buttocks. Contract the buttock muscles (gluteals) and slowly lift them off the floor as high as possible. Do not raise your back off the floor above the waistline, and do not allow your lower back to arch. Hold the raised position then slowly return to the start position.

gluteal muscle
One of the muscles of the buttocks, attached to the pelvic girdle and the thigh bone. The gluteus maximus is possibly the best known; it is the large buttock muscle on which one sits. It is used to swing the leg powerfully backwards. The muscle can work better if the body is bent forwards at the hip (e.g. in a crouch start of a sprint race). It is generally inactive during walking. The gluteus medius and gluteus minimus are smaller muscles, largely covered by the gluteus maximus. They are involved in hip movements, and help to steady the pelvis during walking and running, preventing the body from falling to one side. They come under particular stress during downhill running when their contractions help to control movement and to resist the pull of gravity.

gluten
A mixture of two proteins, gliadin and glutenin, gluten is a major component of rye and wheat flower, imparting springiness into wheat products. Gluten is not present in oats, barley, or maize. *See also* **coeliac disease**.

gluten intolerance: *See* coeliac disease.

glutenin: *See* gluten.

gluteus maximus: *See* gluteal muscle.

gluteus medius: *See* gluteal muscle.

gluteus minimus: *See* gluteal muscle.

glycaemic index
A measure of the relative increase in blood glucose levels after eating similar amounts of different carbohydrate-containing foods. Pure glucose is given a glycaemic index of 100 per cent and all other foods are compared with it. Carrots, for example, have a glycaemic index of 80–90 per cent while peanuts have a glycaemic index of only 10–19 per cent. Foods with a high glycaemic index result in rapid changes in blood glucose levels. The glycaemic index was devised to help diabetics manage their diet, but it can also be used by athletes. Many sports nutritionists recommend that exercisers eat complex carbohydrates such as wholewheat pasta, which have a glycaemic index of less than 50 per cent. A meal with a low glycaemic index should release its glucose slowly during exercise and allow the body's carbohydrate stores

to last. Cyclists who eat a meal with a low glycaemic index (lentils) one hour before a cycle endurance test may be able to prolong their time to exhaustion by up to twenty minutes. However, most athletes would find it too uncomfortable to exercise so soon after eating a high fibre meal.

GLYCAEMIC INDEX (%)	FOOD
100	pure glucose
80–90	carrots, cornflakes, honey, maltose, parsnips
70–79	wholewheat bread, white rice, new potatoes
60–69	bananas, white bread, brown rice, raisins
50–59	sweet corn, frozen peas, digestive biscuits
40–49	wholewheat spaghetti, dried peas, oranges
30–39	butter beans, apples, milk, ice-cream, yoghurt
20–29	lentils, kidney beans
10–19	peanuts, soy beans

The above glycaemic index applies to single foods. It will change when a food is consumed with other foods as part of a meal.

glycerol

A sugar alcohol which is a component of fats and is released in the gut when fats are digested. Glycerol has a hot, sweet taste (about half as sweet as table sugar) and is added to certain foods (e.g. chewing gum, marshmallows, and other sweets) as a sweetener. It also reduces the tendency of these foods to dry out.

glycine

An amino acid that acts as a transmitter of nerve impulses in parts of the spinal cord and eye. It inhibits the action of spinal nerves supplying skeletal muscles. Blocking its action with large doses of strychnine results in uncontrolled muscle spasms, convulsions, and respiratory arrest (breathing stops!); partial blockage with small doses of strychnine can act as a stimulant, enabling muscles to work more efficiently. Glycine is sweet and it is sometimes added to soft drinks to mask the bitter aftertaste of saccharin.

glycogen (animal starch)

The main carbohydrate store in the body; the liver and muscles are the main storage sites. Glycogen is a complex carbohydrate (polysaccharide) made of glucose units that are released when it is digested or metabolized. It is the major energy source for muscles. Compared with other fuels, proportionately more glycogen is used during power activities (e.g. weight lifting, sprinting, and jumping) than during endurance activities. The muscle stores can be loaded above their normal capacity by carbohydrate loading (see separate entry), sometimes known as glycogen supercompensation or glycogen overshoot.

The first scientific evidence that low muscle glycogen levels cause fatigue were provided by studies of cyclists from the volunteer Stockholm firemen. They pedalled until they were exhausted, at which time their muscle glycogen levels had fallen to zero.

glycogen overshoot: See carbohydrate loading.

glycolysis

Literally 'sugar breakdown'; the first stage of respiration when sugar is broken down in the body into pyruvic acid. Oxygen is not needed for the process, but only a small amount of energy is generated.

glycosuria

Presence of glucose in the urine; a condition associated with diabetes mellitus.

GO: See gamma-oryzanol.

goal

The specific target towards which a person is striving. Well-defined goals play an important part in the motivation of exercisers and dieters, enabling individuals to direct their energies towards something tangible. Goal setting (choosing specific, objective, concrete targets) is regarded as very important by coaches and leaders of diet, health, and fitness groups.

In exercise and sport, well-defined goals improve the performance and quality of practice; in both weight control and exercise, achievable goals clarify expectations, relieve boredom, and increase pride and self-confidence. Ideally, goals should be specific, short term, and realistic but challenging. Sports scientists have shown that as goal difficulty increases, performance improves but only up to a critical point, after which performance deteriorates. Goals should not be set so high that they become impossible to attain, nor should they be set so low that they are not challenging. Generally, individually prescribed goals are more effective than one goal set for all members of a group. Occasionally, goals become a disincentive and detract from the original aims of a person. This happens when the process of attaining important goals becomes an end in itself (a condition known by sports psychologists as goal displacement). For example, swimmers who perform time trials in preparation for a major competition may expend more energy on the trial than the actual competition; consequently, they often exhaust themselves both physically and psychologically, and underperform when they want to do well.

goal displacement: See goal.

goal setting: See goal.

golf
Golf is a competitive sport, and a very popular recreational activity played by people of a wide range of age and ability. Unlike many other activities, golf retains its players throughout their lifetime. Golfers in their eighties claim that the game helps them to keep physically and mentally fit. Golf strengthens the back and shoulders, and helps to maintain spine rotation, necessary for a healthy back.

There are two contrasting parts to the game. On the tee, power is used to hit the ball as close to the hole as possible. The tee shot requires considerable strength in the upper body, and flexibility in the back and legs. When on the green, great muscle control and accuracy are needed to putt the ball delicately into the hole.

Golf is generally regarded as a gentle aerobic activity that does not require superb fitness to play. A reasonable level of fitness, however, is essential to reduce the risk of injury. Good levels of stamina and flexibility also enhance performance and enjoyment.

Each of the four phases of the golf swing (backswing or take away, downswing or acceleration, impact, and follow through) imposes stress on specific areas of the body, particularly the wrists, lower back, and outside of the elbow. Stretching exercises for the upper body, back, and legs improve flexibility and reduce injuries caused by rotational stresses. Strengthening exercises for the shoulders reduce the chance of rotator cuff injuries (the rotator cuff muscles help to retain the upper arm within the shoulder socket). Weight training to strengthen the forearm and wrist enables the wrist to cope with the impact forces produced when the club hits the ball. Flexibility and strength training should involve both sides of the body because the golf swing tends to develop one side of the body more than the other. Consequently, right-handed golfers suffer more injuries down the left side of their body. Golfers should also be aware of the dangers of developing overuse injuries (see **golfer's elbow**). This especially applies to older golfers whose powers of recovery are limited.

In addition to flexibility and strength training, golfers should also do aerobic exercise (e.g. jogging or cycling) so that they have sufficient endurance to walk 18 holes on a hot day. Competitive golfers commonly have to play two rounds in a day. They may be on the course for more than 6 hours and walk over 10 miles.

golfer's elbow (javelin thrower's elbow; medial epicondylitis)
An overuse injury that commonly occurs on the medial (inner) surface of the right elbow of a right-handed golfer. Moving a golf club while applying a tight grip strains the tendons of the flexor muscles which curl the wrist and close the fingers into a fist. Most strain is produced when the club is at or near the top of the backswing, and as it goes through the downswing until just before it hits the golf ball. The strain may be so great that, in youngsters, it may pull off a piece of bone or damage the epiphyseal plate (the

region of bone growth). Golfers who make large divots following a chip shot are more likely to develop golfer's elbow. Treatment consists of reducing the pain and swelling (usually by the application of ice), strengthening the muscles, and correcting any faulty swing technique contributing to the strain. A similar overuse injury occurs in javelin throwers; it can also occur when a weight-lifter rotates the arm during a snatch lift. *Compare* **tennis elbow**.

golfer's toe
An acute inflammation of the big toe which may lead to arthritis and a painfully rigid joint. It usually develops on a foot which has structural imbalances.

goniometer
A device containing a 180 degree protractor for measuring the angle of a joint; it is used in tests of flexibility. Some goniometers can only measure the angle of a static joint, but an electrogoniometer can record continuously the changes in the angle of a joint during movements.

gout
A defect in metabolism resulting in an excessive build up of uric acid crystals in the bloodstream and joints. Crystals may be deposited in the kidneys (where they may contribute to the formation of kidney stones), tendons, and joints. Usually, the first symptom of gout is an intense pain felt in the first joint of the big toe. There are a variety of causes, but the main one is poor excretion of uric acid. High intakes of alcohol or fructose can increase the risk of gout.

graded exercise test (GXT)
A test that evaluates an individual's physiological response (e.g. heart rate, blood pressure, and oxygen consumption) to exercise, the intensity of which is increased in stages. These tests can be performed using a bench (for step-ups), a cycle ergometer, or a treadmill. A typical test on a treadmill starts with a subject walking gently on a revolving belt, which is accelerated at three minute intervals until the subject is running at maximum pace or until the subject experiences any discomfort or irregularities (e.g. of heart-

beat). Heart rate and oxygen consumption are monitored continuously. Blood pressure is measured at rest, during exercise, and after exercise. GXTs provide estimates of the ability of the lungs, heart, and blood vessels to deliver oxygen to respiring tissue; therefore they are measurements of aerobic fitness or cardiorespiratory fitness. The American College of Sports Medicine, which validates a number of courses for fitness instructors, recommends that all men over 40 years of age and all women over 50 years of age have a medically supervised, maximal graded exercise test before starting a programme of moderate-intensity exercise (i.e. exercise which is 60–80 per cent of the aerobic capacity).

grapefruit pills
It has been claimed that pills made of concentrated grapefruit contain enzymes or acids which digest fats. Consequently, dozens of grapefruit diets have been devised in the belief that they can reduce fat levels in the body. Grapefruit pills are usually sold with a diet plan, which probably explains the weight loss observed among some users of the pills. There is no generally accepted scientific evidence that grapefruit, or any other kind of food, contains enzymes that increase the rate of fat digestion. However, grapefruit is rich in vitamin C, and the pith lining the fruit contains high levels of pectin, a form of fibre, so the natural fruit is a valuable component of a balanced diet.

grazing
Eating whatever takes your fancy, wherever, and whenever you feel like it. Grazers do not have set meal times and usually eat food for pleasure rather than health. Grazing is a major contributor to obesity. In the UK, new regulations were introduced in 1995 to stop advertisers encouraging children to graze on junk food instead of eating proper meals.

gripping aids
Methods of helping a weight-lifter grip a bar more firmly. They include using powdered chalk, gloves, and training straps. Most competitive weight-lifters prefer chalk, which helps to prevent the bar from slipping and, unlike gloves, enables

the lifter to retain direct contact with the bar. Gloves have the advantage of preventing calluses from forming. Training straps are made from cotton webbing wrapped around the lifter's hands and bar. They make it easier for lifters to retain a grip on the bar and to perform a few more repetitions when they are beginning to tire.

groin
The region of the body including the upper part of the thigh and the lower part of the abdomen. Groin muscles include the adductors which pull the thighs together. These muscles rotate the hip during running and are essential for maintaining a grip on the saddle when horse-riding.

Overextension of the adductor muscles results in groin strain. It can be caused by forceful kicking movements in football, bringing the free leg forward in skating, or intensive sprint training. Groin strain can be avoided by strengthening the adductor muscles and by improving their flexibility. A good exercise for doing this is holding and then compressing a football between the knees.

Groin pain (either osteitis pubis or inguinocrural pain) results from a loosening of the ligaments holding the pubic bones together. It often occurs in football players and others who overload one leg more than the other (by repeated kicking, for example).

groin pain: See groin.

groin strain: See groin.

growth
Growth of human tissue may result from an increase in the number of cells (hyperplasia), or an increase in the size of individual cells (hypertrophy), or a combination of the two. Growth is often confused with development and maturation. Development is the process by which a person or body structure becomes more specialized. Physical development usually results in an increase in the complexity of body structures; intellectual development arises largely from learning and is characterized by more complex behaviour. Maturation refers to

the physiological and psychological ripening of a person or body part; its change towards the relatively stable, adult condition. See also **muscle growth**.

growth hormone
Body growth is greatly influenced by a protein hormone secreted by the anterior pituitary gland. This growth hormone (also known as human growth hormone, GH, or hGH) can now be manufactured by a genetic engineering technique called recombinant DNA technology. The growth hormone gene is cut out of human DNA and spliced into bacterial DNA. The bacteria are fermented and secrete growth hormone (sometimes called recombinant GH) identical to that produced in human cells. Growth hormone is used clinically to treat people with stunted growth. Until recombinant GH became available, the only source of growth hormone was human pituitary glands. This source is extremely expensive and was used almost exclusively for treating people of severely restricted growth (those with severe undersecretion of GH). Growth hormone from pituitary glands was also associated with a number of cases of Creutzfeldt-Jakob disease. The production of recombinant GH has meant treatment is safer and easier to obtain, so that those with less severe growth restriction can be treated. Unfortunately, its wider availability has been abused. It is used by body-builders and participants in power sports to accelerate muscle growth. Other sports people use it to accelerate the healing of musculoskeletal injuries. People concerned about their looks use it to decrease body fat. However, although growth hormone may increase the muscle bulk of inactive individuals, it probably has no significant effect on the muscle growth of young individuals who are engaged in an intense weight-training programme. Intense exercise combined with an adequate diet is sufficient to stimulate maximum protein synthesis in most individuals. In addition, excessive use of growth hormone may cause gigantism in prepubertal individuals and acromegaly (increase in size of the bones in hands, feet, and face) in adults. Other potential adverse effects include muscular

weakness, arthritis, impotence, diabetes, and heart disorders. Use of growth hormone supplements is banned by the International Olympic Committee and some other sports federations, but it is very difficult to detect it.

guar gum
A plant gum used in the treatment of diabetes because it slows down the absorption of sugars. *See also* **appetite suppressant**.

gumshield
A protective device which fits around the teeth and gums to reduce the likelihood of concussion during a contact sport. Gumshields also reduce the risk of serious jaw injuries. They should be fitted by a dental surgeon; poorly fitting gumshields can damage the mouth and cause dental injury.

gut: *See* **alimentary canal**.

gut bacteria (enteric bacteria)
The gut of a healthy person contains a large population of bacteria. Not only are these bacteria normally harmless, they actually benefit us by carrying out fermentation of undigested foodstuffs in the large intestine. Several nutrients are made during the fermentation, including vitamin K and biotin. The bacterial population can be depleted by antibiotics. People wishing to recruit more gut bacteria can now take them in the form of a health food pill, but there is little evidence that this does anything useful. In 1994, there were worrying reports that some of the pills contained the potentially dangerous bacteria, *Enterococcus faecium*. This has been called a 'lethal superbug' by the press because if it gets into the bloodstream it may cause a serious infection. In addition, some of the bacteria are resistant to the antibiotic vancomycin, known as the 'antibiotic of last resort' because it is held in reserve by doctors to treat people who do not respond to conventional antibiotics. Medical researchers are worried that the artificial introduction of large populations of *E. faecium* may spread vancomycin resistance into the general population and increase the number of untreatable infections. The US

Food and Drug Administration has been asked to investigate the sale of health food pills that contain these potentially dangerous bacteria.

GXT
Abbreviation sometimes used for graded exercise test.

gymnastics
Gymnastics is a graceful and artistic sport requiring a combination of strength, suppleness, and muscle coordination. It is increasingly popular at the recreational level and is particularly good as flexibility training. Competitive gymnastics requires very high levels of dedication and all-round fitness, including stamina.

Gymnastics is classified as a noncontact sport, but it is a high impact activity. Injuries can occur due to heavy landings, falls, or striking apparatus. Injuries tend to be most common among those with the greatest skill, because they have to practice longest, have the highest expectations, and perform the most dangerous routines.

In the past decade, gymnastics has become the fastest growing female sport in the United States. Participation usually starts at a young age, but the length of time that girls can take part in competitive gymnastics at a top class level is very short, and becoming shorter. The modern equipment that enables girl gymnasts to perform fast, complex, and very dynamic moves, is designed for short, light people. In 1972, the average female Olympian was 18 years old, weighed 7.5 stones (46.8 kg) and measured 5 feet 2 inches (1.57 m) tall. In 1994, she was two years younger, 1.5 stones (8.6 kg) lighter, and 5 inches (12 cm) shorter. This emphasis on leanness has put a lot of pressure on girl gymnasts to keep their weight down so that they can emulate the achievements of Olympians, like Olga Korbut, Nadia Comaneci, and Mary Lou Retton. Studies have shown that about 75 per cent of female gymnasts use at least one kind of extreme weight control technique (fasting, vomiting, laxatives/diuretics, severe calorie restriction, excessive exercise, diet pills) that may make them susceptible to eating disorders such as anorexia nervosa

and bulimia. These girls also have a high
risk of overuse injuries, particularly to
the shoulders, wrists, and back, because
their bones are still growing. Some training routines encourage hyperflexibility
which can cause joint disease (*see* **hypermobility**). Many of these problems are
not shared by male gymnasts because
their sport places more emphasis on
strength than dynamic flexibility.

Although gymnastics is an excellent
activity for developing fitness and self-
confidence, care must be taken to coach
youngsters properly, and to minimize the
physical and psychological risks associated
with the sport.

gymnast's fracture
A fracture of the elbow resulting from
overextension or excessive flexion of the
arm.

gynoid fat distribution
Distribution of excess fat predominantly
around the hips, thighs, and buttocks.
If sufficient, it results in 'pear-shaped'
obesity (figure 29). It is more common in
females than males. This type of fat
responds to female sex hormones which
makes it easier for the fat to be broken

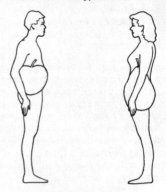

Figure 29 Gynoid fat distribution. Comparison
of the two main types of fat distribution

down into fatty acids during pregnancy
and lactation. Pear-shaped people, men as
well as women, seem to be less prone to
the harmful consequences of moderate
obesity than apple-shaped people (*see*
android fat distribution). This may be
because fat around the hips is less likely
to be mobilized during stress than fat
around the waist. Therefore, the fat
remains in the hips and does not enter
the bloodstream where it can become
deposited in the walls of blood vessels. *See
also* **waist-hip ratio**.

H

haematoma

Haematomas are common sports injuries, often resulting from a collision. A haematoma consists of a swelling caused by accumulation of clotted blood in tissues. The swelling may be inside a muscle (intramuscular haematoma) or outside (intermuscular haematoma). Intramuscular haematomas may be caused by muscle strain, a tear, or bruising. The swelling may press against adjacent nerves, causing pain. It also limits the ability of a muscle to contract and stretch. Intermuscular haematomas cause greater loss of function and a more persistent swelling than intramuscular haematomas. Haematomas require quick treatment by RICE: Resting the affected limb, applying Ice, Compressing the damaged area, and Elevating the damaged limb above the level of the heart.

haematuria

A discharge of blood into the urine (haematuria) can be very frightening, especially if the victim has a little knowledge of medicine and realizes that haematuria is associated with a number of serious diseases. However, it may also be a relatively harmless condition, and is quite common in those who exercise intensively. Cases of haematuria are so common in long-distance walkers and runners that the innocuous occurrence of haemoglobin in the urine is sometimes called march haemoglobinuria, runner's haematuria, or runner's haemolysis. One theory is that haematuria is caused by the soles of the feet pounding against a hard surface and breaking open red blood cells; haemoglobin is released and eliminated in the urine. Another theory is that myoglobin (the special oxygen-carrying red pigment in muscles) may be released into the bloodstream from muscles in the legs. Myoglobin is smaller than haemoglobin and can pass through the kidney filter into the urine.

No treatment is needed if the haematuria is benign. In some cases of haematuria associated with sports, the internal organs (especially the kidneys and bladder) may suffer chronic agitation and shaking, which damages the walls of the organs. The organs usually repair themselves if the exerciser takes sufficient rest. Nevertheless, anyone noticing blood in their urine should consult a physician so that it can be diagnosed professionally and, if necessary, treated.

haem iron

Dietary sources of iron vary in their usefulness to us. Haem iron, the iron within myoglobin and the blood pigment haemoglobin, is the type most easily absorbed by the body. It constitutes a high percentage of the iron in red meats.

haemoglobin

A large, complex protein molecule containing four iron groups onto which oxygen can become attached and detached with relative ease. Haemoglobin is usually confined within red blood cells. Attachment of oxygen takes place in the lungs; the oxygenated red blood cells are pumped by the heart through the arteries and capillaries to respiring tissues; in the tissues, the oxygen is unloaded and used to release energy from food stores. Without haemoglobin, almost no oxygen can be transported to the tissues. *See also* **anaemia**.

haemorrhoids (piles)

Swollen veins, connective tissue, and muscle in or around the anus. Haemorrhoids can be itchy, and bleed. It is a very common condition in the West. The build up of high pressures within the body (for example, when straining on the toilet) may cause haemorrhoids to form by forcing blood to accumulate in the veins. Weight-lifters, pregnant women, and people who have constipation or diarrhoea are at particular risk. Although often irritating, haemorrhoids are rarely dangerous. However, victims should seek a medical evaluation because some of the symptoms (especially anal bleeding) may mimic those of more serious conditions. Haemorrhoids can be avoided or the symptoms alleviated by drinking plenty of fluids and eating a high fibre diet rich in fruits, vegetables, legumes, and whole grains. Haemorrhoids are almost unheard of in countries that traditionally have high fibre diets. Regular exercise, by improving gut mobility, reduces the need to strain on the toilet and also reduces the risk of piles. The condition can be exacerbated by cycling or horse-riding, but piles do not preclude vigorous physical activity. Haemorrhoids which have become very enlarged and painful may require surgical removal.

hair

Hair condition may be affected by a person's diet and health. Bouncy, shiny hair is usually a sign of a well-nourished person in good overall health. Dry, dull, and lusterless hair often belongs to malnourished people in poor health.

Beauticians claim that more than fifty nutrients are needed for healthy hair. A deficiency of proteins (e.g. in anorexics) can lead to hair loss. Lack of vitamin A or linoleic acid (an essential fatty acid found in sunflower oils) may reduce oil secretion from sebaceous glands attached to hair follicles, leaving hair dry and lifeless. Lack of vitamin C causes hair to split and become dry. Copper deficiency sometimes causes hair to lose colour. However, hair condition is affected by so many other environmental factors (e.g. wet weather, smoke, hair sprays, and shampoos) that it is not a reliable indicator of nutritional status.

half-squats

A simple exercise to strengthen the muscles of the thighs and hips, and to improve general fitness (figure 30). The exercise can be performed with or without weights.

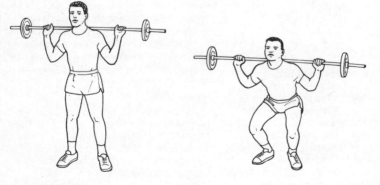

Figure 30 half-squats

■ Stand upright, feet placed firmly on the ground about shoulder width apart, and with arms in front of you for balance (or with a barbell resting behind your neck, on your shoulders). Keeping your back straight, squat down as if you were about to sit in a chair. Do not squat lower than the point which brings your thighs parallel to the ground. Hold the squat position for a few seconds then slowly stand upright. Perform about 10 repetitions to start with, progressing gradually to about 50 over a number of months.

Do not perform this exercise if you have weak or injured knees. Use only light weights until you have thoroughly learned the technique.

hammer toe
A deformity in which the big toe is in a permanently flexed position. It is commonly caused by a weakness of the transverse arch of the foot and by wearing ill-fitting shoes. A painful corn may develop over the affected area.

hamstrings
The term 'hamstrings' properly refers to the prominent tendinous cords at the back of the knee which attach the rear thigh muscles to the lower leg, but it is more commonly applied to the muscles themselves. In the latter sense, the hamstrings consist of a group of three large muscles (biceps femoris, semitendinosus, and semimembranosus). They extend and rotate the hip, and flex the knee. They are very susceptible to pulls and strains, especially when a runner tries to sprint without a sufficient warm up. Such pulls can be very dramatic, being accompanied by a loud 'pop' if the muscle is actually ruptured. Hamstring strains should be treated initially with ice and compression (*see* **RICE**).

hamstring stretcher
A flexibility exercise that stretches the muscles at the back of the thigh and behind the knee joint (figure 31).

Figure 31

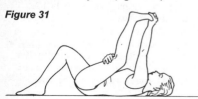

■ Lie on your back with your knees bent. Lift your right leg so that you can grasp the toes with your right hand. Place your left hand at the back of the right thigh, bring your knee towards your chest, and push your right heel upwards. Hold for a few seconds, lower to the start position and repeat with the left leg.

handicapped
Term used to describe individuals with some form of disability. Use of the term is regarded by some as a form of negative stereotyping that prevents those with physical or learning disabilities from achieving their full potential. As disability can be defined as '. . . any partial or total, mental or physical inability to perform any activity (sporting, social, or occupational) the affected person wishes to perform . . .' very few people are truly free of any disability and everyone is, to some extent, handicapped. *See also* **adapted physical exercise**.

hand injuries
The hands are very sensitive parts of the body, containing many bones, ligaments, tendons, and muscles which may suffer fractures, strains, and sprains. These injuries are often difficult to distinguish and require X-ray diagnosis. Important nerves cross the palm of the hand close to the surface where they can easily be damaged by compression and laceration.

A common compression disorder of cyclists is called handlebar palsy. It is caused by continually pressing against the ulnar nerve (a nerve which controls movements of the flexor muscles of the wrists and the hands). Damage to the nerve weakens the muscles it supplies. Handlebar palsy can be prevented by protecting the hands with specially padded cycling gloves, and frequently changing the position of the hands on the handlebars.

The nerves of the hand are so important and so vulnerable to damage as they cross the palms, that the central area of the palm is known medically as 'no man's land'. It is especially vulnerable to damage. Any laceration or penetrating injury to this area is regarded by a physician as being potentially very serious and should be examined with extreme care.

handlebar palsy: *See* **hand injuries**.

Harvard step test: *See* **step test**.

Hawthorne effect

When individuals are made to feel special their physical and intellectual performance improves. Psychologists call this the Hawthorne effect. Successful coaches, fitness trainers, and instructors often use this effect by providing members of their group with as much support and sense of importance as possible.

HCG: *See* **human chorionic gonadotrophin**.

headache

Headaches have a variety of causes. Most are relatively trivial including those associated with alcoholic hangovers, exertion, fatigue, emotional stress, and poor posture. Some headaches have more sinister implications and may be associated with food poisoning, very high blood pressure, or brain damage after a blow to the head.

Headaches encountered during or after vigorous physical activity are sometimes called exercise-induced headaches. Typically the headache is benign, occurs suddenly, and produces a throbbing pain. Other headaches, more severe in intensity, may develop after prolonged exertion in heat, high humidity, or at altitude. These effort headaches usually last about one hour and are probably due to acute dehydration. Not surprisingly, footballers sometimes develop headaches and other unpleasant symptoms after heading a ball. These 'footballers' migraines' are more likely if the ball is not headed properly. Another common exercise-induced headache is called weight-lifter's headache. This occurs when a person lifts a heavy weight while breathing in or holding breath (*see* **Valsalva's manoeuvre**); pressure in the brain increases, precipitating an intense, incapacitating pain.

Headaches may also be diet related: food allergies, low blood sugar levels, and very salty foods can provoke headaches and migraines.

Migraines are severe, throbbing, disabling headaches that usually affect only one side of the head. The pain often starts behind one eye and is accompanied by nausea, vomiting, and visual disturbances (variously described as 'auras', 'shimmering lights', or temporary 'blind spots'). Doctors reassure us that migraine is a medically harmless condition, but this is little comfort to those whose lives are periodically disrupted by excruciatingly painful attacks. These usually last from 4 to 72 hours. About 10 per cent of the population in Britain suffer from a migraine attack some time during their life. Women are about three times more likely to suffer from these debilitating headaches than men. A woman's migraine often coincides with the sudden drop in oestrogen levels that occurs just before menstruation. Although there are many theories, the exact cause of migraine is unknown. Migraineurs (migraine sufferers) often attribute their attack to dietary triggers such as coffee, cheese, chocolate, citrus fruits, and red wine. They may be reacting to chemicals in these foods (such as tyramine and phenylethylamine in chocolate, octopamine in citrus fruits, and 5-hydroxytryptamine in tomatoes, bananas and pineapples). An elimination diet is sometimes successful in identifying triggers which can then be avoided. However, for many migraineurs, no obvious trigger can be found. During an attack, most sufferers lie down in a dark room, drink plenty of watery fluids, and keep themselves warm with blankets and hot water bottles. Treatment includes antimigraine drugs, self-hypnosis, and acupuncture.

Those suffering from persistent headaches or severe chronic headaches should seek medical advice. It is especially important to see a doctor if a child has a headache which starts suddenly and is accompanied by a rash, vomiting, high temperature, or a stiff neck.

head injuries

A number of sports such as boxing, horse-riding, and cycling, carry a high risk of head injury. A blow to the head can result in brain damage and should be treated with great caution. Other injuries, such as those to the face, may be potentially disfiguring or disabling. If a head injury causes numbness, an inability to move the limbs, or a pins-and-needles sensation, it should be treated very seriously and medical advice sought. *See also* **concussion**.

health
A state of complete physical, mental, and spiritual well being. Health is not merely freedom from disease and infirmity. Healthy individuals are able to mobilize all their physical, mental, and spiritual resources to improve their chances of survival, to live happy and fulfilling lives, and to be of benefit to their dependents and society.

health-related fitness
Aspects of physical fitness associated with improving health. Emphasis is usually on aerobic endurance, flexibility, muscular condition, and body composition (especially percentage body fat).

health risk
Any factor that increases the chance of disease or injury. Health risks are usually expressed in terms of probabilities and percentages. These can be difficult to interpret. In the 1980s, for example, there were press reports that taking high-dose oestrogen oral contraceptives increases the risk of a heart attack by a factor of almost five. This appears to be a dramatic increase, but it is not meaningful unless the initial risk of heart attack, and the relative risk of unwanted pregnancies, are known. Assuming a woman is between 20 and 24, the risk of a heart attack will be less than 1 in 500 000. A five-fold increase will mean that the risk is 5 in 500 000. This is much less dramatic than the reports suggested, and is offset by the even greater risk of death resulting from pregnancy. It is not possible to predict whether a particular woman taking the contraceptive will fall into the lucky 99.999 per cent who do not have a heart attack, or the unlucky 0.001 per cent who do. It can also be very difficult to show that a particular factor is the true cause of a disease. A cause–effect relationship should be claimed only where all the following conditions are satisfied: the factor and disease are experienced by the same person; the experience of the factor immediately pre-cedes the occurrence of the disease; and the disease is unlikely to have happened without the factor being present. If these criteria are not met, the factor and disease may exhibit a close association, but not a cause–effect relationship.

health risk appraisal
An assessment tool used by health promoters to evaluate a person's health. The appraisal usually takes the form of an extended questionnaire that enquires into personal lifestyle, and personal and family medical history. The appraisal may also include a physical examination, laboratory tests of blood chemistry (e.g. of cholesterol level), blood pressure, and physical fitness levels. The outcome is a profile identifying specific risks (e.g. heavy smoking and sedentary lifestyle) with strategies and targets for reducing the risks.

health screening
A procedure used to establish whether a person is healthy enough to undertake strenuous exercise. Its main objectives are to find out about the current state of fitness and any abnormalities likely to present a risk of sudden death or injury, and to detect any condition that would be seriously aggravated by exercise. Health screening may be relatively informal and consist of a self-report questionnaire. Medical screening is a more formal procedure carried out by a medically qualified person. Routine medical screening prior to sports participation is not common in the UK (except for boxing), but in the USA there is an increasing demand for medical certificates before people are allowed to participate in some sports and recreations.

healthy lifestyle
A lifestyle which includes activities and habits that encourage the development of total physical, mental, and spiritual fitness, and which reduces the risk of major illness. Healthy activities and habits include regular exercise; a balanced, nutritious diet; adequate sleep and relaxation; abstaining from smoking and taking nonessential drugs; and moderating the intake of alcohol.

heart

The heart is an amazing pump. It maintains the circulation of blood by beating approximately 70 times a minute, more than 36 million times each year. The heart is about the size of a clenched fist and lies in the chest cavity between the two lungs. Its walls consist mainly of cardiac muscle. It is divided into a left side and a right side, each of which has two chambers: an atrium and a ventricle. Deoxygenated blood from the veins enters the right atrium and is passed through the tricuspid valve into the right ventricle. This contracts and pumps blood through the pulmonary artery into the lungs. Oxygenated blood returns through the pulmonary vein into the left atrium and then into the left ventricle. This contracts forcefully to pump oxygenated blood to the rest of the body. The unidirectional flow of blood is maintained by heart valves.

The heart is a very active organ, and it needs a good supply of oxygen to keep it alive. Some of the oxygenated blood pumped out of the left ventricle goes directly to the heart through the coronary arteries. These branch out to supply the thick heart muscle with oxygen and nutrients. Disease of these arteries causes a heart attack.

heart attack (myocardial infarction)

Blockage of one or more of the arteries that deliver blood to a portion of the heart muscle. The blockage may be caused by a clot or by a narrowing of the coronary arteries. The section of the heart which has its blood supply cut off will die, causing severe pain in the centre of the chest. Other symptoms, such as feeling faint, sweating, extreme tiredness, and breathlessness, may or may not be present. If the blockage is towards the beginning of the coronary artery, the heart attack may be very severe causing the heart to stop beating. If the blockage is towards the end of the artery the heart attack may be less severe since the amount of heart tissue deprived of oxygen would be minimal. Heart attacks are the most frequent cause of premature death in Western countries. In Britain, one person dies of heart attack every three minutes, and one in five men will have a heart attack before the age of 65. Most heart attacks are preventable. There are now many volumes of research evidence to indicate that a healthy lifestyle (which includes regular, moderate aerobic exercise and a well-balanced diet, and excludes smoking and excessive alcohol consumption) can reduce the risk of heart attack. *See also* **coronary heart disease risk factor**.

heartburn (pyrosis)

A burning pain felt behind the breastbone that often seems to rise from the stomach into the throat. It is usually caused by the regurgitation of acidic stomach contents into the oesophagus. It is a very common complaint and is usually nothing to worry about. However, repeated regurgitation of the stomach contents can damage the lining of the oesophagus, causing oesophagitis (inflammation of the oesophagus). Heartburn may be alleviated or prevented by increasing fluid and fibre intake, and limiting fat intake. Smoking, wearing tight clothes, and eating before lying down can all cause heartburn.

heart overload

A condition that occurs when the body's demand for the oxygen carried by blood exceeds the ability of the heart to pump blood around the body.

heart rate

The number of times the heart contracts per minute to pump blood around the body. It is often, but not always, the same as pulse. Heart rate at rest is usually between 60–80 beats per minute; males tend to have a lower rate than females, and the resting rate tends to fall with age. Resting heart rate is also generally lower in those who are physically fit; rates of less than 50 beats per minute are relatively common in endurance athletes. A sharp increase in resting heart rate is usually a sign that something is wrong. It may indicate illness, injury, emotional stress, or overtraining. Many elite athletes regularly monitor their resting heart rate and stop or reduce training if it increases significantly. This method of assessing fitness is not, however, very reliable.

During exercise, heart rate rises dramatically, and is a good indicator of exercise intensity. Maximal heart rate is usually assumed to be 220 minus the person's age in years, but actual measurements indicate a wide variation (*see* **maximal heart rate**). *See also* **pulse and training heart rate.**

heart test

A simple test which gives a rough estimate of aerobic fitness.

■ Lie on your back and relax for about 5 minutes. Take your pulse. Slowly get up and, after standing for 10–15 seconds, take your pulse again. The difference between your lying or supine pulse and your standing pulse indicates your fitness: a difference of 0–7 is good; 8–11, average; and 12–19, poor.

heat acclimatization

If you give your body sufficient time, it will gradually become adapted to living and working in a hot environment. The process by which you become physiologically more tolerant to high environmental temperatures is called heat acclimatization. During the process, resting pulse rate decreases, blood flow to the skin improves, and sweating increases. Sweat becomes more watery so that heat loss from the body can be maximized without losing too much salt. Heat-acclimatized individuals suffer less from nausea, dizziness, and discomfort in hot conditions. Exercisers who train exclusively in cool weather perform badly when suddenly exposed to much hotter conditions. If they stay in a warm environment, continue to exercise at a moderate level, and maintain an adequate fluid intake, they should gradually become acclimatized, be less susceptible to heat injury, and perform better. Acclimatization usually takes 7–10 days. Once established, it is retained for about 2 weeks.

heat balance

A condition reached when the heat gained by a body is equal to the heat lost from it. The amount of stored heat does not change and the body temperature remains constant. It is particularly impor-

tant that the temperature around the vital organs of the human body is kept at about 37°C because this is the temperature at which they work most efficiently. Mechanisms within the body maintain a constant internal temperature by ensuring that heat gained from body activities and the environment equals heat losses. Considerable heat is generated by the body's activities. During exercise, the metabolic rate can increase as much as 25 times the basal rate. Only about 30 per cent of this energy is used in movement, the rest is converted to heat which could produce a theoretical increase in body core temperature of 1°C every 5 minutes. In order to prevent overheating, the excess heat must be lost. Evaporation of sweat and convection by air currents of the heat and water vapour away from the body surface is an important cooling mechanism. This is one reason why exercisers should wear comfortable, loose-fitting clothes and drink plenty of watery fluids. Conversely, in cold environments it is important to insulate the body surface to prevent hypothermia.

heat collapse

Loss of consciousness associated with hot environmental conditions or exercising in clothing that restricts heat loss and causes overheating. Excessive sweating and an increase in the flow of blood to the skin and muscles reduces blood flow to the brain to cause fainting. Heat collapse is one of the most common medical conditions on a hot day. Nevertheless, its dangers should not be underestimated since it can lead to heat exhaustion and heat stroke. Uncomplicated heat collapse often occurs when a person stands for long periods in very hot conditions. Sufferers usually respond rapidly if they lie down, elevate their legs, drink plenty of fluid, and are sponged down with tepid water. However, if loss of consciousness continues heat stroke should be suspected and medical advice sought.

heat cramps

Painful muscular contractions caused by prolonged exposure to hot conditions. The contractions probably result from electrolyte and water imbalances. Leg muscles and abdominal muscles seem to be particularly vulnerable to heat cramps.

Heat cramps can be prevented by drinking plenty of fluid and, if necessary, a weak electrolyte solution to replace salts.

heat equivalence (caloric equivalence)

The energy released by the combustion of food in 1 litre of oxygen. The heat equivalence of a particular food varies according to its proportions of carbohydrate, fat, and protein. One litre of oxygen releases 5.0 kilocalories of energy from carbohydrates; 4.7 kilocalories from fats; and 4.5 kilocalories from protein. Thus, carbohydrates provide the most energy per litre of oxygen. In addition, for a given level of energy expenditure, more oxygen has to be inhaled if fat, rather than carbohydrate, is used as an energy source. See also **metabolic equivalent**.

heat exhaustion

Fatigue caused by prolonged exposure to environmental heat. Sufferers of heat exhaustion usually have a normal body temperature but their pulse rate is accelerated, their skin is cold and sweaty, and they often experience drowsiness and vomiting. The condition can be prevented by drinking plenty of water. Heat exhaustion is usually relieved by rest and cooling, but if it persists there is a risk of heat neurasthenia developing. Heat neurasthenia is a progressive condition characterized by feelings of apathy, hysteria, and aggression. It can lead to chronic behaviour disorders. Compare **heat stroke**.

heat neurasthenia: See heat exhaustion.

heat stroke

A potentially fatal condition caused by overexposure to heat. Heat stroke is characterized by high body core temperature and hot, dry skin, usually flushed. Sufferers show signs of mental confusion and loss of muscular coordination. They may collapse into unconsciousness. There is an urgent need to reduce the body temperature rapidly by loosening clothing, fanning, and tepid sponging. However, iced fluids and iced baths should not be used because they may constrict blood

vessels, reducing the blood supply to the skin and the means by which heat can escape. Medical attention is necessary; hospitalization may be required as there is a danger of kidney failure. During June 1995, there was an unprecedented heat wave in Chicago when more than 400 fatalities were attributed to very high temperatures and humidities.

heat syncope

Fainting or sudden loss of strength due to overheating. See also **heat collapse**.

heat treatment

The use of heat to treat injuries and accelerate recovery. The heat is usually applied to induce feelings of relaxation and comfort, and to increase blood flow through damaged tissue. It is particularly useful for treating injuries that reduce the range of joint movement (e.g. muscle stiffness), but the heat should not be applied immediately after an acute injury because it may increase internal bleeding. Also, heat treatment should not be used while inflammation persists. In addition to treating injuries, heat, sometimes in the form of hot wax or mud packs, is used to reduce weight by inducing perspiration. However, as the weight loss is mostly in the form of water, it will be regained quickly. See also **sauna baths**.

heel raise: See calf raise.

hernia

The protrusion of an organ or other body structure through a weakness in the wall of the cavity that usually confines it. One of the most common hernias associated with sport is an inguinal hernia (commonly called a rupture). This occurs in the lower abdomen when a sac made from the membrane (peritoneum) lining the abdominal wall and organs passes through the abdominal wall into the inguinal canal, an opening that leads, in males, into the testes. Inguinal hernias are often caused by lifting heavy weights, but they are also associated with obesity. Some hernias are quite easy to return to their normal site (reducible hernias) but others (irreducible hernias) may be impossible to replace. Some unresolved hernias, particularly in those who weight train and exercise vigorously, are potentially dangerous. An increase in the intra-abdominal pressure that accompanies exertion can cause strangulation, stopping blood flow and resulting in gangrene. In these cases, surgical repair is usually recommended. However, there is a tendency not to perform surgery on hernias that are causing no symptoms. Physicians usually evaluate each case individually before offering sufferers advice about participating in particular physical activities. *See also* **fascial hernia**.

herniated disc: *See* **prolapsed intervertebral disc.**

hexagon test
A test of agility, coordination, and balance sometimes used by gymnasts (figure 32).

Figure 32 Hexagon test. The footprints indicate where you should land

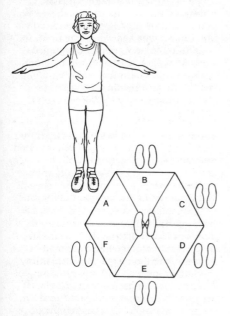

■ Using masking tape, make a hexagonal shape on a level, firm floor with each of the six sides measuring 65 centimetres (see figure). Stand at the centre of the hexagon facing side F. Jump with both feet over side A. Jump back to the centre and then jump

over side B and so on round the hexagon, returning to the centre to face side F between each jump. Time how long it takes you to complete three circuits of the hexagon: 12 seconds or less is excellent; 13–17 seconds, good; 18–22 seconds, fair; more than 22 seconds, poor.

hexose
A simple sugar, such as glucose, in which each molecule has six carbon atoms.

hidden fat
Fat occurring in some processed foods which are usually assumed to be low in fat because the fat cannot be seen. Packaged dried potato, frozen vegetables in a sauce, and crackers are examples of unlikely foods in which fats may lurk. The term is also used for fat in cakes and biscuits because it is not visible.

hidrosis
Sweating; especially applied to excessive sweating.

high altitude pulmonary oedema
A serious, often fatal condition in which fluid accumulates in the lungs of some individuals who ascend heights exceeding 2400 metres (7874 feet). *See also* **altitude.**

high-density lipoproteins: *See* lipoprotein.

high protein diet
High protein diets are marketed as body-building diets because muscle is made mainly of protein. They are often ineffective because excess protein is not stored within the body (*see* **body building**), and insufficient energy is the usual factor limiting muscle growth, not lack of protein. High protein diets are also marketed as weight-loss diets on the basis that proteins are complex molecules that need a lot of energy to be digested. It is claimed that up to 30 per cent of the energy content of protein is required for its digestion, but this claim is disputed. It is generally accepted that protein yields about the same amount of energy as carbohydrates (approximately 4 kilocalories per gram). Furthermore, many high protein diets (especially those using

animal protein) are rich in saturated fats and cholesterol, which carry a health risk and make a significant contribution to obesity.

High protein diets are potentially dangerous. The excess protein has to be broken down and eliminated. This puts a strain on the excretory system, particularly if the dieter does not drink sufficient quantities of watery fluids. High protein diets include the 'Complete Scarsdale Medical Diet', the 'Doctor's Quick Weight Loss Diet', the 'Miracle Diet for Fast Weight Loss', the 'New You Diet', and the 'Women Doctor's Diet for Women'.

hill training

One of the best ways to increase exercise intensity for running and walking. It is better than training with additional weights, because hill training uses the same muscles as normal running or walking. A 10 degree incline can almost double the energy demands of a run. An equivalent exercise intensity on level ground would necessitate running much faster, increasing the risk of injury from the mechanical stress produced as the feet hit the ground on each stride. Hill training is particularly good at developing the buttock muscles, which drive the legs backwards during the climb.

hip and thigh diet: See spot theory of fat reduction.

hip stretch

A simple warm-up and stretching exercise for the hamstrings, buttock muscles and hips.

■ Lie on your back. With your left leg slightly bent, slowly and gently draw your right leg towards your chest and hold it there for about 10 seconds. Repeat on the other side.

histamine

Histamine, a chemical derived from the amino acid histidine, has been implicated in a number of disorders. It is a transmitter of nerve impulses secreted by the hypothalamus in the brain. In addition to its function in the nervous system, it is released from body tissues during allergic reactions. Release into the skin causes nettle rash; release in the lungs contributes to asthma. Certain foods, such as chocolate, fish, and strawberries may stimulate immune cells (mast cells) to secrete histamine in sensitized individuals. This may be responsible for some cases of food intolerance.

histidine

An amino acid. Histidine was once thought to be an essential nutrient only for infants and children. Since 1975, it has been recognized as essential for adults as well.

hockey

Hockey or field hockey was once played exclusively on grass and was a relatively slow, tactical game in which players tended to confine their activities to certain areas of the pitch. The introduction of artificial turf has transformed the game, making it much faster with play moving quickly from one end of the pitch to the other. Players require high levels of fitness to keep up with the game and to ensure that their ball-hitting skills do not break down when they become tired. So, in addition to improving individual skill work (dribbling, shooting, and passing), hockey players need to develop agility, coordination, flexibility, running speed, and stamina. See also ice hockey.

hollow sprints

Training in which one sprint is separated from the next by a so-called hollow period involving either jogging or walking.

homeostasis

The maintenance of a constant physical or chemical state. Many processes in the body are under homeostatic control: deviations of output from a normal level (set point or norm) activate corrective mechanisms to bring the level back to normal.

Temperature regulation is an example of a homeostatic mechanism. The usual set point for the core temperature is 37 degrees Celsius (37°C): body temperatures above this norm result in sweating and an increase in blood flow to the skin to cool the body; low body temperatures result in an increase in basal metabolic rate (more fuel is burnt by the liver) and shivering to generate heat.

Other, homeostatic mechanisms include those controlling blood glucose levels, blood acidity, and hormone secretions. There are also suggestions that percentage fat composition and body weight have similar control systems (*see* **adipostat** and **set point theory**).

hormone

A chemical produced in one part of the body (an endocrine gland), which has its effects in another part (the target structures). Hormones are chemical messengers transported in the bloodstream; they regulate and coordinate the activity of many organs in the body.

hormone replacement therapy: *See* menopause.

horse-riding

Horseriding is not generally regarded as the most physically demanding activity, but it can be good exercise and an activity that can be enjoyed by all ages. It is recognized as an excellent therapy that can help to improve numerous mental and physical disabilities. The health, condition, and fitness of the horse is usually given much more attention than that of the rider. However, riders, whether recreational or international competitors, will gain maximum pleasure from horse-riding only if they have also reached a suitable level of fitness. A rider should improve general fitness by taking regular aerobic exercise (e.g. jogging, swimming, walking, or cycling). Stair-walking is particularly good for strengthening the muscles in the thighs. Particular attention should be given to exercises that promote suppleness, especially of the hip adductors. These muscles are used to grasp the horse's flanks and help to manoeuvre the horse. Stretching exercises can be performed on or off the horse. The adductor stretch, leg swings, and riding without stirrups, all help stretch and strengthen the adductors. Press-ups can also be useful exercises for strengthening the arm muscles, essential if you ride a very hard-pulling horse. However you train, it is important to increase your riding time gradually if you wish to avoid excessive stiffness and strains.

housemaid's knee (prepatellar bursitis)

An inflammation of a bursa (a fluid-filled sac) overlying the kneecap. It can develop when the knee is damaged after being knocked. Although it can interfere with physical activity, housemaid's knee is relatively harmless.

HRmax: *See* maximal heart rate.

hug

A simple stretching exercise that improves the flexibility of the shoulders and upper back.
■ Stand upright, wrap your arms across your chest and hug yourself as tightly as possible. Hold the hug for about 10 seconds, relax, and repeat.

human chorionic gonadotrophin (HCG)

A hormone secreted by the placenta during pregnancy. HCG stimulates the production of the sex hormone, testosterone. Artificial preparations have been misused by athletes to boost performance levels by increasing their testosterone levels.

HCG has also been used as a slimming agent. In the 1950s it was claimed that a low calorie diet combined with a course of injections of HCG mobilizes fat, enabling the body to use fat as a fuel more easily. The treatment was reported to have been successful in removing fat from those parts of the body, such as thighs and hips, where excesses tend to accumulate. However, the success is probably attributable to the low calorie diet (as low as 500 Calories per day) and not to HCG. There is little scientific evidence to support the use of HCG as a slimming aid.

hunger

A need for food that is usually experienced as an unpleasant sensation. Hunger develops under conditions of food deprivation and the physiological need for nutrients. It may also be provoked by psychological factors. A child who eats lunch regularly at midday will probably feel hungry if the meal is delayed by an hour, even if there is no real physiological need.

Hunger is usually non-specific: the desire is to satisfy the need for energy, and most foods will do. However, under some circumstances of vitamin or mineral deficiency (especially salt deficiency) hunger may be very specific and result in a search for a particular food (this may explain some of the peculiar feeding behaviours of pregnant women).

Subjectively, the sensation of hunger appears to be localized in the stomach, appearing and disappearing as the stomach empties and is refilled. In the nineteenth century a North American hunter, Alexis St. Martin, suffered a gunshot wound to his side which left a hole (fistula) leading into his stomach. The fistula enabled his physician to perform some remarkable experiments, one of which demonstrated that food placed directly in the stomach reduced hunger sensations. However, subsequent experiments have shown that people given food directly in the stomach develop a strong desire to taste, chew, and swallow food. Much to the relief of restauranteurs, the mere physical presence of food in the stomach is not as satisfying as the complete process of eating!

Hunger, it seems, cannot be explained by purely local effects in the stomach and mouth. There is good evidence that the brain contains hunger mechanisms. Receptors in the brain are believed to monitor the availability of glucose for use by cells. As glucose becomes less available, hunger sensations develop. Animal experiments indicate that centres in the hypothalamus (a structure at the base of the brain) play a role in eating behaviours: one centre (the feeding or hunger centre) seems to be responsible for initiating eating, the other (the satiety centre) for stopping. However, it is not clear how important these centres are in determining feeding behaviour in people who have free access to food.

Clearly, hunger is a complex sensation. Whatever mechanism is responsible for hunger, the desire for food may become so intense that it dominates every thought and action. *Compare* **appetite**.

hurdle stretch

A stretching exercise that helps to improve the flexibility of the hips. It is quite difficult to perform and you need to be supple before you attempt it. It is not suitable for beginners.

■ Sit on the floor with your back straight, one leg stretched behind so that the heel is touching your buttocks. The other leg is extended forwards with toes pointing upwards. Stretch your arms straight out in front of you and slowly arch forward until you can grab your toes with your hands. Hold for 5 seconds and return to the start position. Repeat on the other side.

hyaluronic acid: *See* **hyaluronidase**.

hyaluronidase

An enzyme which contributes to the break down of hyaluronic acid, a constituent of connective tissue. Hyaluronidase occurs naturally in many tissues. Preparations are injected into the skin of patients undergoing liposuction. The enzyme assists in breaking down the connective tissue so that the fat can be sucked out more easily. Hyaluronidase has also been used successfully to treat bruises.

hydrafitness: *See* **omnikinetic resistance machine**.

hydrocollator

A hot, moist pack used to treat bruises, sprains, and muscle spasms. A pack is heated to about 65°C and applied to the injured region. Dry towels are placed between the pack and the skin to prevent burning. The heat reduces pain by increasing blood circulation at the body surface. *See also* **heat treatment**.

hydrocortisone

A steroid hormone secreted by the outer part of the adrenal gland. It is released during stress reactions and has strong anti-inflammatory actions. It has been used in the treatment of sports injuries, but injection directly into a damaged structure (e.g. an inflamed Achilles tendon) can do more harm than good. Consequently, injections are administered around rather than into tendons and ligaments. There is an increased risk of ligament and tendon rupture if vigorous physical activities are performed within 48 hours of a steroid injection.

Hydrocortisone is on the International Olympic Committee's list of restricted substances.

hydrogenation
The process of adding hydrogen to another substance. Food manufacturers often hydrogenate vegetable oils to convert them to solid fats so that they can be incorporated into spreads. Hydrogenated fats have less susceptibility to slow oxidation, which would cause them to turn rancid. However, artificially saturated vegetable fats are as unhealthy to eat in excess as saturated animal fats.

hydrolipodystrophy: *See* **cellulite**.

hydrostatic weighing
Weighing a person fully submerged in water. The difference between the person's mass in air and in water is used to calculate body density and then from this estimate the proportion of fat in the body. Although one of the most accurate methods of estimating body composition, hydrostatic weighing is usually not very practical or convenient. *See also* **bioelectrical impedance** and **skinfold measurements**.

hydrotherapy
Hydrotherapy, the use of water to treat disorders, has been popular since the time of the ancient Romans. It continues to be used to treat sprains, strains, and other muscle injuries. Injured athletes often rehabilitate by exercising in swimming pools. *See also* **aquarobics** and **flotation therapy**.

hydroxyproline: *See* **muscle soreness**.

hyperbaric oxygen therapy
A medical treatment in which oxygen under high pressure is inhaled. For several years, it has been used to treat a wide range of medical conditions, including carbon monoxide poisoning, gangrene, and decompression sickness. Recently, there have been several trials of hyperbaric oxygen therapy (HBO) on patients with sports injuries. Several English football teams have used it to treat players with damaged ligaments. The treatment was apparently successful, with significantly accelerated recovery rates. HBO is thought to stimulate white blood cell activity in the damaged tissues. The therapy also has effects on the heart and circulation, reducing blood flow to the injured parts, which become less swollen. However, HBO appears to have limited application. It is effective on only certain types of injuries. In addition, there are concerns that the high levels of oxygen within the tissue after HBO may increase the level of free radicals. Free radicals are destructive chemicals that attack cell membranes.

hyperglycaemia
An abnormally high level of glucose in the blood. It may occur acutely and transiently as a result of a binge on carbohydrate-rich foods (such as sweets and pastries), or it may be related to a disease such as diabetes mellitus.

hypermobile joint disease: *See* **hypermobility**.

hypermobility
Gymnasts and dancers train hard so that they can move their joints much more than is normal. If they train properly, their high level of flexibility is not associated with increased risks of injury to muscles and joints (a condition known as benign hypermobility). However, if they overemphasize their flexibility training to the exclusion of other aspects of fitness (especially strength training) they are likely to suffer from hypermobile joint disease, a condition in which the joints are excessively mobile ('double-jointed'). Some so-called double-jointed individuals may suffer growing pains as children. As they mature, they may develop osteoarthritis, joint pains and degenerative joint changes, recurrent dislocations, and other musculoskeletal complaints.

hypernatremia
The presence of an abnormally high sodium concentration in the blood plasma. It may occur as a result of excessive sweating and inadequate fluid intake.

hyperplasia: *See* **growth**.

hypertension

Chronic, persistent, high blood pressure. Approximately one in four adults in the United States suffers from hypertension. Hypertension increases the risk of heart attack, stroke, and kidney failure because it adds to the workload of the heart, causing it to enlarge and, over a period of time, to weaken. In addition, it may damage the walls of the arteries. It is regarded as the silent killer because it can develop without symptoms. It is estimated that half of those with hypertension are not even aware of their condition. In adults, hypertension occurs when the blood pressure of a resting person is equal to or greater than 140/90. Regular, vigorous aerobic exercise at a safe level can help to prevent hypertension and reduce blood pressure. Moderating the intake of fat, salt, and alcohol also has beneficial effects. Smoking tobacco adds to the risk of hypertension.

hyperthermia

An abnormally high body core temperature (more than 41°C). *See also* **heat stroke**.

hypertonic drink: *See* **electrolyte drink**.

hypertrophy: *See* **growth**.

hyperventilation

Heavy breathing. Hyperventilation may be voluntary or result from lack of oxygen. Some people voluntarily hyperventilate the lungs in an attempt to supersaturate their blood with oxygen so that they can improve their performance in physical activities. Hyperventilation may improve the oxygen-carrying capacity of blood, but only to a very small extent and for short periods only. It may be advantageous before a sprint but not before an endurance activity. Underwater divers sometimes hyperventilate in order to increase their diving times. This is a potentially dangerous practice. The hyperventilation removes carbon dioxide from the lungs, reducing the stimulus for breathing. The divers may feel that they do not need to breathe even when their blood oxygen levels get so low that they are in danger of fainting. It is not a good idea to faint underwater!

hypervitaminosis

A disorder caused by the intake of excessive quantities of certain vitamins, such as the fat-soluble vitamins A and D and the water-soluble vitamin B_6. In very high doses these vitamins are toxic.

hypnotherapy

The use of hypnosis to treat behavioural disorders, to induce relaxation, or as an aid to motivation. Hypnosis is an artificially-induced, trance-like mental state in which the hypnotized person is more than usually receptive to suggestions. It has been used in sport for a variety of reasons. It has helped to relax elite athletes prior to major competitions; it has enabled others to deal with phobias associated with performing in public; and it has been used to improve self-confidence in boxers.

Hypnotherapy has also been used extensively by qualified hypnotherapists to treat eating disorders. Although its effectiveness is questioned by many psychologists, it has assisted some people to overcome food aversions and adopt healthier eating habits. It seems to be particularly helpful to those with a long-standing weight problem who need to boost their self-confidence in order to lose or gain weight.

hypoglycaemia

Hypoglycaemia is an abnormally low blood sugar level. It is characterized by loss of coordination, muscular weakness, sweating, and mental confusion. Mild hypoglycaemia can occur, paradoxically, by eating too much refined sugar (*see* **insulin rebound**). It can also occur after vigorous exercise. Towards the end of a marathon race, the muscle glycogen stores of an overambitious runner become completely exhausted and blood sugar levels drop. The brain is deprived of vital glucose. The runner becomes completely disorientated and may even lose consciousness before reaching the finish line. However, a few minutes after being given a sugary drink, the runner usually makes a rapid recovery.

Severe hypoglycaemia is rare and dangerous; it may lead to unconsciousness and coma. It can be caused by a severely decreased food intake, an alcoholic binge, certain diseases, or by taking medicines containing insulin. Diabetics who take an overdose of insulin suffer hypoglycaemia which is relieved rapidly by the administration of glucose.

hypokinetic disease

A disease related to, or caused by, insufficient activity and lack of regular exercise. Coronary heart disease, diabetes, high blood pressure, lower back problems, joint disorders, and obesity are all thought to be hypokinetic diseases.

hyponatremia

A condition characterized by abnormally low sodium ions in the blood plasma. It may be caused by drinking too much water, particularly after some salt has been lost through sweating. See also **water intoxication**.

hypotension

An abnormally low arterial blood pressure. It occurs after excessive fluid losses and bleeding. It can also occur transiently when a person stands up from a lying position. Moderate hypotension is an indication of good health but can, in rare cases, signify an underlying disease. See also **postural hypotension**.

hypothermia

A condition characterized by an abnormally low body core temperature. It results in rapid, progressive mental and physical collapse. Hypothermia is caused by exposure to cold when a person is suffering from physical exhaustion, and lack of food. It can be aggravated by wet and windy conditions. Victims have a weak pulse, become increasingly irrational, slow to respond, are cold to the touch, and have speech and visual disturbances. Hypothermia can occur all year round even when the weather is not particularly cold. Those involved in water sports are at particular risk, as are cyclists after hard hill climbs. During the climb they are in danger of overheating, but on the descent they are no longer generating much heat but losing it rapidly due to evaporation accelerated by an increase in relative wind speed. Hardened veterans of the Tour de France can be seen at the top of alpine climbs stuffing newspapers down their front in an effort to reduce heat loss. A person with hypothermia should be warmed in a controlled manner. For mild or moderate hypothermia, warm blankets or a warm bath may be all that is required. Those with severe hypothermia will require professional medical attention. Under no circumstances should the body surface be rubbed or alcohol given; although both may make the victim feel warmer, they can cause further heat loss.

hypotonic drink: See **electrolyte drink**.

hypotonic hydration: See **water intoxication**.

hypoxia

An inadequate supply of oxygen to the tissues.

ibuprofen

A painkilling drug often used to treat sports injuries. As well as reducing pain, it also reduces swelling and accelerates recovery from soft-tissue injuries (e.g. of muscles, tendons, and ligaments).

iceberg profile: See Profile of Mood States.

ice hockey

Ice hockey was played by Native Americans as long ago as the 1600s, but the first recorded match in its modern form took place in Montreal in 1875. Today, there are more than 300 000 ice hockey players in North America. It is an extremely fast and tough sport demanding high levels of all round fitness. Professional players can skate at speeds in excess of 30 mph and even young skaters reach speeds of 20 mph. Puck speeds range from 50 mph to more than 120 mph, producing impact forces greater than 1250 pounds (567 kg). To minimize the damage caused by collisions with other players, the boards, or the puck, hockey players wear so much protective gear that they look like armoured gladiators. Nevertheless, ice hockey is still a high-risk sport. It is made even more dangerous by fans who expect fights and violence during a game, and by officials who do not enforce the rules strictly. Ice hockey is regarded by many sports medicine experts to be the most dangerous sport in the USA for non-fatal catastrophic injuries (i.e. injuries that are severely incapacitating). Statistics show that 2.55 non-fatal catastrophic injuries occur per 100 000 player hours in ice hockey, compared with 0.68 per 100 000 player hours for American Football. In recent years there has been an alarming increase in the number of cervical spine injuries. Some neck injuries resulted from players skating head first into the boards or another player, but most resulted from illegal checking from behind. Although the risk of injury can be reduced by strengthening neck muscles, ice hockey can be made a much safer sport only by better enforcement of the rules, and by coaches, players, and spectators not tolerating or promoting intentional violence. Ice hockey is an exciting game demanding high levels of skill and speed; these are the features to emphasize, not violence.

ideal weight

In medicine, ideal body weights are usually described for groups of people (classified according to height, age, and sex) and are expressed as weight ranges associated with optimum health. Ideal weights for individuals are specific and difficult to define. Some tables of ideal weights refer to the average weight for persons of a given height and sex, but this average may not be the ideal weight for the good health of a particular person. Some coaches refer to the ideal competitive weight for a particular sport, but this may be quite different from the desirable weight for health. For example, long-distance runners usually do best when they are significantly underweight for their height.

In the past, coaches used to determine by eye whether an athlete should lose or gain weight. The technique was sometimes called the binocular scanning method. Despite its impressive name, the method is very subjective and unreliable. In the modern, highly competitive world of sport, coaches use the latest scientific knowledge and techniques to determine and maintain ideal weight.

Ideal weight is specific to a particular individual and his or her sport. It should be considered in conjunction with body composition. Athletes striving for optimal performance should have just the right weight, and the right combination of carbohydrate energy stores, fat, muscle, and bone to give them sufficient size, strength, power, and endurance to meet the specific demands of their sport. *See also* **body mass index**.

iliopsoas stretcher

A stretching exercise that improves the flexibility of the iliopsoas (a composite of two muscles that cross the hips and insert onto the thigh bone) and relieves some lower back problems (figure 33).

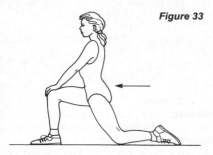

Figure 33

■ Stand upright; extend your left leg backward so that the knee touches the floor; and bend your right leg so that the knee is above the ankle. Press your pelvis forwards and downwards, but do not bend your right knee more than 90 degrees. Hold for a few seconds then return to the starting position and repeat with the other leg.

Illinois agility run: *See* agility.

imagery relaxation

A relaxation procedure in which you imagine being in a relaxing, comfortable environment. It is a technique used by many people faced with stressful situations. Jackie Stewart, former Formula One world champion racing driver, used to sit·in his car for several moments before a race and imagine his body

inflating like a balloon. Then he would let the air out gradually and feel himself relax. This helped him to prepare mentally for a race.

imaging: *See* **visualization**.

immune system

The system of internal defence mechanisms which enables the body to resist disease. The body's first line of defence is the skin and lining of the cavities (especially the gut and lungs). They act as a barrier to the entry of unwanted substances and foreign cells. If foreign bodies penetrate through these defences, the immune system is activated. Cells and proteins within the blood and lymph attack, disarm, destroy, and remove the foreign bodies. Special white blood cells (B-cell lymphocytes) are able to recognize the chemicals (called antigens) associated with foreign bodies and produce antibodies, proteins which attack them. The immune system seems to be able to remember previous encounters with a specific foreign substance, so that if confronted again with the same substance it can mount a prompt and effective defence. This is the basis of immunity.

People with allergies may have an overzealous immune system that attacks harmless substances or fails to attack harmful ones. Sometimes the immune system breaks down and starts to attack the body's own cells. This condition is called autoimmunity and is implicated in the development of a number of diseases, including rheumatoid arthritis.

The immune system can function efficiently only if it is supplied with adequate nutrients. Energy from carbohydrates and fat is needed to mobilize the army of white cells that fight off attacks. Vitamins and minerals are essential components of many chemicals produced to defend the body (*see* **antioxidant**). A deficiency or an overdose of any nutrient is likely to harm the immune system.

The immune system is also affected by the physiological and psychological stress of exercise. Although the results of scientific investigations are not clear, it appears that low to moderate levels of exercise are generally beneficial, activating the immune system and improving its ability to defend the body against disease. Exercise may boost the production of natural killer cells. One of their main duties is to destroy cancer cells before they can develop into full-blown tumours. However, there seems to be a critical level of exercise, specific to each individual, above which the immune system becomes increasingly compromised (*see also* **general adaptation syndrome**). Many athletes preparing for a major competition push themselves to their mental and physical limits, exceed their critical level, and succumb to illness. Elite athletes walk a tightrope between supreme physical condition and a breakdown of health. A new test that uses saliva samples is being devised for monitoring the competence of the immune system. This should help athletes and others know when they should take particular care to avoid overtraining.

impingement exostosis: *See* footballer's ankle.

incentive
A factor that motivates a person to achieve a particular goal. People need positive incentives to encourage them to exercise regularly and to eat healthily. Incentives are especially important for competitive sports people who have to train intensively and strictly regulate their diets to achieve success. Incentives vary from individual to individual, but most people are attracted towards activities which offer the following:

- pleasant sensations (sensory incentive)
- novel situations, providing varied and exciting stimuli (curiosity incentive)
- reassurance and support from a group (affiliation incentive)
- an opportunity to work independently (independence incentive)
- a feeling of self-control and not being dominated by others (power incentive)
- low levels of frustration and hostility (aggression incentive)
- a strong sense of achievement and success (achievement incentive).

A particular incentive will direct a person's immediate behaviour towards a particular goal only if it is the strongest of all competing incentives. Sport

psychologists generally agree that the achievement incentive is often the greatest driving force for competitive athletes. Psychologists also recognize that in order to reach long-term goals, a sense of achievement must be reinforced continually by successful completion of short-term intermediate goals.

incline bench
A bench with an adjustable back that can be inclined at different angles to suit different weight-training exercises. Many exercises, such as the incline bench press, are performed against an incline angle of 45 degrees. It is very important to make sure that an incline bench is safely anchored before using it.

incomplete proteins
An old-fashioned term used to describe foods such as legumes, nuts, and cereals, that may be protein-rich but are low in one or more essential amino acids. For example, cereals are low in the amino acid lysine, and leafy vegetables are low in methionine. It should not be implied that a vegetarian diet is incomplete. Mixtures of vegetable proteins can be as 'complete' as animal proteins.

incontinence
An inability to control the passage of urine or faeces. *See also* **stress incontinence**.

incremental run
A run that increases in intensity at predetermined, fixed levels. Incremental runs are used in training, and are performed on treadmills as part of tests for aerobic fitness.

indigestion (dyspepsia)
A pain felt in the upper abdomen (usually just below the breastbone or sternum) after eating. Indigestion may be psychological in origin and associated with stress. It is sometimes due to food intolerance: spicy or fatty foods often cause abdominal discomfort. It may also be a symptom of another disorder (e.g. an ulcer) or, in rare cases, of general disease (e.g. heart failure).

Some physical activities carried out in a crouched position, such as cycling, encourage the build up of gas in the stomach which presses against the diaphragm. Antacids (e.g. a weak solution of sodium bicarbonate) may help to bring up wind, releasing the gas and relieving the symptoms.

Anyone with severe, persistent indigestion should consult their physician.

indisposition: *See* **run down**.

individual differences principle
A principle of training which states that optimal benefits are achieved by devising training programmes to suit the specific needs of individual athletes. The principle applies equally well to exercisers. Ideally, each exerciser should have an individualized exercise programme. This would ensure that the exercises are tailored to meet the requirements of the individual, and would minimize the risk of overtraining and overuse injuries.

infancy
The first two years of a child's life. During infancy growth is irregular and occurs in spurts. The different parts of the body grow at different rates. Some bones are only just becoming hardened by ossification and are therefore susceptible to deformation if too much stress is put on them. Swimming under expert supervision is an excellent activity for developing heart, lungs, and muscles in infants, without putting too much strain on bones and joints. There is unanimous agreement among paediatricians that stimulation of the infant through simple playful exercises, such as rolling, kicking, and throwing a ball, is a tremendous help in the infant's physical and mental development.

inflatable belt: *See* **elastic belt**.

infraspinatus: *See* **rotator cuff**.

inguinal hernia: *See* **hernia**.

inguinocrural pain: *See* **groin**.

injury: *See* **sports injury**.

inosine monophosphate
An organic chemical. Like adenosine triphosphate, it belongs to the chemical group called nucleotides. Much of the information available about its effects is anecdotal and comes from weight-lifters and body-builders who have taken it as an ergogenic aid (performance booster). They have reported that it delays the onset of fatigue, helping them to accelerate strength development. They believe that it also helps to metabolize sugar, improves protein synthesis, and facilitates oxygen transport, but there is little scientific evidence to support these beliefs.

inositol
A water-soluble sugary substance present in cereals as phytic acid. Inositol is sometimes included in the Vitamin B complex. However, it is not a vitamin because it can be synthesized in the body. It may help to control blood cholesterol levels by promoting the transport of fats to the liver and their utilization once there. It is also claimed that inositol acts as a mild anxiety-reducing factor and that it helps to maintain healthy hair. There is little evidence to support these claims.

insoluble fibre: *See* **fibre**.

insomnia
The ability to sleep can be affected by diet and exercise. The nervous anticipation experienced before a major sports competition commonly causes insomnia. People who consume certain foods and drinks (e.g. those which contain caffeine or high levels of salt) may also suffer from the condition. On the other hand, certain foods and drinks (e.g. warm milk) seem to be conducive to a good night's sleep. Also, a vigorous bout of exercise taken during the day (but not immediately before going to bed) may be sufficiently tiring physically to help a person get to sleep.

Many insomniacs resort to taking drugs ('sleeping tablets') to induce sleep, but frequent use should be discouraged. Some drugs, such as the benzodiazepines, are habit forming and have side-effects such as inducing drowsiness when awake, which adversely affect physical performance. Moderate exercise, a change of diet, and relaxation techniques (*see* **progressive muscle relaxation**) may help a person overcome insomnia.

instructor: *See* coach.

insulin

A hormone secreted by cells within the islets of Langerhans, in the pancreas. Insulin is released into the bloodstream in response to raised blood glucose levels. It stimulates the liver, muscles, and fat cells to remove glucose from the blood, and to store it as glycogen and fat in cells. It also promotes the conversion of glucose to fat and stimulates protein synthesis in muscles. Inhibition of insulin production (e.g. by adrenaline or exercise) results in increased blood glucose levels. Although insulin secretion is reduced during exercise, sensitivity to insulin increases in well-trained individuals. Lack of insulin or progressive loss of sensitivity to insulin, can result in diabetes mellitus.

insulin-dependent diabetes: *See* diabetes.

insulin-independent diabetes: *See* diabetes.

insulin rebound (rebound hypoglycaemia)

A physiological response to eating too much sugar. The resulting high blood sugar causes an exaggerated insulin response so that the blood glucose level, after initially rising, actually falls to a level lower than it was before eating the sugar. Thus, less glucose than normal is available to respiring muscles. Insulin rebound can be exacerbated by alcohol, for example, drinking gin and tonic can cause a marked abnormal hypoglycaemia.

intelligence

Although there is no universally accepted definition of intelligence, it is generally regarded as an ability to act purposefully, to think rationally, and to deal effectively with new situations. There have been many attempts to measure intelligence, the best known being the standardized test which scores an individual's intelligence quotient (IQ). An IQ is the ratio of mental age to actual age (usually expressed as a percentage). It is often used as an index of intellectual development.

In recent years much research has been conducted on the possible influence of vitamins and minerals on intelligence. It has been claimed that vitamin supplementation can significantly improve a child's learning ability. It is generally accepted that vitamin and mineral deficiencies may retard intellectual development (e.g. iron-deficient children have reduced verbal ability, perform poorly in IQ tests, and have lower powers of concentration). However, the claim that supplements can increase the intelligence of children who show no clinical signs of vitamin or mineral deficiency, are hotly disputed. Until we are all able to agree on a definition of intelligence and on a universally accepted means of testing it, the controversy will continue.

intensity of exercise

One of the four main exercise variables that affect the attainment of cardiovascular fitness. The others are duration, frequency, and mode of exercise. *See* **training intensity**.

International Olympic Committee

The governing body of the Olympic Games. The International Olympic Committee (IOC) is a permanent committee entrusted with the control and development of the modern Olympic Games. It is responsible for ensuring that the Olympic Games are celebrated in the spirit that inspired their revival in 1894. The IOC elects its own members. Each member speaks either French or English and lives in a country with a National Olympic Committee, approved by the IOC, to promote the Olympic movement and amateur sport in that country. In 1966, the IOC created a body, the International Olympic Committee Medical Commission, to combat doping. It is now divided into four subcommissions with responsibilities that include: combating doping; helping athletes to improve their performances without contravening basic principles; enabling athletes to avoid injury; and disseminating information, such as a code of ethics, to physicians treating athletes and to other interested people.

intertrigo: *See* chafing.

interval sprinting

Training during which a runner sprints 50 metres and jogs 50 metres for a distance of up to 5000 metres.

interval training

A system of training for aerobic fitness that alternates spurts of intensive exertion (work interval) with periods of lower intensity activity (relief period) in one exercise session. By carefully spacing the periods of exertion and relief, more total work can be accomplished than with continuous training. High intensity exercise can also be achieved with less stress and strain than in one continuous session.

Each session is usually described in terms of an interval training prescription indicating the number of sets or repetitions, training distance, training time, and relief time. Thus, a running session may have the following prescription: one set of six repetitions of 200 metres each run at a pace of about thirty seconds, with a relief period between each run of 1 minute 10 seconds. This can be abbreviated as:

Set 1 6×200 at 0:30 (1:10)

Interval training for elite athletes was pioneered by the German coach, Gerschler. It is now used by many people as an effective way of becoming fit. Often, the intensity of the work intervals and relief periods are strictly controlled.

A typical session for a well-conditioned 20-year-old 1500 metre runner might consist of stretching and other warm-up exercises to raise the pulse rate to about 120. Then running 400-metre repetitions at a pace sufficient to raise the pulse to between 170–180 beats per minute, with the recovery between each repetition consisting of a walk or jog continued until the pulse rate goes down to between 120–140. Often 20 repetitions are planned for a session, but it should be terminated with cool-down exercises when recovery takes longer than 90 seconds.

Interval training is infinitely variable and can be adapted to the needs of the total beginner as well as to the prospective world champion. As fitness improves, the length and intensity of each session can be increased gradually. Of course, the principles of interval training can be applied equally well to cycling, swimming, and exercising on machines.

intervertebral disc: *See* disc.

intrinsic factor

A factor (a glycoprotein) secreted in the stomach that is essential for the absorption of vitamin B_{12} across the wall of the gut into the bloodstream. (Vitamin B_{12} is known as an extrinsic factor because it is provided from an external source, the diet). A lack of the intrinsic factor results in a deficiency of vitamin B_{12} because of malabsorption and a decrease in the number of red blood cells, and degeneration of the spinal cord (pernicious anaemia). The anaemia reduces the ability of blood to carry oxygen and decreases aerobic fitness.

intrinsic motivation: *See* motivation.

inversion

Turning the sole of the foot sideways so that it is pointing inwards. Inversion during running or walking results in the body weight being applied mainly to the outer edge of the foot.

inverted U hypothesis

An hypothesis applied to sport, which states that performance improves as arousal levels increase up to an optimum point, beyond which it deteriorates. In practice, this means that a little excitement and stress associated with competition or performing in public can have a positive effect, but a situation that is too stressful is detrimental. The optimal levels vary between people doing the same task and for the same person doing different tasks. Optimum arousal levels tend to be lower for more complicated tasks. *See also* **catastrophe theory**.

involuntary muscle

Muscle, such as smooth muscle of the gut and cardiac muscle, not usually under voluntary, conscious control.

iodine

A trace element present in fish, iodized salt, and vegetables grown in iodine-rich soils. Iodine is an essential ingredient of thyroid hormone, which helps to regulate growth, development, and metabolic rate. The Reference Nutrient Intake for adults is 140 micrograms each day. An excess of iodine can be poisonous; a deficit leads to an underactive thyroid gland.

iodized salt: *See* table salt.

IQ: *See* intelligence.

iron

Iron is essential to good health. Most iron in the body is contained in haemoglobin and myoglobin, the red pigments that carry oxygen. It also occurs as part of enzymes involved in energy production. A deficiency of iron results in anaemia, a lowering of haemoglobin concentration in the blood. The muscles and tissues are starved of vital oxygen, we feel tired and lethargic, and less inclined to exercise. Other more specific problems may include a sore tongue, cracks at the corner of the mouth, and nails that lack their usual pink flare. Heavy endurance training and bleeding (including menstrual bleeding) can increase the risk of iron deficiency and the need for iron therapy (increased iron intake by dietary adjustment and supplementation). Ten to fifteen percent of women between the ages of 13 and 45 lose more iron in menstrual bleeding than they acquire throughout the month from foods. Therefore, they probably require iron supplements to prevent iron deficiency.

The best sources of iron are meats, legumes, and watercress. Watercress and some other vegetables may have higher concentrations of iron than some meats, but iron from meat is mainly haem iron, which is easier to absorb than non-haem iron. Meat also contains a factor (not yet identified, but named MFP factor) that increases by four times the absorption of non-haem iron from other foods eaten with the meat. Cooking with traditional cast iron pans or a steel wok significantly increases the iron content of food as the surface releases fine particles, but little (if any) of this iron is absorbed. Vitamin C improves iron absorption, while tannic acid in teas, and phytic acid in many vegetables, interfere with it. (This is why you are advised not to drink large volumes of strong tea with a meal.) Large doses of other minerals (particularly calcium, copper, and zinc) in supplements may also reduce absorption. The recommended daily intake varies, but is about 8–10 mg for men and 15 mg for women of child-bearing age, increasing in physically active people.

Too much iron is toxic. It can damage the liver, heart, and pancreas, and irritate the stomach and gut, causing constipation or diarrhoea. If you take iron supplements, therefore, you should be careful not to overload your body.

irritable bowel syndrome

A digestive disorder characterised by irregularities in the muscle contractions that normally propel waste through the large intestine to the rectum. This may result in diarrhoea or constipation, or alternating bouts of both. Other symptoms often include abdominal pain, flatulence, excess mucus, nausea, and heartburn. It is not certain what causes irritable bowel syndrome but anxiety, lack of fibre, high fat diets, and smoking tobacco may be contributing factors. Treatment usually involves reducing anxiety, making dietary adjustments (e.g. eating more fibre), and taking regular exercise to improve gut mobility. Sometimes a doctor may prescribe drugs that alleviate the pain and control the muscular contractions.

isokinetic contraction: *See* muscle contraction.

isolation stress

A form of training that was used by coaches in Eastern Europe to adapt their international athletes to the stress of competition. Isolation stress involves placing the competitor in a situation that requires self-coaching for a period. It was imposed prior to major competitions when a top competitor was shifted to a new team and coach, unfamiliar with the athlete. It was hoped that the voluntary break from the usual coach, under controlled conditions, might make an enforced break during the international competition less traumatic.

isoleucine
An essential amino acid that can be obtained only from the diet.

isometric contraction: *See* muscle contraction.

isometrics
Exercises in which muscle tension is produced without moving a joint (for example, when pushing against an immovable object). Isometric exercises (figure 34) produce good strength gains at the specific angle of contraction. Best results are obtained when maximal contractions are held for about 5 seconds or longer. These exercises have the advantage that

Figure 34 Isometrics. Two simple exercises

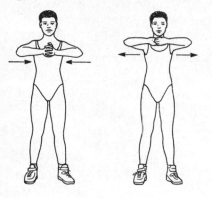

they can be performed almost anywhere, anytime. However, they do little for cardiovascular fitness. In fact, such exercises are inadvisable for people with heart disease because isometrics increase the pressure within the abdomen, raise the blood pressure, and put the heart under stress.

isotonic contraction: *See* muscle contraction.

isotonic drink: *See* electrolyte drink.

Italian football diet
A diet based on simple Italian country food consisting mainly of pasta, bread, olive oil, plenty of fruit and green vegetables, small amounts of meat (mainly poultry and fish), helped down with moderate amounts of red wine. The diet has been popularized in a book (*The Italian football diet and fitness programme*, written by Jane Nottage and Dr Claudio Bartolini and published by Thorsons in 1993). It has been endorsed by Beppe Signori, a striker for the Italian national football team. The diet is designed to provide ample energy (as much as 4000 calories a day are needed by professional footballers) and all the essential nutrients needed for an active lifestyle. It is especially high in carbohydrates and vitamins, but low in saturated fats. *See also* **Mediterranean diet**.

J

"Orandum est ut sit mens sana in corpore sano."
(You should pray to have a sound mind in a sound body.)

Juvenal, AD *c*.60–*c*.130, from Satires X 356. Quoted in (1979)
The Oxford dictionary of quotations. Oxford University Press, Oxford.

javelin thrower's elbow: *See* golfer's elbow.

jaw wiring
An extreme method of controlling the food consumption of obese compulsive eaters. Apparently, despite being prevented from chewing by having their jaws wired together, some patients still manage to consume their favourite foods by liquidizing them and drinking them through a straw. Jaw wiring is usually successful only when used in combination with expert counselling and the patient is given sound nutritional advice following removal of the wires.

jiu-jitsu: *See* **martial arts**.

jock itch
A fungal infection (often of the fungus, *Tinea cruri*) of the groin area, relatively common among rugby players who wear sweaty jockstraps. Jock itch is very contagious and spreads quickly if towels and clothing are shared. *See also* **fungal infections**.

jogger's nipple
Soreness of the nipple due to chafing, commonly experienced by male and female long-distance runners. Jogger's nipple may be quite painful and accompanied by bleeding. It can usually be avoided by the application of petroleum jelly to the nipples before running.

jogger's trots: *See* **food transit time**.

jogging
Slow, relaxed continuous running is an excellent exercise for cardiovascular fitness and weight control. Many people regard jogging as the foremost aerobic activity. It requires no special skill, little expenditure, and can be done almost anywhere. It strengthens the heart and helps to burn off excess fat. In the 1970s, it caught the imagination of the public and made exercise generally acceptable. However, reasonable caution should be observed. Excessive jogging, especially on hard surfaces, can result in injuries to the joints and muscles. The mechanical stress and shock associated with jogging can be moderated by wearing appropriate footwear (*see* **training shoes**). Regular jogging and distance running tends to shorten and tighten muscles because movements take place through a restricted range and are repeated many times. It is important therefore to perform stretching exercises to maintain the flexibility of muscles at most risk: the calf muscles, quads, hamstrings, and the muscles of the lower back.

Individuals (particularly those over 35 years old) who have not exercised for a long time should check their fitness with their physician before jogging. A physician's approval should also be obtained by those with arthritis, osteoporosis, and heart and circulatory problems.

The following suggestions will help you to maximize the benefits and minimize the injury risks associated with jogging:

- perform slow, static stretching exercises before and after jogging
- if you are a beginner, alternate walking with jogging during a session, and jog no more than three times a week
- increase your weekly mileage slowly, by no more than 10 per cent to 20 per cent every 2 weeks

- allow yourself plenty of time to recover. Alternate hard weeks with easy ones. Never run hard on two consecutive days. Have at least one rest day each week. (Risk of injury is greatest for those who jog every day.)
- alternate running with other activities, such as cycling and swimming, so that you reduce stress on your legs.

joint injury

Physical damage (such as a sprain, dislocation, or stiffness) to a joint. Sometimes an injury may result in loose bodies, called joint mice, occurring in a joint. These can cause locking and may require surgery. Joint injuries, unlike many muscle injuries, may require absolute rest and immobilization (fixation of the joint to prevent movement). In such cases, any damaged ligaments are kept unstressed while the joint is moved passively by someone else to keep the surrounding muscles fit.

joint mice: *See* **joint injury**.

joint stability

The ability of a joint to withstand mechanical shocks and movements without being dislocated or otherwise injured. Stability depends on a number of factors, including the strength of the ligaments that bind the bones together, and the strength of muscles associated with the joint. Excessive flexibility training, especially without appropriate strength training, may reduce stability making an individual more prone to dislocations.

joint stiffness

A condition characterized by difficulty in moving a joint. It is usually accompanied by pain and discomfort. Stiffness often follows a joint injury when muscles go into a spasm that reduces movement in order to protect against further damage. It should be treated cautiously and no attempt should be made to move the joint forcibly. Persistent, painful stiffness requires medical investigation and treatment.

jostling: *See* **massage**.

joule

Unit of energy; approximately 4.2 joules (J) equal one calorie. One kilojoule (kJ) equals 1000 J and is the amount of heat required to raise the temperature of 239 g of water by 1°C; and 1 megajoule (MJ) equals 1000 kJ.

judo: *See* **martial arts**.

judo elbow

A tear in the ligaments either side of the elbow. It occurs in judo when a player resists an armlock by clenching the fists extremely tightly.

jumper's heel

An injury to the heel that causes pain between the Achilles tendon and the back of the ankle bone. It is commonly associated with explosive jumping, stamping down, blocking the foot as a ball is kicked, or any other action that compresses the fat pad between the heel bone and shin bone. If an os trigonum (an extra bone in the ankle) is present, the compression may press the bone against a nerve resulting in considerable pain.

jumper's knee (patellar tendinitis)

Inflammation mainly of the patellar tendon, but which may also involve the quadriceps tendon. Jumper's knee is thought to be due to tiny lesions in the tendon that develop as a result of constant, repetitive jumping. It is quite common in participants of basketball, long jump, triple jump, and high jump.

jump height

A measure of the difference between the height of a person and the height he or she can jump. Jump height is usually recorded by the jumper making a mark with chalk-covered fingertips against a board.

Jumping is an anaerobic activity that relies exclusively upon high energy phosphates (mainly ATP) stored within muscles. Jump height, therefore, can be used as an indicator of instantaneous power or elastic strength. In order for the jumps of two or more people to be compared fairly, the type of jump must be standardized. For example, the heights attained if a person bobs down before jumping or drops down from a specific height before jumping are usually higher than if the jump is made from a static squat position (*see also* **Sargent jump test**).

A more sophisticated measurement of power can be made using a force platform that records the actual force exerted by a jumper at take off.

jumping

Jumping forms an integral part of the training programme of many athletes, particularly those who compete in explosive events requiring very powerful legs. Athletes may perform a wide variety of jumps, including long jumps from a 40 metre run-up, short jumps using a shorter approach, and drop jumps from the top of benches. Jumping facilitates the stretch reflex in muscles and helps to strengthen ligaments, tendons, and connective tissue in and around the joints. However, it is a risky activity because it imposes a lot of mechanical strain on joints and muscles. Care should be taken not to overtrain. Overuse injuries are common among jumpers. *See also* **plyometrics**.

jumping jack

A simple exercise for the whole body.

■ Stand upright with your hands at your sides and legs almost together. Bend your knees to the half-squat position (your thighs should be above the level of your knee caps). Then jump upwards, clap your hands above your head, and land with your feet together. Repeat about five times.

junk food

A pejorative term for food high in calories, low in nutrients and usually quick to prepare. Pasta, burgers, pizzas, fish and chips, crisps, and sweets have all at some time been classified as junk foods. Some nutritionists condemn all such foods with a zeal bordering on fanaticism; but most nutritionists believe that there are no bad foods, only bad diets. So-called junk foods can provide valuable nutrients and, if taken in moderation as part of a balanced diet, do little harm and can be of psychological benefit. Fish and chips, for example, if prepared properly to minimize the fat content, provides a nutritionally rich meal high in vitamins D and B_{12} as well as some minerals. There is no doubt, however, that it would be extremely difficult to design a balanced diet based exclusively on junk food since most have a high fat and salt content.

juvenile-onset diabetes: *See* **diabetes**.

K

karate: *See* martial arts.

kayaking: *See* canoeing and kayaking.

kelp

A group of large, brown seaweeds with the scientific name *Laminaria*. Kelp is used for human food, especially by the coastal populations of China and Japan. It is very rich in iodine, consequently it is sometimes prescribed to treat deficiencies of that trace element. Some manufacturers of dietary products containing kelp claim that their high levels of iodine act as a weight-reducing agent by increasing the production of thyroid hormones (of which iodine is an essential component) and raising metabolic rate. This would result in excess fat being consumed as an energy source. The claim is unlikely to be true for people who are not iodine deficient. An excessively high iodine intake can be toxic.

ketogenic diet

A diet (e.g. a low carbohydrate diet) resulting in the production of high levels of ketone bodies. Ketones are energy-containing organic chemicals formed as a result of the incomplete breakdown of fat. As these materials accumulate, acetone is also produced. This gives the breath a very recognisable smell, similar to nail varnish.

Ketosis, the production of large amounts of ketones, is a normal response to fasting lasting 4 to 12 hours (e.g. between meals). The ketones are produced from fat reserves to provide fuel for muscle and so spare glucose for use by the brain. A more extreme form of ketosis occurs during starvation, and when the diet is low in carbohydrates and high in fats. Persistent ketosis is associated with muscle wasting; it may also have some other harmful side-effects. Acetone cannot be metabolised and is toxic in high concentrations. The ketones can form acids that upset the acid-base balance in the blood.

Ketogenic diets are sometimes used to reduce weight in obese people. Some depend on the idea that ketones impair appetite, so you eat less. The effectiveness of a ketogenic diet can be monitored by measuring the amount of ketones in urine; the more ketones, the more effective the diet. Simple kits are available from some pharmacists for doing this. However, most dietitians advise against using these diets.

Ketogenic diets may have a place in the therapy of people with potentially life-threatening obesity, but they should be used only under medical supervision. They are not really suitable for others; they definitely should not be used by diabetics.

The best form of weight- and fat-loss diet is one that is balanced, calorie controlled, rich in carbohydrates, and does not cause muscle loss.

ketone bodies: *See* ketogenic diet.

ketosis: *See* ketogenic diet.

kidney stones (nephrolithiasis; renal stones)

Concretions of calcium salt and uric acid or oxalic acid that form irregularly shaped stones in the kidney. Kidney stones can cause excruciating pain and obstruct the passage of urine. If they present problems, they are usually surgically removed or broken down with ultrasound, but they sometimes pass out of the body spontaneously. Those prone to developing kidney stones should ensure that they drink adequate amounts of water, especially before, during, and after physical exertion. Excessive amounts of protein in the diet can lead to high levels of calcium and increase the risk of developing kidney stones. Body-builders in particular should be aware of this risk. It has been suggested that high intakes of vitamin C cause kidney stones, but this suggestion has been hotly disputed by some nutritionists.

kinaesthesis

The sense by which motion, weight, and the position of various body parts are perceived. Kinaesthesis depends on the sense organs (proprioceptors called muscle spindles and golgi tendon organs) that monitor the state of contraction of muscles, skin receptors, and the balance receptors in the ear. These all pass information to the brain so that a person is aware of body and limb position during movements. This awareness, known as kinaesthetic perception, is important for many physical activities, especially those involving gymnastic movements.

Kinaesthetic perception can be determined by testing the ability to distinguish between different weights when blindfolded, or by timing how long a blindfolded person can maintain balance while standing on one leg (*see* **blind stork test**).

kinesiology

The study of the anatomical and mechanical basis of human movement. Kinesiology includes anatomy, mechanics, and physiology of muscles and skeleton. There is considerable overlap between the disciplines of kinesiology and biomechanics.

kneading: *See* massage.

knee

The knee joint combines mobility with strength. Mobility is required so that we can move our legs freely, and strength so

that we can cope with the tremendous impact forces produced during running and jumping. The knee is the largest joint in the body. It is formed between the thigh bone (femur) and tibia (shin bone). It is a complex joint containing the patella (knee bone), semi-lunar discs of cartilage (menisci), and several ligaments that criss-cross between the tibia and femur (*see* **cruciate ligaments**).

Although the knee appears to be a hinge joint, it moves in more than one plane. In addition to flexion (bending) and extension (straightening) it can rotate slightly. This is essential during walking and running. Its ability to rotate makes it susceptible to injury during physical activities. Between one quarter to one third of all sports injuries involve the knee. Zipper-like scars decorating the knees of many professional sports people (especially body-builders and weightlifters) is evidence of the high rate of injury. Many knee disorders involve the patella. There are a number of anatomical factors (for example, flat feet and unequal development of thigh muscles) that predispose a person to patellar injury, but most injuries are due to overuse (*see* **chondromalacia patellae** and **patellar tendinitis**). Flexibility exercises; correction of foot deformities with orthotics; and knee exercises which improve the alignment and coordination of leg muscles, can minimize patellar problems, but sometimes surgery is needed to realign the forces on the patella. Other knee injuries include dislocations, ligament tears and strains, bursitis (*see* **housemaid's knee**), and torn cartilage (more correctly called a meniscus tear). Because the knee is such a complex joint involving so many structures, diagnosis of injury is notoriously difficult.

The following exercises are often performed after recovery from a knee injury to minimize the risk of recurrence (figure 35).

■ **Knee exercise 1** Lie flat on your back with your legs extended and feet turned slightly outwards. Lift your right foot about 10 centimetres (3 inches) off the ground. Hold for about 10 seconds, relax, and repeat with the left foot. Do this exercise about 10 times.

Three exercises for improving knee mobility. They are commonly performed after knee injury to minimize the risk of recurrence

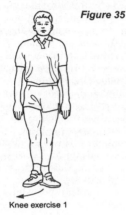

Figure 35

Knee exercise 1

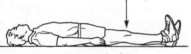

Knee exercise 2

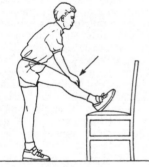

Knee exercise 3

- **Knee exercise 2** Lie on your back with your legs straight. Push your right knee into the floor by tightening the quads (the muscles at the front of your thighs), pull the toes and ankles of your right leg towards you. This should result in your heel being lifted off the floor. Hold for 10 seconds, relax, and repeat with the left leg. Do this exercise about 10 times.

- **Knee exercise 3** Stand about 60 centimetres (2 feet) away from a stable surface that is about the same height as a chair.

Keeping both legs straight, place your right heel on the surface (e.g. chair seat). Put both your hands on your right knee and lean gently into it, holding it firmly and steadily for 30 seconds. Do not rock. Relax. Repeat using the left leg. Do this exercise about five times.

See also **leg extension**.

kneecap (patella)

A small, lens-shaped bone at the front of the knee. It develops within the tendon which attaches the quadriceps muscles (the four muscles on the front of the thigh) onto the tibia. The kneecap has two major functions: first, it protects the front of the knee joint; second, it provides a low friction surface, improving the efficiency of the thigh muscles that straighten the lower leg. The kneecap is in a very vulnerable position and it is poorly nourished, making it susceptible to injury. *See also* **knee**.

knee disorders: *See* **knee**.

kneeling kickback

An exercise that develops the muscles at the back of the thighs (hamstrings) and buttocks (gluteals).

- Go down on your hands and knees, keeping your back rounded and chin tucked in. Bring your right knee forward so that it can almost touch your head. Push your right leg slowly and gently backwards so that it is fully extended and parallel to the floor. Hold the extended position for a few seconds. Return to the starting position, pause for a few seconds and repeat the exercise with your left leg. Throughout the exercise, take care to ensure that your back is not arched and that your hips remain facing the floor.

knee raises

A basic, simple strength training and stretching exercise for muscles in the lower back and buttocks.

- Lie flat on your back with your hands by your sides. Slowly and smoothly, bend your knees up towards your chest. Hold the position for a few seconds. Return gently to the starting position and repeat the exercise.

knockout: *See* **concussion**.

Krebs cycle (citric acid cycle)
A series of reactions named after the
1953 Nobel prize winner, Sir Hans Krebs,
its discoverer. The Krebs cycle is an integral part of aerobic respiration in which
acetyl coenzyme A, a product of carbohydrate, fat, and protein metabolism, is broken down in the presence of oxygen to
release energy.

kung-fu: *See* martial arts.

kwashiorkor
A protein and energy deficiency disease
that occurs only in young children. It is
characterized by oedema (swelling of
tissues, typically in the abdomen). It is a
complicated disease, not, as once
thought, due simply to a lack of protein.
It is not known what triggers the disease,
but it is thought that oxygen radical damage superimposed on general malnutrition is important. There is some evidence
that fungal toxins (known as aflatoxins)
in mouldy food may play a role in the
development of some cases of kwashiorkor. The toxins damage the liver which
is then unable to manufacture albumin
(a protein found in plasma). Improved
food storage may reduce the incidence of
aflatoxin-related kwashiorkor.

laceration

A cut that may be superficial or deep. Long, shallow lacerations usually cause no great problems, but there is a risk of tetanus with any penetration of the skin by a foreign object. Until recently, it was a relatively simple job to treat a laceration. Cleaning and closure were often all that was required. With the onset of AIDS, people are much more aware of the dangers of blood-borne diseases. Even small cuts, if bleeding, should be dealt with carefully. The bleeding person must be removed from contact with others. The carers should wear gloves, and any area contaminated with blood should be disinfected. Lacerations contaminated with gravel or some other substance may have to be scrubbed clean.

lactase: *See* lactose.

lactate: *See* lactic acid.

lactate threshold: *See* lactic acid.

lactic acid

An organic acid formed during energy production from the breakdown of glucose when there is not enough oxygen available for the complete breakdown of glucose, or when there are insufficient mitochondria to take up pyruvate, an intermediate breakdown product of glucose. Mitochondria are the components of the cell which can use oxygen to break down the pyruvate completely and release energy by aerobic respiration or aerobic metabolism. The energy production system which relies mainly on the partial breakdown of glucose to lactic acid, is called the lactic acid system. It takes place without oxygen and is therefore a form of anaerobic metabolism or anaerobic respiration. The lactic acid system provides energy for high intensity activities lasting up to two or three minutes. Lactic acid accumulates in the blood and tissue fluids where, like any acid, it dissolves in water to produce hydrogen ions (protons). The accumulation of protons contribute to muscle fatigue. In addition to protons, lactic acid also produces lactate ions, but these do not have a detrimental effect on muscle activity. When intensive exercise is completed and more oxygen becomes available, the lactic acid is broken down to release more energy, or is converted into glucose which may be stored as glycogen. Lactic acid production increases with exercise, as does the production of lactate ions and protons. During low intensity exercise, lactate concentration is usually less than 2 mmol. per litre of blood but this may rise to 25 mmol. per litre during high intensity exercise.

There appears to be a critical level of exercise above which lactate increases dramatically. This has been called the lactate turnpoint and the onset of blood lactate accumulation (OBLA). It has been assumed that the lactate turnpoint represents the anaerobic threshold, the transition between aerobic metabolism and anaerobic metabolism. Below the turnpoint, oxygen supply is sufficient to satisfy energy demands, above it the supply is insufficient. Recent studies have questioned this assumption. Improved mathematical analysis suggests that lactate levels rise as a continuous function of exercise intensity, and therefore the lactate turnpoint does not indicate an anaerobic threshold. Nevertheless, the turnpoint is very useful, indicating the exercise intensity above which the production of lactic acid exceeds the body's capacity to eliminate it. It can be used to establish optimum endurance training intensities: exercising at an intensity just below the turnpoint prevents a large accumulation of lactic acid in the muscles so that performance is not impaired. In addition, endurance training between 85–90 per cent maximum heart rate tends to raise the lactate turnpoint, indicating that training improves the body's ability to deal with lactic acid production.

lacto-ovo vegetarian diet
Diet consisting of plant foods supplemented with milk, milk products, and eggs. See also vegetarian.

lactose (milk sugar)
A sugar found in milk. It is a disaccharide made by the combination of galactose and glucose. Milk goes sour because the lactose is converted by bacteria into lactic acid. Lactose is an energy-rich food but some people suffer from lactose intolerance in which the consumption of milk (or other foods containing lactose) causes cramps, flatulence, and diarrhoea.

Lactose intolerance is due to a deficiency in the production of lactase, an enzyme that digests lactose into glucose and galactose. It most often affects people who consume few milk products, but since lactase production tends to reduce with age, a large proportion of the population may suffer some degree of lactose intolerance as they grow older. In fact, most ethnic groups (apart from Caucasians) do not retain lactase past adolescence so most adults are lactose intolerant. A few sufferers can still eat some fermented dairy products, such as buttermilk and yoghurt, or they may be able to obtain lactase-treated products. Others may have to avoid dairy products altogether. These people have to find alternative sources of the nutrients, such as calcium and riboflavin, that they would otherwise obtain from milk or its products.

lactose intolerance: See lactose.

laetrile
A water-soluble compound first extracted from apricot kernels in the 1950s. Its full scientific name is laevo-mandelonitrile-beta-glucuronoside but it is also known as amygdalin. It is often present in foods with vitamin B complex. This has led to laetrile being marketed by some producers as vitamin B_{17}, but it is not a vitamin and has no known function in the body.

Laetrile is a source of organic cyanide. Cancer cells are believed to convert this into inorganic cyanide that destroys the cells. Consequently, laetrile has been used in cancer therapy. However, its use is very controversial. Excess laetrile is toxic to normal cells and causes cold sweats, headaches, nausea, lethargy, breathlessness, and low blood pressure. Consequently, the sale of laetrile has been restricted in some countries due to its potential toxicity. In the UK it is available only on prescription. Its use in the USA is illegal because of its toxicity, and because there is not enough convincing evidence that it is beneficial.

lateral arm raise
A weight-training exercise that develops the shoulder muscles.

■ Stand with feet slightly apart. Hold a dumbbell in each hand. Your palms should be facing inward and your arms hanging down at your side. Raise the dumbbells sideways to head level, hold briefly, lower, and repeat.

The exercise is often done sitting to stop the tendency of using parts of the body other than the shoulders to lift the dumbbells.

lateral pull-down
An exercise performed at the pull-down station of a weight-training machine. It strengthens the shoulder muscles and the biceps (figure 36).

■ Sit or kneel on the floor. With your arms extended and your hands more than shoulder width apart, use a pronated grip (palms facing forward) to grasp the pull-down bar. Pull the bar down behind you to the base of your neck. Return to the starting position and repeat.

Figure 36 Lateral pull-down

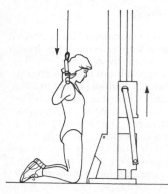

laxative

A substance that increases the frequency of bowel movements. It may also be used to encourage the formation of a softer or bulkier stool. Common laxatives include castor oil, senna (and its derivatives), magnesium sulphate, and some bulking agents (e.g. bran and methyl cellulose). Some common laxatives, such as castor oil and senna, irritate the gut lining and can cause severe cramps. They are sometimes used by people trying to lose weight but they can result in dehydration and malabsorption of nutrients, leading to nutrient deficiencies. Most experts agree that taking such laxatives is a dangerous and ineffective way to lose weight.

lean body mass

The total body mass minus the non-essential stores of fat. In a fully grown adult, changes in lean body mass are usually due to growth or wasting of muscle tissue (for example, associated with ageing), but lean body mass is also affected by fluctuations in body fluid and bone density.

lecithin

A compound consisting of two fatty acid chains, a phosphate group, and a base (choline), present in egg yolk and soya beans. It is also called phosphatidyl-choline. Lecithin usually contains a high proportion of linoleic acid. It is often added to processed foods as an emulsifying agent, binding food components together and making them more soluble. In the body, lecithin is a component of cell membranes, including the myelin sheath around nerves, and it is involved in fat metabolism. It has been claimed that lecithin helps cholesterol bind to the high density lipoproteins that remove the cholesterol from tissues. The involvement of lecithin in fat mobilization has led to it being sold as a slimming aid, but there is no evidence that it helps weight reduction. On the contrary it is probably just as fattening as other vegetable oils. Some coaches prescribe lecithin in post-competition diets because they believe it accelerates recovery.

lectins

Toxic substances found in most pulses, especially butter beans and kidney beans. Their toxicity is destroyed by cooking but if kidney beans, for example, are eaten raw or undercooked then the lectins they contain may upset digestion and cause vomiting, diarrhoea, and nausea.

leg curl

An exercise that helps to strengthen the hamstring muscles. It is best performed on a fixed-weight machine with a leg extension unit (figure 37).

■ Lie on your stomach. Hook both your feet under the leg extension unit so that the bottoms of your calf muscles are resting against the bar. Pull the unit upwards, moving your heels towards your buttocks. Hold for a few seconds then slowly lower the leg unit; repeat about four times.

If, like many exercisers, you have neglected the hamstrings in your strength-training programme, start with light weights, progressing gradually to heavier ones.

leg extension

A weight-training exercise that strengthens the quadriceps (the muscles at the front of the thighs). It is often used to rectify knee problems caused by weak quadriceps. Leg extensions can be performed on a weight bench that has a special attachment or by sitting at the end of a table and lifting ankle weights (figure 37). The exercise is sometimes performed with one leg at a time to prevent the stronger leg from doing most of the work.

Figure 37 Leg curl, leg extension, leg press, and leg raise

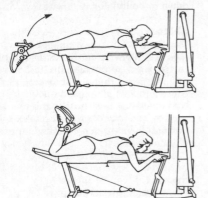
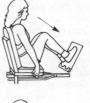

Leg curl

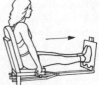

Leg press

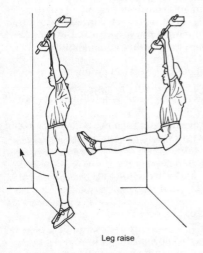

Leg raise

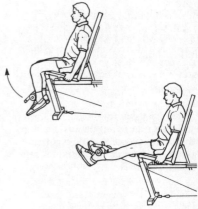

Leg extension

■ Begin with one leg extended with the foot behind the padded bar of the leg extension attachment. Hold the bench with your hands, and slowly lower your leg about 45 degrees before lifting again. Avoid lowering it all the way down because this puts too much strain on knee ligaments. Do not assist the movement by swinging your upper body. Repeat with the other leg.

Aim to do about three sets of ten repetitions for each leg, about three times a week.

leg lift

An exercise performed lying on your back on the floor. Both legs are raised simultaneously above the ground and held in the raised position for a few seconds. It is designed to strengthen the abdominal muscles, but it is not a good exercise for most people because it puts too much strain on the lower back.

leg press

1 A simple exercise that strengthens the quadriceps muscles at the front of the thigh and improves leg mobility.

■ Sit on the floor with your hands supporting you and your knees bent at a comfortable angle. Keeping both knees bent, slowly bring your right knee towards your chest, then straighten that leg so that it is fully extended. To minimize the risk of injuries during the movement, do not allow your lower back to arch, contract your abdominal muscles, and ensure correct alignment by pointing your legs straight in front of you.

A typical session for beginners is three sets of 10 repetitions. Increase the number of repetitions as fitness improves. If the exercise becomes too easy, use ankle weights or an exercise band for additional resistance.

2 A strength-training exercise done at a leg press station on a weight-training machine (figure 37). It is popular among sprinters and other runners because it puts little strain on the back. The muscles worked include the quadriceps, gastrocnemius, soleus, and gluteals.

■ Place your feet flat on the foot rests. Your legs should be bent at 90 degrees at the knee, and your hands should be grasping the seat handles. Fully extend your legs and thighs then return to the start position. Keep your backside on the seat and your back against the backrest throughout the exercise.

leg raise

1 An exercise that strengthens the muscles at the back of the thighs (hamstrings), buttocks (gluteals), and lower back (erector spinae).

■ Lie face down with your head resting on your hands. Lift your right leg, hold it for a few seconds in the raised position, and then lower it. Repeat the exercise with your left leg. Throughout the raises, make sure that you keep your hips on the floor.

2 An exercise that strengthens the trunk muscles (figure 37).

■ Grip an overhead bar with palms facing forward. Slowly lift your legs until they are parallel to the ground. Lower the legs and repeat.

lentils

A highly nutritious pulse, especially rich in carotene and some B vitamins. Lentils contain high amounts of phytates and lectins. Phytates can interfere with mineral absorption and lectins can be toxic. The phytate content is reduced by soaking in water and the lectin is broken down by boiling for 10 minutes.

libido

The sex drive. A large number of psychological and physiological factors interact to determine an individual's libido. It is often difficult, therefore, to pinpoint the cause for a loss of sexual desire. Nevertheless, a healthy diet and regular exercise can improve a person's sex drive; overindulgence in food, alcohol, or exercise can reduce it.

Loss of sexual desire in middle age may be linked to lowered levels of sex hormones. This can be alleviated by hormone replacement therapy in females and, possibly, testosterone treatment therapy in men. (Testosterone treatment remains controversial and its effectiveness needs to be tested by clinical trials.) However, reduced sex drive is more likely to be due to non-hormonal causes, such as boredom, domestic or job worries, and mental and physical fatigue. The following advice may help a person cope with the stresses of life and maintain a healthy libido:

● avoid overindulgence in food or alcohol
● eat a healthy, balanced diet
● take regular (but not excessive) exercise
● incorporate relaxation exercises into your daily routine to reduce stress.

See also **sex and exercise.**

lifting

If you do not lift a heavy object properly, you may suffer a serious injury, particularly to your back. More man-hours are lost in industry because of accidents resulting from faulty handling of heavy objects than from any other cause. Similar accidents occur when exercisers use the wrong technique to lift weights. An electronic strain gauge can be used to compare the stress imposed on the back during different activities. The most stressful activity is lifting with the knees straight. The strain on the back is reduced considerably if the body is correctly positioned during the lift. To minimize the risk of injury, it is important to lift objects in a controlled manner, with the minimum of effort and the maximum efficiency and skill.

- Stand with your feet about a hips' width apart; this should be a comfortable and stable position from which to make a lift.
- For most weight-lifting exercises, point your toes forwards, but if you intend carrying an object to a new location, point the toes in the direction in which you want to go.
- Lower your body by slowly bending your knees.
- Make full use of your leg muscles and other large muscle groups when lifting an object.
- Make full use of momentum to produce a smooth, controlled lift; avoid snatched or jerky movements.
- Keep your back straight, but not stiffly vertical, throughout the lift. Avoid bending your back because this can impose unnecessary strain on the lower back and abdomen.
- Tuck your chin in during the lift. This helps to keep your back straight by shortening the sternocleidomastoid muscles (large muscles at the front of the neck that lock the upper region of the spine, reducing the tendency for the buttocks to move out of alignment).
- Ensure you have a broad, even grip on the object by using the full palmed surface of your hands and fingers. Do not interlock your fingers; this can be dangerous because the pressure of heavy weights may prevent you from unlocking your fingers making it difficult to get rid of the load in an emergency.
- When lifting a heavy weight, keep your arms as close as possible to the centre of your body. Keep your elbows tucked in; do not allow them to wing outwards as this imposes unnecessary strain on your shoulders and may cause you to lean backwards.
- Use both sides of your body. Avoid regularly lifting or carrying weights on one side of your body. This imposes unilateral strains which can upset a number of body processes and impose mechanical strains which can damage the joints, particularly those in the spine and hips.

liniment
A liquid applied to the skin to warm and protect muscles or to relieve muscle pain and stiffness. Applied externally, liniments certainly provide a warm sensation (very warm if a man carelessly rubs the liniment into the more sensitive regions of his body!). Apart from the psychological benefit of feeling warm, liniments do not seem to have much effect on muscles (except, possibly, to divert blood from the deep muscles to the superficial muscles) and they are no substitute for a proper warm-up routine.

linoleic acid
An essential polyunsaturated fatty acid which must be obtained from food. It belongs to the family called omega–6 fatty acids, obtained in the diet principally from vegetable seeds and polyunsaturated margarines. Linoleic acid is the raw material for a number of compounds vital for health (e.g. arachidonic acid which is involved in the inflammation response). Linoleic acid is especially important for the proper growth and development of infants. It was once known as vitamin F but is no longer regarded as a vitamin.

lipid
An organic compound, insoluble in water, but which dissolves readily in other lipids and in organic solvents such as alcohol, chloroform, and ether. Lipids contain carbon, hydrogen, oxygen, and sometimes phosphorus. They are classified according to their solubility and include neutral fats (triglycerides), phospholipids, and steroids. *See also* **fat**.

lipid deposit theory
A theory suggesting that regular aerobic exercise can reduce lipid deposits and atherosclerosis, and so reduce the risk of heart disease.

lipolysis
The breakdown of lipids into fatty acids and glycerol.

lipoprotein
A combination of a lipid and protein (figure 38). Lipoproteins serve as transport vehicles for fatty acids and cholesterol in the blood and lymph. They are classified according to their density as high-density lipoproteins, low-density

Figure 38 A lipoprotein

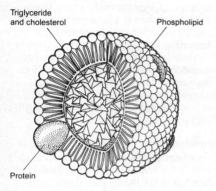

Triglyceride
and cholesterol

Phospholipid

Protein

lipoproteins, and very-low-density lipoproteins. Health care workers are interested in the concentration of the different types of lipoproteins in the blood because it has implications for health: a high concentration of low-density lipoproteins appears to present a health risk and is associated with a high incidence of heart disease.

High-density lipoproteins (HDLs) have the highest proportion of protein, are the smallest in size, and carry the least amount of lipid. They transport cholesterol from tissues to the liver where cholesterol is broken down and excreted or used to manufacture other substances. Thus, HDLs seem to accelerate the removal of cholesterol from blood, reducing the likelihood of cholesterol becoming deposited in arterial walls where it can cause blockages. Although many experts think that high levels of HDLs provide some protection against heart disease, the relationship between HDLs and the disease is not simple. The composition of HDLs in an individual varies, and some components seem to be more effective at mopping up cholesterol than others. To further complicate matters, heart disease is absent in some families that have almost no HDLs.

Low-density lipoproteins (LDLs) contain a larger proportion of cholesterol than HDLs. They release the cholesterol where it can be used but continue to carry it in the blood if it is not used. High concentrations of LDLs enable more cholesterol

to be transported in the circulatory system. It may be deposited in the walls of blood vessels and cause cardiovascular diseases such as atherosclerosis. Many medical practitioners agree that it is desirable to have LDL-cholesterol levels below 130 milligrams per decilitre of blood. Raised LDL concentrations (more than 160 milligrams per decilitre) are a sign of a high heart attack risk.

Very low-density lipoproteins (VLDLs) are the largest type. They transport cholesterol and fat in the blood, dropping off these chemicals at sites where they are used. When they unload their contents, VLDLs break down into smaller LDLs that continue to carry cholesterol in the bloodstream.

Regular aerobic exercise can raise the concentration of HDLs. This is one reason why most medical practitioners regard such exercise as a potent preventative and therapeutic tool against heart disease.

liposis (adiposis)
The accumulation of abnormally large amounts of fat in the body. See also **obesity**.

liposuction
A body 'sculpturing' technique. It involves surgically removing fat from the adipose layers under the skin. Enzymes are injected into the tissue to help loosen and break down the fat. Then a needle is inserted to suck the fat out of the body. It is a relatively quick technique made popular by a number of film stars who have used it to improve their appearance. According to the American Society of Reconstructive Surgeons, liposuction is the country's third most common form of cosmetic surgery. It is estimated that more than 100 000 liposuctions are performed each year.

Some advertisements for liposuction claim that the technique is simple, safe, and has a permanent effect. But if not carried out properly, the procedure can be unpleasant, ineffective, and sometimes dangerous. Older people with inelastic skin may be left with skin that sags and appears flabby. Blood loss and blood clots can occur during surgery, which may also cause severe bruising. In addition, liposuction is usually carried out under general anaesthetic. This can be traumatic for anyone, but obese people are two to three times more likely to die under general anaesthetic than lean people, and they have a higher risk of post-operative complications.

It is generally agreed by doctors that liposuction is not an effective long-term treatment for obesity. However, if someone wants liposuction, it should be performed by a reputable, fully qualified surgeon.

liposurgery
A form of cosmetic surgery in which fat and skin are cut away from the adipose layers beneath the skin. Liposurgery can be painful and dangerous if not carried out properly. *See also* **liposuction**.

liquid protein diet
A diet in the form of high-protein drinks. Such diets were very popular in the 1970s until some forms were blamed for several sudden, unexpected deaths. The deaths were never satisfactorily explained, but they might have been due to high sodium:low potassium levels, plus an imbalance of essential amino acids needed for muscle growth and repair. Since the heart is mainly muscle, this would have had serious and sometimes fatal consequences. *See also* **high protein diet**.

listeria
A type of bacteria (*Listeria monocytogenes*) found in soil, water, and certain foods, such as unwashed vegetables, some soft cheeses (Brie and Camembert often contain listeria), and chilled foods (especially chicken and any kind of paté) not kept at the correct temperature. Listeria is peculiar in being able to multiply in temperatures as low as $-2°C$ and as high as $42°C$. The bacteria are often present in the gut with no ill-effects because the body's defence mechanisms keep the bacterial population within tolerable limits. However, in some susceptible individuals (especially pregnant women and elderly people), listeria can multiply and cause a form of food poisoning called listeriosis. Symptoms range from those like mild influenza to severe inflammation of the membranes of the brain and spinal cord. In pregnant women, listeriosis can terminate pregnancy or damage the foetus.

listeriosis: *See* listeria.

loafer's heart theory
The proposition that the heart of an inactive individual is less able to cope with physical stress and an increase in workloads, making it more susceptible to a heart attack.

local cross-fibre stroke: *See* massage.

locking
An inability to move a joint through its full range because of a mechanical defect or obstruction within the joint, or because the joint is fixed in one position. Locking can result from extreme pain caused by a muscle spasm, from interference by a foreign body, or from a torn cartilage. Locking of the knee joint, for example, may be due to a spasm of the hamstring muscle, a loose body in the joint capsule, or a torn lunar cartilage.

locomotives
A form of pyramid training used especially in swimming. A typical session in a 25 metre pool might consist of swimming four lengths fast, four lengths slow; three fast, three slow; two fast, two slow; one fast and one slow. Then back down the pyramid starting with one fast length, one slow; two fast, two slow; etc.

longevity
If you want to have a long life, choose the right parents. Although genetic factors seem to affect our longevity more than any other, exercise and diet can also have a significant effect.

There are hundreds of well-respected studies showing that diet and exercise influence a number of health-risk factors, such as blood cholesterol levels, hypertension, and obesity. Those who take moderate levels of exercise (expending more than 2000 extra Calories a week on vigorous physical activity) may live up to two years longer than sedentary people who expend less than 500 extra Calories per week. A 150 lb (68 kg) man burns about 500 Calories walking six miles (9.6 km).

The beneficial effects of exercise seem to continue with energy expenditures of up to 3500 Calories, but diminish above this level.

Many comparative studies of diet and disease have implicated poor diet in the development of heart disease and certain cancers. Although a balanced diet increases the chances of enjoying a long and healthy life, and certain special diets may help control the development of some diseases, there is no unequivocal evidence that diet can cure chronic disease.

long-slow distance training

A form of endurance training consisting of continuous, extended low-intensity activity, usually running. During the training, the heart rate is raised to levels of 60–80 per cent maximum, but the emphasis is on maintaining a continuous effort for at least one hour. This form of training is intended to strengthen the heart and therefore increase aerobic fitness. It also improves the body's ability to use fat as an energy source.

loose bodies: *See* joint injury.

lordosis

An accentuated inward curvature of the lumbar region of the spine. It may result from rickets (vitamin D deficiency disease), but it is more often caused by poor posture or an unequal muscle pull on the spine. It tends to affect people who have to carry a large mass in front of the body (e.g. pregnant women, and men with a 'pot-belly'). It may also occur during a growth spurt in adolescents. There is wide ethnic variation in the shape of the back, and lordosis might be quite marked and normal in some people.

low back stretcher

An exercise that helps to prevent backache (figure 39).

Figure 39

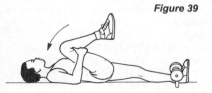

■ Lie on your back with your legs fully extended. Draw one knee up to your chest and grasp the thigh (not the knee) so that you can pull the knee tightly down with your hands. Keep the other leg extended and, if possible, stabilized by a partner, weight, or strap. Return to the starting position and repeat with the other leg.

low carbohydrate diet

Low carbohydrate diets are often designed for fast weight loss. This is rarely effective in the long term because it is achieved mainly by loss of water and lean mass. The water is rapidly regained when normal eating is resumed. As well as being ineffective, these diets produce ketones (*see also* **ketogenic diets**) which can be harmful. Therefore, such diets should only be taken under medical supervision. Low carbohydrate diets can also increase blood cholesterol levels, cause hypoglycaemia, and disrupt the balance of minerals. The diets rarely provide sufficient nutrients and are usually difficult to follow.

Some people reduce their carbohydrate intake in the mistaken belief that carbohydrates are as fattening as pure fats. However, less fatty tissue is made by eating 2000 Calories of carbohydrates than by eating 2000 Calories of pure fat. Fat overeaters tend to put on weight more easily and to be overweight for longer than carbohydrate overeaters. Stated simply, excess fats are more fattening than excess carbohydrates.

Far from reducing the proportion of carbohydrate in the diet, most people would benefit from increasing it so that it contributes at least 50 per cent of food energy. Carbohydrate is a better source of energy for exercise than fat. Many dietitians recommend a diet rich in complex carbohydrates as the foundation of a weight-reducing diet, a sports diet, and healthy eating for all.

low-density lipoprotein: *See* lipoprotein.

lower leg lift

An exercise that develops the inner thigh muscles (figure 40).

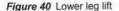

Figure 40 Lower leg lift

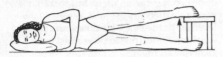

■ Lie on your right side with your left leg supported in a raised position by resting the foot on a bench. Slowly raise and lower your right leg about five times. Repeat on your left side.

low fat diet

Most dietitians advocate a low fat diet, This has often been misinterpreted as meaning very little fat of any kind. However, a very low fat diet (one which contributes less than 7–10 per cent of food energy) may not provide sufficient essential fatty acids or provide the amount of fat required to absorb enough fat-soluble vitamins. Such a diet may also make it difficult to meet energy requirements. So, fats should not be avoided, but they should be restricted so that they contribute no less than 10 per cent of food energy. The average contribution of fats in western diets is 40–45 per cent, and health guidelines generally recommend that this should be reduced to less than 35 per cent. It is also recommended that saturated fats and trans fatty acids should contribute no more than 10 per cent and 2 per cent respectively. Trans fatty acids occur in margarines that have been hydrogenated to improve their spreading quality. Some polyunsaturated fats and monunsaturated fats are essential to health, but only in moderate amounts.

low impact activity

An activity that does not impose high impact forces on joints. Swimming is one of the best low impact activities. A swimmer has to use large muscle groups of the upper and lower body, so it can be a strenuous activity, excellent for improving aerobic fitness. It has the added advantage that there is little jarring of the joints because the body is supported by water. Walking is another good low impact exercise that does not impose the mechanical stresses of high impact activities, such as running.

lunges

A lunge is a position assumed when standing with one leg to the front, knee bent, and the other leg stretched out backwards. When the body is inclined forwards, most of the weight is on the front leg and the muscles of the rear leg are stretched. Lunges are performed as a warm-up exercise for the legs and buttocks.

■ Stand upright with your feet slightly apart and with your back straight. Take a step forwards with the left leg and bend the knee forwards so that it is directly above the foot. The right leg should be extended backwards with the knee touching (or almost touching) the floor as a result of the movement. The knees should be bent only to a 90° angle. Put your left hand on your left knee and lower your buttocks slightly to increase the stretch in the muscles of the extended leg. Swap legs and repeat.

lung volume

The volume of air inspired into, expired from, or contained within the lungs during breathing.

One of the most useful measurements of lung volume is vital capacity: the maximal volume of air that can be forcefully exhaled after taking the deepest breath. Values vary from 3 litres to 6 litres. The actual value is not a very good indicator of fitness because it tends to vary for a number of reasons, including the size and sex of each individual. However, among individuals of the same size and sex, the vital capacity tends to be greater in those who exercise regularly. Usually, relatively fit and healthy individuals can exhale at least 83 per cent of their vital capacity in the first second of exhalation (*see* **forced expiratory volume**).

At rest, only about half a litre of air is drawn into the lungs with each breath; this is known as the tidal volume. It increases with exercise until it reaches the vital capacity. The total amount of air inhaled each minute (ventilation rate) depends on both the depth and frequency of breathing. At rest, about 12 breaths per minute are taken so that the total volume of air inhaled is about 6 litres. During very strenuous exercise, this can increase to more than 100 litres a minute.

luxation: *See* **dislocation**.

lysine

An essential amino acid found in all proteins. Its concentration is relatively low in certain vegetables, such as cereal crops, so lysine is likely to be deficient in poorly designed vegetarian diets, but mixed vegetable diets are as good as meat. Low levels of lysine can slow down protein synthesis, resulting in poor muscle growth and repair.

M

"The trouble with Italian food is that six days later you're hungry again."
Marathon runner, Frank Miller. Quoted in Hazeldine, R. and McNab, T. (1991)
Fit for rugby. Kingswood Press, London

macrobiotic diet

An oriental dietary system based on the view that all life, including nutrition, is a balance between two energies: yin, representing negative life forces, and yang, representing positive forces. Followers of the diet believe that in order to live naturally and healthily, they must eat only natural foods. Generally, meat, eggs, and fish are classified as yang foods; dairy produce, fruits, and sugar are yin types; and cereals, nuts, and vegetables are in between. However, the terms are relative. Apples, for example, are fruits and therefore belong to the yin group, but they are the most yang of the fruits. Since the aim of a macrobiotic diet is to have a correct balance of yin and yang, cereals and vegetables form a bulk of the diet. The diet has been criticized because it discourages the consumption of fruits and because it can be difficult to obtain sufficient calories. For this reason, a macrobiotic diet is often unsuitable or inadequate for infants and young children.

macrocycle: *see* cycle training.

macromineral

A mineral, such as calcium or magnesium, required by the body in relatively large amounts. *Compare* **trace element**.

macronutrient

A category of nutrients, including carbohydrates, fats, and proteins, that are present in foods in large quantities.

mad cow disease: *See* bovine spongiform encephalopathy.

magic formula

Some purveyors of diets claim that their product contains a 'magic formula' to help you lose weight without any need to diet or exercise. These claims appeal to a desire for easy answers to difficult problems. The only 'magic formula' for weight loss with significant scientific backing is a balanced diet and exercise regime that results in a person expending more energy than is consumed. A high carbohydrate, low fat diet, and an exercise regime such as the one below, should help most people lose fat and stay healthy.

- carbohydrates (mainly complex) — 50% of calories consumed
- protein (lean) — 15%
- fat (mainly unsaturates) — < 35%
- water — equivalent of eight glasses per day
- vitamins and minerals — five or more servings of fruit and vegetable per day
- exercise (e.g. brisk walking) — 30 minutes/session, four to five times per week

The actual calorific intake should be individually determined, but (unless medically supervised) should not be less than 1000 Calories per day. For those who are overweight, the aim should be to lose no more than 1 kg (2 lb) per week. Do not forget to include fruit and vegetables in the calorie count. *See also* **advertisements**.

magnesium

A metallic element essential for life and which has a number of indispensable roles in exercise. Magnesium is an important component of some of the chemicals that aid respiration (the release of energy from food). It also plays a role in the function of nerves, and the contraction of heart and other muscles. Good sources are milk, dairy products, wholegrain cereals, nuts, legumes, and leafy green vegetables, which contain magnesium within their green pigment, chlorophyll. After being absorbed, magnesium is stored in the bones. Excessive intake may cause diarrhoea. A deficiency is rare, but it can lead to neuromuscular problems. High fat diets may reduce magnesium absorption. Not all the fat can be absorbed through the small intestine. Fat remaining in the gut may bind with magnesium to form insoluble soaps which cannot pass through the intestinal wall. The magnesium may be absorbed from the colon after fermentation of the soaps by gut bacteria. However, if these are not functioning properly, serious losses of magnesium may occur. Very high calcium intakes may also interfere with the absorption of magnesium. Magnesium supplements are taken in the belief that they can offer some protection or relief from atherosclerosis, insomnia, premenstrual tension and other menstrual problems, alcoholism, insomnia, heart disorders, and, in children, hyperactivity. Magnesium has been used in some hospitals to reduce the recurrence of a heart attack. The magnesium is given as salts in solution directly into a vein during the first 24 hours after a heart attack.

making weight

Jockeys, boxers, and wrestlers are among sports people who compete within strict weight categories. They often have to lose weight quickly. Traditionally, if a boxer was slightly overweight immediately prior to a match, he would sweat it off by exercising. This, combined with severely restricting fluid and food intake, would usually enable him to make weight. Then he could take in a large volume of fluid to rehydrate. Unfortunately, the dehydration–rehydration regime leaves a boxer weakened. The dehydration reduces the blood volume which cannot be restored completely in a short time by the rehydration. This reduces the ability of the blood to carry oxygen, and lowers endurance.

Some sports people resort to taking diuretic drugs (sometimes called water pills) to lose weight, even though the drugs are banned by the International Olympic Committee. Diuretics help to eliminate water but leave a person prone to dehydration and its harmful effects.

If you need to make a particular weight category, it is best to adopt a long-term strategy. Eat sensibly and exercise so that if you need to lose weight, you do so gradually without harming your performance or putting your health at risk.

malabsorption

A condition in which the uptake of one or more nutrients from the small intestine is reduced. *See also* **coeliac disease**.

male menopause: *See* viropause.

mallet finger

An injury that occurs when the tip of a finger is bent forcibly backwards, stripping a tendon from its bony attachment, and leaving the victim unable to extend the finger. The tendon is so strongly attached to the bone that a bony fragment is sometimes torn away with the tendon. Mallet finger commonly occurs when a hand is slightly closed before a ball is caught. The ball strikes the end of the finger, forcing it backwards.

malnutrition

Condition caused by an unbalanced diet with certain foods being deficient, in excess, or in the wrong proportions. *See also* **kwashiorkor**; **marasmus**; and **obesity**.

maltose

A double sugar (disaccharide) consisting of two glucose molecules. Maltose forms when starch is broken down in the gut. It is digested readily into its component glucose molecules in the presence of the enzyme maltase.

mammaplasty (breast reduction)

A complicated, major operation which may remove 1.3–1.5 kg (2–3 lb) of tissue from each breast. It is usually performed for health rather than cosmetic reasons because oversized breasts can cause severe, chronic backache and other disorders. The operation sometimes leaves surface scarring, but most patients are more concerned with the alleviation of discomfort than minor effects on physical appearance.

manganese

A metallic element, essential in the diet but required in very small amounts. It is a component of a number of enzyme systems, including those involved in the synthesis of cartilage. Good sources of manganese include nuts, legumes, wholegrains, leafy vegetables, and fruit. Deficiency is unknown in humans, therefore there are no recommended intakes.

manipulation

Any technique using the hands to produce a desired movement of a part of the body, or to return bones and joints to their normal position after displacement (*see* **dislocation**). Physiotherapists sometimes use manipulation to relieve stiffness in joints. It is a more rigorous procedure than mobilization.

marasmus

Malnutrition caused by lack of food. It is characterized by general wasting (body weight is less than 60 per cent of that expected for the age), apathy, and lethargy. Unlike some forms of malnutirition (for example, *see* **kwashiorkor**), it affects adults as well as children.

march fracture

A stress fracture, typically of one of the small bones of the foot, that causes pain when walking or running. March fractures were originally described as occurring in military recruits who had to march great distances, but they are a common overuse injury among road runners. Treatment is immobilization and rest.

march haemoglobinuria: *See* haematuria.

marijuana

A drug sometimes called cannabis or grass. It is obtained from the hemp plant *Cannabis sativa*, which contains the active ingredient tetrahydrocannabinol. The psychological effects of marijuana include sedation, relaxation, and euphoria. It may disturb the sense of balance and reduce aggression. Persistent marijuana smoking is incompatible with serious training because it tends to demotivate exercisers.

Many people argue that, compared to alcohol, marijuana is harmless and should be legalized. But its harmless nature has been seriously questioned recently. Chronic over-indulgence has been linked to a number of disorders and possible addiction.

martial arts

The martial arts were originally concerned with preparing men for battle. They no longer have a military role, but still retain an aggressive element. There are many forms, including aikido (meaning 'way of harmony'); hapkido (a Korean form of martial art, very similar to aikido); jiu-jitsu ('compliant techniques'); judo ('compliant way'); karate ('way of the empty hand'); kung-fu (a form of Chinese boxing); and tae kwon do ('foot, hand, way'). Many of the techniques in martial arts have developed from jiu-jitsu which was first used in Japan as a ruthless means of self-defence involving throws, strangleholds, arm- and wrist-locks, kicks, punches, and chops. However, each modern form of martial art requires its own particular combination of skills. Some emphasize dynamic, precise, and direct movement (e.g. karate); others utilize softer, slower, and more continuous movements (e.g. aikido). Each martial art also has its own fitness requirements including strength, flexibility (especially around the pelvis), muscle coordination, and endurance.

Martial arts are performed by males and females of a wide age range. Karate and tae kwon do have more than 200 000 participants in the USA, including 40 000 children. People choose to study martial arts for a variety of reasons: to acquire self-defence techniques; to improve cardiovascular fitness, strength, flexibility, and self-esteem; and to enjoy the artistic expression of the sport.

Although martial arts are contact sports, injuries are relatively rare. This is probably due to the excellent supervision in most clubs and the insistence on high levels of self-discipline. In a comparison of injuries per 100 000 participants, martial arts came bottom of the list (16.9) with the most common injuries being bruises, contusions, sprains, and strains. Basketball was top of the list (188.0) and even dancing (18.8) had a higher injury rate than martial arts. Unlike most dancing injuries, however, some of the injuries sustained doing martial arts can be serious. These include concussion, fractures, and paralysis. On at least three occasions, blows to the front of the abdomen or chest have resulted in fatalities because of damage to soft organs. However, fatalities are very rare. A more common serious risk is an injury to the head from kicks, punches, and chops (prohibited in some martial arts, such as judo). Repeated head injuries, even if there is no concussion, can cause brain damage (*see* **punch-drunk syndrome**). Because of the potential dangers, both physical and psychological, it is important that prospective participants join reputable clubs with competent instructors.

massage

Rubbing, kneading, and tapping of body parts. It has been called the world's oldest therapy. It is used by exercisers to warm, stretch, and relieve tension in muscles prior to and immediately after strenuous activity. Massage may increase blood flow through muscle, helping the body to remove lactic acid that has built up during strenuous exercise. Many people also use massage to relieve fatigue and pain caused by injury to muscles and soft tissues. Massage may orientate collagen fibres in scar tissue so that subsequent stretching is less likely to result in an injury. Many experts believe, however, that massage has little beneficial effect on recovery and, if used immediately after injury, can be harmful.

Massage often forms part of a weight-reducing regime in health clinics. Some masseurs claim that, by stimulating circulation, massage can decongest tissue and help remove fat. A special form of massage, called connective tissue massage, is directed at pummelling surplus flesh in an attempt to break up hard, adhesive fat, and flatten unsightly bulges. However, the massage itself will not reshape or slim the body.

Other common forms of massage used by exercisers and slimmers are:

- CROSS FRICTIONAL MASSAGE, in which the masseur applies firm pressure for short distances across the line of the muscle or tendon growth. It is thought to break down scar tissue

- DEEP MASSAGE, in which a firm pressure is applied to treat deep muscle injuries

- DEEP STROKING, performed by moving the pads of the thumbs along the length of a muscle, starting from the point farthest from the heart and moving towards it. Deep stroking moves blood and lymph through the muscle, removing fluid built up during exercise. This type of massage can be painful, causing tension that can be relieved by another form of massage called jostling

- EFFLUAGE (OR EFFLEURAGE), consisting of superficial or deep stroking movements, administered with the flat of the hand and fingers. It stimulates circulation of the blood and lymph

- FANNING, in which the masseur begins with hands together, then spreads them out to cover a muscle by moving away from a central point out to the edges of the muscle. Fanning is applied to muscles such as those of the chest and abdomen which radiate from the body's centre. It provides equal pull and pressure over the whole muscle to improve circulation

- JOSTLING, in which a relaxed muscle is grasped at its fixed attachment point (the origin) and shaken gently back and forth. The stroke continues all the way down the muscle to the opposite point of attachment (insertion) and then back again

- KNEADING, in which groups of muscles are held between the thumb and fingers of both hands and squeezed. Each hand works alternately in a rhythmical way up and down the muscle in a manner reminiscent of kneading dough. Kneading is used to assess the state of muscle tension. It may also help to pump blood and tissue fluids through muscle, accelerating recovery by helping to remove the waste products of exercise

- LOCAL CROSS-FIBRE STROKE, is a gentle but deep massage applied with the thumb or fingertips across muscles in which there are problem areas that feel hard. It is used during rehabilitation but not on newly injured areas

- TAPOTEMENT, massage technique in which the fingertips, palms, and sides of the hands create tapping and slapping movements. It stimulates circulation and helps to remove the waste products of exercise.

Although massage may be beneficial, it can also be harmful if applied incorrectly: massage of recently damaged tissue may disturb a clot and cause further internal bleeding. People suffering from heart, circulatory (e.g. varicose veins), or skin problems should not subject themselves to a massage.

massager

An electronic device that vibrates and is used to massage the body.

mat burn: *See* friction burn.

maturation: *See* growth.

maximal heart rate (HRmax)

The highest heart rate that can be achieved during exercise. It can be determined directly on a heart rate monitor when running to exhaustion, but this is not always a safe or practical procedure. It should be attempted only with a doctor's approval. Therefore it is usually assumed that the absolute maximal heart rate is 220 and that it decreases by a value of one beat per year of life. Thus, an individual's maximal heart rate (HRmax) can be estimated using the formula:

HRmax = 220 − age (in years)

The estimate may be subject to errors of 10 per cent or more and actual values may exceed the theoretical limit. For example, maximal heart rates of 250 beats per minute have been recorded in cross-country skiers subjected to intense workloads. Values vary according to the type of exercise performed: for example, HRmax is about 13 beats per minute less for an activity which uses mainly upper body muscles (e.g. swimming), than for an activity which uses mainly lower body

muscles (e.g. cycling). Maximal heart rate is often used as a guide to exercise intensities. Exercise physiologists recommend that unconditioned people train at a heart rate of between 60–70 per cent maximal heart rate. Thus a forty-year-old person with a maximal heart rate of 180 would maintain a training heart rate of between 108 and 126 beats per minute. The generally recommended training heart rate for a moderately fit person is between 70 and 80 per cent HRmax, and that for a highly-conditioned, competitive athlete is more than 80 per cent HRmax.

maximal oxygen consumption

Maximal oxygen consumption (often abbreviated to VO_2 max) is the maximum volume of oxygen consumed per minute. The fitter a person is, the more oxygen he or she can draw from the blood. Oxygen is extracted from air in the lungs, transported in the blood, and then utilized by respiring tissues to release energy from food. The energy that is released is used to synthesize ATP, a high energy compound which is the only direct source of energy for the body's activities. Maximal oxygen consumption is therefore a measure of a person's ability to use aerobic respiration as a source of energy. As such, it also reflects a person's aerobic work capacity, endurance capacity, and maximal aerobic power.

Maximal oxygen consumption is usually expressed in units of millilitres of oxygen consumed per kilogram body mass per minute. It is determined during a large muscle group activity (e.g. cycling or running). The intensity of the activity is progressively increased until exhaustion. Sometimes maximal oxygen consumption is expressed as litres of oxygen consumed per minute, to indicate total work capacity. The average value for a 20-year-old female is between 32–38 ml/kg/min; for a 20-year-old male it is 36–44 ml/kg/min.

Maximal aerobic capacity can improve with training. The amount of improvement is highly individualized and inversely related to the initial level of fitness. A sedentary person may experience as much as a 25 per cent increase in VO_2 max after only 8 weeks training; someone used to aerobic exercise may experience 5 per cent improvement or less in the same time. There is an upper limit of oxygen consumption beyond which training has no effect. This limit seems to be genetically determined and may be reached after 18–24 months of intensive endurance training.

maximum passive range: *See* range of movement.

McCutchen's weeping lubrication theory

The theory that when a joint is moved during a load-bearing exercise, the fluid within the joint cavity (synovial fluid) is squeezed in and out of the articular cartilage (cartilage lining the ends of the bones forming the joint). Synovial fluid contains nutrients that nourish the cartilage, and help it to grow and repair itself. This may be one reason why moderate exercise is beneficial to joint mobility. Of course, excessive exercise may wear down the cartilage faster than it can be repaired and reduce joint mobility.

meal replacement diet

An artificial diet especially formulated to replace food eaten at a normal meal. Meal replacement diets are designed to replace one or two meals per day as part of a calorie controlled diet. They usually come in the form of milkshakes, soups, biscuits, bars, and drinks. Most are made from sugar and milk, and contain a filler or bulking agent (e.g. plant fibre or gum; *see* **guar gum**) which helps you to feel full, as well as sufficient vitamins and minerals to meet or exceed requirements. Some manufacturers claim that the cellulose they use as a filler also reduces appetite. This claim has not been substantiated to the satisfaction of the food authorities in the United States, who have banned the use of cellulose in over-the-counter diet products. Some meal replacement diets incorporate additional substances that are claimed to aid weight loss, for example, by reducing appetite or increasing metabolism.

Meal replacement diets may be effective if used properly because they provide fewer calories per day than the average person requires to maintain weight. It is, however, important to follow the instructions carefully and include real meals in your eating plan. A major criticism of most meal replacement diets is that they do not help overweight people adopt good eating habits that would enable them to maintain weight loss without continually returning to the diet.

Some meal replacement diets that include fillers or bulking agents are not suitable for certain groups of people (e.g. those with high blood pressure) because they may cause problems similar to those caused by very low calorie diets (e.g. fatigue and heart irregularities). Many of the problems seem to be due to dehydration associated with consuming the fillers and bulking agents. The problems can be avoided by drinking plenty of water. You are, nevertheless, advised to consult your doctor before starting a meal replacement diet. Remember, doctors do not recommend diets of less than 1000 Calories per day without medical supervision. *See also* **formula diet**.

meal tolerance test

A measure of the response of blood sugar levels to normal dietary intake. *See* **glucose tolerance test**.

medau

A combination of music and gentle gymnastics that uses the entire body, firming up the muscles, and improving suppleness. Medau instructors try to encourage free movement, and a sense of balance and rhythm. It is a non-competitive aerobic activity recommended by a number of osteopaths and physiotherapists because of its fitness benefits and its low risk of injury.

medial epicondylitis: *See* golfer's elbow.

medical screening: *See* health screening.

medicine ball

A large, heavy ball used for physical training. Different throwing and lifting exercises have been devised to improve the flexibility and strength of the shoulders, arms, hips, or legs. A medicine ball offers extra resistance to movements usually performed explosively with a pre-stretching phase. As with weight training, the exercises are usually done in sets and repetitions, the number of which will differ for each individual. A typical session for one exercise in which the ball is thrown from a standing position, would consist of five sets of 10 repetitions with one minute rest between each set.

Mediterranean diet

Typically, a diet rich in pasta, bread, fruit, and vegetables, with moderate amounts of poultry and fish, cooked in olive oil and washed down with red wine. The Mediterranean diet is reputed to be among the healthiest in the world. Epidemiological studies show that Mediterraneans suffer less heart disease than people from northern Europe. Nutritionists believe that the typical Mediterranean diet reduces fat and increases the level of natural antioxidants such as vitamins C and E, significantly reducing the risk of heart attack.

Some people question the wisdom of a having a diet in which up to 40 per cent of the calories come from fat, and which encourages the use of alcohol. However, the fats in a Mediterranean diet are of a particular kind. Olive oil, the main fat in many meals, is very rich in monounsaturates. These are believed to protect cell membranes against the harmful effects of free radicals. The oily fish used in a Mediterranean diet (e.g. sardines and mackerel), are rich in long chain fatty acids, such as eicosapentaenoic acid (ESA). This acid apparently makes the blood less likely to clot and also makes the heart less prone to dangerous irregular contractions. The Mediterranean diet (especially of Cretans) often includes a salad made of walnuts and purslane. This is rich in alpha-linolenic acid, a fatty acid known to protect heart attack patients from further attacks. In moderate amounts, red wine is believed to reduce the risk of heart attacks by making blood less likely to clot. (This effect of wine is thought also to explain the 'French paradox'; the relatively high longevity of French people despite their notoriously high alcohol consumption.)

The benefits of a Mediterranean diet could, therefore, be due to any of a number of dietary factors. Some researchers think that the lifestyle of Mediterraneans also has health benefits. Many Mediterraneans still tend crops and livestock. This will give them the same benefits as regular, vigorous aerobic exercise.

medium chain triglycerides: *See* fatigue.

megadoses

Applied to supplements that provide 10 or more times the Recommended Daily Amount (RDA) of particular vitamins and minerals. They may be used to treat nutrient deficiencies and are sometimes prescribed to those suffering certain ailments. Megadoses have to be used cautiously because many vitamins and minerals are toxic in large doses. *See also* **megavitamin**.

megavitamin

A large dose of a particular vitamin. Megavitamins are sometimes used under medical supervision to treat specific diseases. Generally, they are not recommended for use except by those suffering from a vitamin deficiency. Some vitamins, for example, vitamin B_6, niacin, and the fat-soluble ones like vitamins A and D, can be poisonous in high doses. However, Linus Pauling, the Nobel Prize winning biochemist, suggested everyone would benefit from taking megadoses of vitamin C. He recommended 1 or 2 grams per day, 20–40 times the Recommended Daily Amount, to protect the body from cold viruses and other diseases. Preliminary tests of Pauling's claims indicate that there are only a few instances in which taking more than 100–300 milligrams per day is beneficial; when more than 100 mg is taken in one day, most of the vitamin is excreted unchanged in the urine. Doses of more than 1000 milligrams (1 gram) per day may be harmful to certain people causing nausea, abdominal cramps, and diarrhoea. Pauling's most controversial suggestion was that megadoses of vitamin C might be effective against certain cancers. There is no doubt that adequate amounts (i.e. between 30 and 100 milligrams per day) of vitamin C are needed to defend the body against the onset of cancer, but there is no evidence that megadoses of vitamin C act as a cancer cure.

menarche
The onset of menstruation defined by the first appearance of menstrual flow. The age of menarche varies from country to country, but in the USA and UK it generally begins at about 12 to 13 years of age. The age of menarch has come down on average over the last two generations, with diets being generally more adequate during childhood. However, girls who exercise strenuously, particularly female athletes with long, lithe bodies, may have their menarche delayed until their late teens. It is not clear whether this has long-term beneficial or harmful effects, but generally the later the menarche the higher the incidence of subsequent menstrual irregularities. *See also* **amenorrhoea**.

meniscus (pl. menisci)
A semi-lunar disc or wedge of cartilage within a joint such as the knee. Menisci may modify the shape of the surfaces of articulating bones and increase joint stability during complex movements. They also improve resistance to large, compressive loads by absorbing energy and reducing the mechanical shock that other joint structures would otherwise have to withstand.

Meniscal injuries are quite common. The inner meniscus of the knee is especially susceptible to damage by rotatory stresses and to excessive pressures (e.g. those produced by a weight-lifter performing full squats). Repeated twisting movements and changes in direction, such as those performed by footballers, may result in a torn cartilage (meniscal tear). The injury can be so painful that it can cause the knee to 'give way'. Movement is restricted because the knee can no longer be fully extended. The injury may also lead to the development of cysts which do not heal.

Meniscal tears may require surgery to remove detached fragments. Once removed, the space occupied by the meniscus is filled by a replacement material, but this is not of the same type or quality as the original meniscus. Consequently, joint stability becomes marginally worse and the likelihood of arthritis in later life is significantly increased.

menopause
Menopause is, strictly speaking, a woman's last menstrual period, but the term is commonly used to refer to the changes that lead up to the last time ovulation and menstruation take place. Menopause usually occurs between 45 and 55 years of age, but may start when a woman is in her thirties. Menopause is associated with changes in hormonal balance, which can lead to some unpleasant emotional and physical effects. Post-menopausal women have lower levels of the reproductive hormones, oestrogen and progesterone. Low concentrations of these hormones are linked to bone loss and osteoporosis (brittle bone disease).

Many post-menopausal women minimize or delay the effects of menopause by taking hormone replacement treatment (HRT) consisting of low doses of oestrogen and progesterone administered in pill form or as a skin patch. John Studd, a gynaecologist at King's College Hospital in London, is quoted as saying that HRT was probably '. . . the most important advance in preventive medicine in the Western world for half a century.' (*New Scientist.* **140**:21. October, 1993.) HRT can slow down bone loss and protect against heart attack. There is also some evidence that HRT may reduce the risk of uterine cancers, but other evidence suggests that some forms of HRT may actually increase uterine cancers. In the UK, the number of post-menopausal women taking HRT doubled between 1990 and 1993, from 9 per cent of women to 18 per cent. However, HRT is not suitable for all women; it is contraindicated for some who have had breast cancer, or who suffer from diabetes, asthma, heart disease, and some other disorders. For these people, and for those not wishing to take HRT, exercise may offer some benefits. Regular load-bearing exercise can increase spinal bone density up to 20 per cent, even in women who do not take hormone replacement treatment. As well as reducing the risk of osteoporosis, moderate exercise enables many women to cope with the psychological stresses of menopause by helping them to relax, and by boosting their self-esteem.

menstruation

The discharge of blood and fragments of the uterine wall at approximately monthly intervals during the menstrual cycle. The cycles begin at puberty and end at menopause. During menstruation, most women experience feelings of lassitude or fatigue. Women who exercise strenuously are particularly susceptible to iron-deficiency anaemia because of blood losses. They need higher than normal levels of haemoglobin to carry the oxygen they require for exercise. Athletes can take hormones, such as oestrogen, proges-terone, and progestogens, to adjust the time of menstruation. Although most sports women perform less well during menstruation, a few perform better. World and Olympic titles have been won at all stages of the menstrual cycle.

The effects of exercise on menstruation varies from one individual to another but reported effects include the following:

- delayed onset of the first menstruation, common in participants in sports such as gymnastics that require a slim physique
- shortening of cycle by up to 4 days
- reduced menstrual pain associated with regular aerobic exercise
- increased failure to ovulate or menstruate in up to 50 per cent of competitive track and field athletes.

See also **amenorrhoea** and **premenstrual tension**.

mental health

A positive state of mind engendering a sense of well being that enables a person to function effectively within society. Individuals who have good mental health are well-adjusted to society, are able to relate well to others, and basically feel satisfied with themselves and their role in society.

Breakdown of mental health is a major problem in Western societies: it has been estimated that at least one in four adults will suffer from some form of mental disorder, such as depression, during their life. Many physicians and psychologists believe that individuals are physical, mental, and spiritual beings and that these aspects are interrelated. Consequently, mental health is not possible without both physical and spiritual health.

Although there is no clear cause-and-effect relationship between exercise and mental health, aerobic exercise can improve self-esteem, lessen anxiety, and relieve depression. Exercise can act as a form of meditation, changing the state of consciousness and providing a distraction from stressful situations. Many doctors believe that exercise improves mental health and prescribe exercise to relieve depression and anxiety. Walking is the most frequently prescribed exercise, followed by swimming, bicycling, strength training, and running.

mental practice

A form of practice in which individuals produce a vivid mental image of actually performing an activity. See also **visualization** and **psychoneuromuscular theory**.

mesocycle: See **cycle training**.

mesomorph

An individual who tends to be stocky and of medium height with well developed muscles. There is a tendency in Western cultures to believe that the most desirable body shape is mesomorphic-muscular with little body fat. This belief, called mesomorphism by sociologists, is reinforced by advertisements in the mass media which portray muscularity and slimness as being associated with health, fitness, and success. This often leads to the assumption that all mesomorphs share these positive characteristics. There is also the implication that mesomorphy can be acquired by a disciplined, controlled, efficient lifestyle. However, body type is determined mainly by inheritance. See also **somatotype**.

mesotherapy: See **cellulite**.

MET: See **metabolic equivalent**.

metabolic acidosis: See **acidosis**.

metabolic equivalent (MET)

A measurement of the energy demands of exercise. At rest, the basal metabolic rate is approximately 3.5 millilitres of oxygen per kilogram body weight per minute; this is regarded as being equivalent to 1 MET unit. Activities are expressed as requiring multiples of the MET unit. Therefore an activity which requires 10 METs would consume 35 ml of oxygen per kg per min. *See also* **heat equivalence**.

metabolism

The sum total of all the chemical reactions that take place in the body. Metabolism includes anabolic reactions which manufacture substances needed for growth and repair, and catabolic reactions which break down substances to release energy. *See also* **basal metabolic rate**.

methaemoglobin: *See* nitrates.

methionine

An essential sulphur-containing amino acid. All meats contain methionine. For vegetarians, grains and soya beans are a good source, but beans belonging to the legumes are not. *See also* **carnitine**.

methyl donors

Chemicals that have a readily transferable methyl group (-CH₃). They are involved in the synthesis of DNA. They include dimethylglycine (DMG) and trimethylglycine (TMG) that are taken as ergogenic aids (performance boosters) by athletes who believe that these chemicals can improve the supply of oxygen to muscles.

microcycle: *See* cycle training.

micromineral: *See* minerals.

microtrauma

A microscopic injury, usually affecting connective tissue (e.g. bone). Cumulative microtrauma can cause a major injury. Running on hard roads, for example, may create microscopic fractures in the shin bone (tibia). If a runner overtrains and does not allow microfractures to heal, they may join together to form deeper

fractures that produce a dull aching pain along the shins. *See also* **shin splints**.

migraine: *See* headache.

milk sugar: *See* lactose.

military press

A strength-training exercise in which a weighted barbell is pushed upwards from the chest a number of times; the up-and-down movement is called a pressing action because it puts pressure on the chest muscles. The military press helps to strengthen the deltoids, pectorals, and triceps muscles (figure 41).

Figure 41

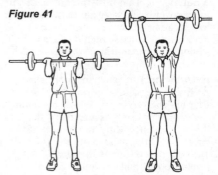

■ Lift the weighted barbell up to your shoulders, breathing in as you do so. As with all lifts, keep your back straight and use your legs to execute the movement. Hold the barbell on your shoulders for a few seconds and breathe out. Then lift the weights above your head by fully extending your arms. Hold for a few seconds. Gently lower the barbell to your chest then immediately push up again. Repeat the pressing action about four times before slowly lowering the barbell to the ground. Remember to continue breathing throughout the exercise; at no time should you hold your breath.

minerals

Natural inorganic substances that are basic components of the Earth's crust. They also occur in the human body where they are essential for the efficient action of many enzymes and hormones. Minerals play a vital role in blood formation; blood clotting; regulation of heart rate; nerve and muscle activity; bone formation; and digestion Soluble mineral salts also help to control the composition of body fluids. Several minerals, known as macrominerals, are needed in large amounts. These include calcium, magnesium, phosphorus, potassium, sodium, and sulphur (mainly present as part of the amino acids methionine and cysteine). Chlorine is also required in large amounts and is obtained mainly as sodium chloride. Minerals required in very small amounts (milligrams or micrograms per day) are called trace elements or microminerals. Trace elements known to be important include chromium, cobalt, copper, fluorine, iodine, iron, manganese, molybdenum, and selenium. A number of other minerals are known to be important for other animals, but their role in humans has not been clearly demonstrated. These include nickel, tin, silicon, and vanadium.

mitochondrion (*pl.* mitochondria)
A sausage-shaped structure within cells that has the specific function of generating energy by using oxygen to break down foodstuffs. Mitochondria are sometimes called the powerhouses of the cell. They contain coloured chemicals (cytochromes) and enzymes needed for aerobic respiration. When mitochondria are tightly packed together, the cytochromes impart a reddish-brown colour to cells (*see* **brown fat**). Mitochondria are particularly dense in slow twitch muscle fibres used for activities of long duration. Regular endurance training increases the density of mitochondria within muscle. In addition, training seems to increase the ability of each mitochondrion to generate energy, further improving endurance capacity.

mixers: *See* emulsifiers.

mobility
The ease with which a joint or series of joints is able to move before being restricted by the surrounding structures. Joint mobility is determined by the ligaments, joint capsule, musculature, and the size and shape of the bones within the joint. *See also* **flexibility** and **range of movement**.

mode of exercise
One of the four main exercise variables affecting the attainment of physical fitness. The others are duration, frequency, and intensity of exercise. Most people exercise to develop or maintain their cardiorespiratory fitness. To achieve this, the exerciser should choose a rhythmical aerobic activity that uses large muscle groups. The exercise should also allow the intensity to be sustained for long periods. Activities that fulfil these criteria include aerobic dance, cycling, jogging, cross-country skiing, rowing, swimming, and walking. Similar cardiorespiratory benefits are gained from each of these activities as long as the intensity, duration, and frequency of each is the same and basic training principles are followed. According to a survey by the National Sporting Goods Association, the most popular mode of exercise in the USA is walking (64.4 million participants), with swimming ranked second (61.4 million).

molybdenum
An essential mineral used in iron metabolism, and needed for normal growth and development. Because deficiency is not known, there is no Recommended Daily Amount (RDA) but the UK and USA estimated safe and adequate daily intake is 0.15–0.5 mg. Cereal crops and meat are good sources. High intakes may disturb copper metabolism and cause gout-like symptoms.

monosaccharide (single sugar)
A crystalline, sweet-tasting, very soluble carbohydrate consisting of a single chain or ring structure. Fructose, glucose, and galactose are monosaccharides. They are the end-products of the digestion of complex carbohydrates (e.g. starches), and disaccharides (e.g. milk sugar and table sugar). Monosaccharides are absorbed through the intestinal wall and carried in the bloodstream to tissues where they may be stored or used as an energy source.

monosodium glutamate (MSG)
A white crystalline substance added to food to enhance its taste. It was originally extracted from the seaweed, *Laminaria*

japonica. Some people may be allergic to MSG. It has a high sodium content and may contribute to hypertension in sodium-sensitive individuals. *See also* **Chinese restaurant syndrome**.

monounsaturated fat
Fat not fully saturated with hydrogen; that is, each molecule contains at least one pair of carbon atoms connected by a double bond. Monounsaturated fats include oils from olives and peanuts. Olive oil, unlike a number of polyunsaturated fats, appears to decrease harmful low-density lipoproteins without reducing the beneficial high-density lipoproteins. Eating monounsaturated fats rather than saturated fats reduces the risk of heart disease.

mood swings
It is common knowledge that what you eat can affect how you feel and, conversely, that how you feel can affect what you eat. Many people feel depressed, agitated, and tense before eating carbohydrate-rich foods, but happy and relaxed afterwards. High protein, low carbohydrate diets are sometimes associated with feelings of depression and an intense craving for foods such as chocolate.

Until about 30 years ago, most nutritional scientists denied that mood can be affected by diet. They believed that the membrane separating the blood from the brain (the blood–brain barrier) effectively kept dietary chemicals out of the brain. More recent research has forced many of these scientists to change their mind. It has been demonstrated that certain chemicals, such as the amino acid tryptophan, can penetrate the blood–brain barrier and affect behaviour. Mood appears to be affected by a complex interaction between diet and other factors, including sex, hormone levels, time of day, and even time of month. After eating carbohydrates, men tend to become calmer and women sleepier. A high carbohydrate meal eaten for breakfast usually has less effect than the same meal taken at lunch. Women tend to have a keener desire for carbohydrates for the 10 days before menstruation than during the 10 days after.

Although most scientists now agree that diet can cause mood swings, they are still unsure about the precise mechanisms involved. As yet they are unable to predict with certainty the effects of specific types of food on the mood of a particular individual. *See also* **serotonin**.

motivation
High motivation is the key to success in any endeavour. It may come from within a person (intrinsic motivation) or from external influences (extrinsic motivation). For example, intrinsic motivation is derived from engaging in exercise for its own sake, for the satisfaction and the sheer enjoyment it brings, and for no external reason. Those who are intrinsically motivated give up less easily and generally achieve higher levels of fitness than those who are solely motivated by external rewards such as praise, money, and trophies.

The motivation to lose weight may also have intrinsic and extrinsic components: the dieter may get a great sense of well being from eating healthily (intrinsic motivation), or may be dieting mainly to acquire a body shape that gains praise and acceptability (extrinsic motivation).

Coaches and trainers recognize the importance of motivation and often adopt special strategies to improve or maintain it. Motivational strategies include providing competition; giving pep talks, praise and constructive criticism; and setting appropriate short-term goals (*see* **goal**). In order to train successfully, exercisers must have sufficient motivation to expend time and energy on their training and be able to endure a certain amount of fatigue, boredom, and discomfort. Many coaches adopt the attitude encapsulated in the phrase 'No pain, no gain!', but this should not be taken as an exhortation to overtrain and become injured or ill.

motivational strategies: *See* motivation.

MSG: *See* monosodium glutamate.

mud treatment: *See* body wraps.

multi-gym
A weight-training machine on which a number of different exercises can be

performed. The weights are confined within a fixed frame and travel on fixed guide bars. This makes multi-gyms very safe. The trainee can assume a starting position without having to support any weights; there is no fear of losing balance or of the weights slipping; and the weights can be released without danger at any time.

Multi-gyms are also simple and convenient to use. Multiple weights enable a trainee to vary resistance almost instantaneously, and it is easy to shift from one exercise to another. Since their introduction, multi-gyms have become very popular in sports clubs, fitness clubs, and even in the home. Because of their safety, simplicity, and convenience, they are especially valuable for the beginner. However, many experienced weight-lifters prefer free weights (barbells, dumbbells etc.) which allow them to perform complex movements. Free weights also allow a much greater variety of exercises than the multi-gym.

multi-poundage system

A type of weight training in which an exercise is performed in sets, with the weights being reduced in each set. Typically, for the first set the weight-trainee performs as many repetitions as possible using the 10 RM (the maximum load that can be lifted for 10 repetitions). In the second set, a weight (usually 5 kg) is removed from the bar and, after a rest, the weight-trainee again attempts as many repetitions as possible. The procedure is repeated for each set, removing the same weight each time.

multi-set system

System of weight training in which several different exercises, each with slightly different effects, are used to strengthen the same muscle group.

multi-weight sets: *See* descending sets.

mumie

A resin-based substance extracted from decaying vegetation within marine sediments, found on the shores of the Black Sea. It contains a number of biologically active chemicals, including salicylic acid (related to aspirin), copper, iron, and magnesium compounds. It was used in former times to treat a variety of ailments. Great claims have been made for its healing powers. It was used to treat radiation poisoning following the Chernobyl disaster. It has recently been introduced into the USA where it is rumoured that athletes are taking it to boost their performance and to accelerate recovery times. There is little evidence about its efficacy or safety.

muscle

There are three main types of muscle: cardiac (heart) muscle, smooth muscle, and striated (or skeletal) muscle. They all contain cells specialized for contraction. The cells convert chemical energy from food into mechanical energy, producing tension and movement.

Cardiac muscle is very odd in that it contracts rhythmically, even when removed from the body. This inherent rhythm is the basis of the heartbeat, variations of which are controlled by signals from nerves and hormones (e.g. adrenaline). Cardiac muscle is unique in never suffering fatigue. However, it will stop contracting if starved of oxygen or nutrients, or if the tissue fluid is of the wrong chemical composition.

Smooth muscle occurs in many parts of the body (e.g. gut and womb lining) where it produces slow, long-term contractions. Although smooth muscles usually contract involuntarily, it is possible to bring them under conscious control by training. Infants learn quite quickly (but probably never quickly enough for parents) to control the smooth muscle of the anal sphincter. Unfortunately, some people, especially elderly women, have great difficulty maintaining control of these sphincter muscles and suffer from incontinence. Special exercises (*see* **pelvic floor exercises**) can help to improve control.

Skeletal muscles are attached to bones (figures 42, 43, and 44). When they contract they pull bones closer together or enable parts of the body to resist external forces. They are responsible for locomotion and movements used in physical activities. Contractions are usually under conscious control, therefore the muscle is sometimes referred to as voluntary muscle. There are approximately 600 skeletal

Figure 42 Muscles: front view

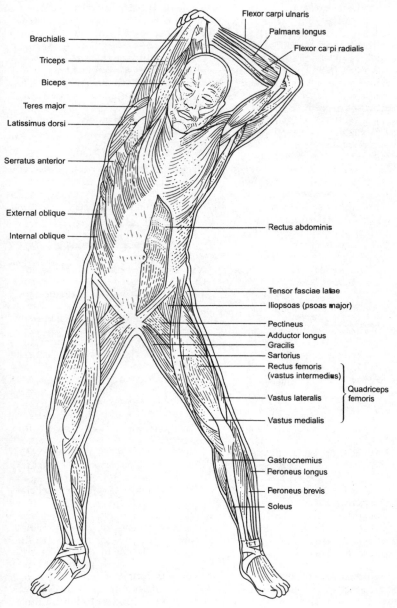

Brachialis

Triceps

Biceps

Teres major

Latissimus dorsi

Serratus anterior

External oblique

Internal oblique

Flexor carpi ulnaris

Palmans longus

Flexor carpi radialis

Rectus abdominis

Tensor fasciae latae

Iliopsoas (psoas major)

Pectineus

Adductor longus

Gracilis

Sartorius

Rectus femoris
(vastus intermedius)

Vastus lateralis

Vastus medialis

Quadriceps
femoris

Gastrocnemius

Peroneus longus

Peroneus brevis

Soleus

Figure 43 Muscles: side view

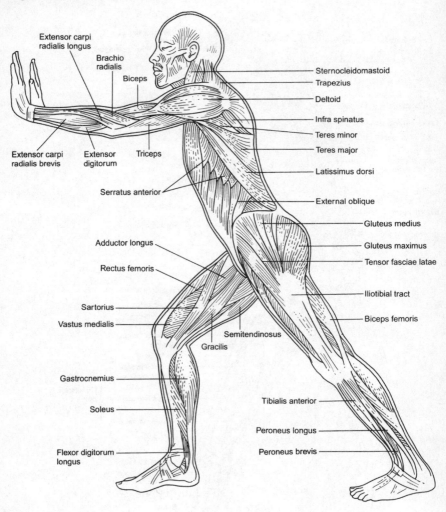

Extensor carpi radialis longus
Brachio radialis
Biceps
Extensor carpi radialis brevis
Extensor digitorum
Triceps
Serratus anterior
Adductor longus
Rectus femoris
Sartorius
Vastus medialis
Gracilis
Semitendinosus
Gastrocnemius
Soleus
Flexor digitorum longus

Sternocleidomastoid
Trapezius
Deltoid
Infra spinatus
Teres minor
Teres major
Latissimus dorsi
External oblique
Gluteus medius
Gluteus maximus
Tensor fasciae latae
Iliotibial tract
Biceps femoris
Tibialis anterior
Peroneus longus
Peroneus brevis

muscles, each consisting of contractile muscle fibres wrapped in connective tissue, and supplied with blood vessels and nerve fibres. A muscle fibre is a cell with many nuclei. Under the microscope, it appears to consist of bands of light and dark fibres. Each muscle block comprises between 10 000 and 450 000 fibres. *See also* **muscle fibre types**.

muscle balance

When weight training, it is good to work muscles on both sides of a joint. This achieves muscle balance. It reduces the risk of injury and improves physical performance. Muscle balance in the upper arm, for example, is achieved by training both the biceps (flexors that straighten the elbow) and triceps

Figure 44 Muscles: back view

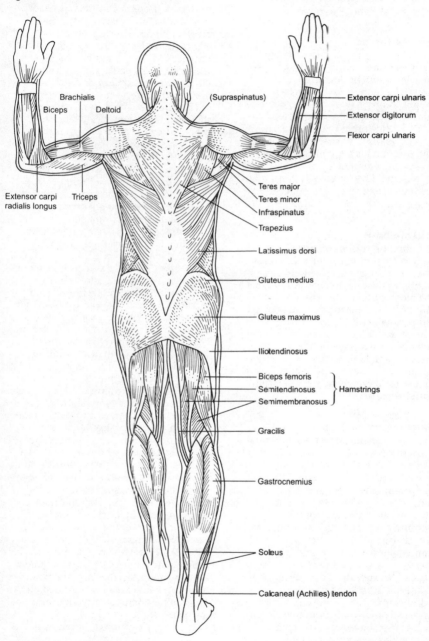

Brachialis

Biceps   Deltoid

(Supraspinatus)

Extensor carpi ulnaris

Extensor digitorum

Flexor carpi ulnaris

Extensor carpi
radialis longus   Triceps

Teres major

Teres minor

Infraspinatus

Trapezius

Latissimus dorsi

Gluteus medius

Gluteus maximus

Iliotendinosus

Biceps femoris

Semitendinosus

Semimembranosus

⎫
⎬ Hamstrings
⎭

Gracilis

Gastrocnemius

Soleus

Calcaneal (Achilles) tendon

(extensors that bend the elbow). *See also* **super-set system**.

muscle-bound

A colloquial term used pejoratively to describe someone with well-developed muscles which limit the range of movement. The term is often associated with weight training. Although large muscles and their tendons can restrict joint movement, the idea that weight training always results in a person becoming muscle-bound is a myth. The risk of muscle bulk developing at the expense of joint mobility occurs only with high-resistance, low repetition exercises that do not incorporate stretching.

muscle bulk

The absolute volume of muscle in the body. A large muscle bulk is advantageous in contact sports both to give protection against opponents and to provide the momentum to dislodge opponents. Muscle bulk tends to decrease with age, but regular aerobic exercise delays this degeneration. It also decreases with inactivity (*see* **atrophy**). Unlike fatty tissue, muscle has a high metabolic activity and people with a large muscle bulk have a higher basal metabolic rate than those with low muscle bulk.

muscle contraction

The electrochemical process of generating tension within a muscle. You would be forgiven for thinking that when a muscle contracts it shortens. This does happen in some types of contraction (concentric contractions), but muscles can also lengthen during a contraction (eccentric contractions), or stay the same length (isometric contractions). Consequently, many exercise physiologists prefer to use the phrase 'muscle action', because this does not imply a change in muscle length.

Concentric contractions occur when a muscle develops sufficient muscle tension to overcome a resistance. The muscle shortens visibly to move a body part. Concentric contractions may be isokinetic or isotonic.

During isokinetic contractions a muscle shortens at constant speed (or constant angular velocity) over the full range of motion. During a full isokinetic contraction, the tension developed by a muscle is at its maximum throughout its whole range. To perform a controlled isokinetic contraction, special equipment is needed which contains a speed governor so that the speed of movement is constant no matter how much tension is produced by the contracting muscle. Training that uses isokinetic contractions is thought to increase the blood supply to skeletal and cardiac muscle, and therefore it improves muscle strength, endurance, and cardiac fitness. Because high muscle tensions are exerted at each phase of movement, isokinetic contractions strengthen the whole muscle. In addition, isokinetic exercises can be designed to mimic the actual speeds of sports-specific activities. This is thought to improve neuromuscular coordination so that more muscle fibres can be recruited and muscles can contract more efficiently. The major disadvantages of isokinetic exercises are that they can only be performed properly on machines which are usually expensive, and the types of movement that can be performed are rather limited.

Isotonic contractions are the most common type of contraction (figure 48). The muscle changes length and takes a joint through a specific range of motion against a fixed resistance; the muscle may shorten (concentric contraction) or lengthen (eccentric contraction). Isotonic exercises often involve raising and lowering a weight. The speed of movement is controlled by the exerciser but the load remains constant. Isotonic exercises are good for developing strength and cardiovascular endurance. Unfortunately, the efficiency of joints vary with joint angles; consequently, unlike isokinetic contractions, a fixed resistance may not provide a sufficient workload over the complete range of motion to give maximum training benefits.

An eccentric contraction causes a muscle to lengthen under tension. Such contractions are used to resist external forces such as gravity. The quadriceps

Figure 45 Muscle contraction

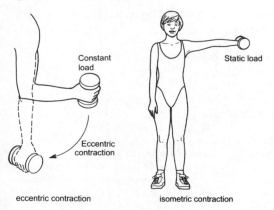
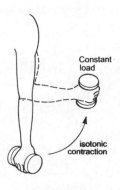

eccentric contraction   isometric contraction   Isotonic contraction

muscles, for example, undergo eccentric contractions when a person walks down steps, runs downhill, or lowers a weight. Eccentric contractions also occur during the deceleration phases of running.

Training in which eccentric contractions predominate tends to cause significantly greater muscle soreness than other forms of training, though it may protect against future muscle soreness. Strong muscle fibres may replace weak ones, and neuromuscular coordination improve, so that forces are distributed more effectively. To get the maximum benefit from weight training using eccentric contractions, the weights must be lowered slowly and in a controlled manner.

Isometric contractions are static contractions during which muscle fibres do not change length. There is no movement of the joint to which the muscle is attached but energy is expended resisting a force that does not move. Isometric contractions occur when a rugby front row forward pushes against opponents in a static scrum, when American footballers perform a block tackle, or when a weightlifter holds a barbell above his head for a few seconds.

Exercises involving isometric contractions are good for developing strength, but poor for developing cardiovascular fitness. People suffering from cardiovascular disease (e.g. high blood pressure)

are advised not to do them (see also **isometrics**).

muscle fibre types

Top athletes should be careful in their choice of parents. Their ability to compete in a sprint or marathon may be determined more by the type of muscle fibre they inherit than by the training they do. Muscle fibres are multinucleated cells responsible for muscle contractions. Each muscle has between 10 000 and 450 000 fibres. There are two main types that can be distinguished by their colour. Red muscle fibres (also called Type 1 or slow-twitch fibres) acquire their colour from their good blood supply and high myoglobin content. They fatigue slowly, and use glycogen and fat as their fuels. White muscle fibres (also called Type 2 or fast-twitch fibres) have a more moderate blood supply, only use glycogen as fuel, and fatigue more quickly than the red fibres. However, they are bigger than the red fibres and their contractions are much more powerful. Red muscle fibres are adapted for aerobic activities of long duration. White fibres are adapted for short bursts of explosive anaerobic activity. Human muscle has a mixture of fibre types, but endurance athletes have a preponderance of red, slow-twitch fibres while sprinters have a preponderance of white, fast-twitch fibres. as the following table* shows:

AVERAGE % COMPOSITION OF FIBRE TYPE IN THE GASTROCNEMIUS MUSCLES OF ELITE ATHLETES

ATHLETE	PERCENTAGE OF FIBRES	
	WHITE (SLOW-TWITCH)	RED (FAST-TWITCH)
sprinter	24	76
middle-distance runner	52	48
marathon runner	79	21

*Data from Costill, D.L., *et al.* (1976) Skeletal muscle enzymes and fiber composition in male and female track athletes. *Journal of Applied Physiology.* **40**:149–54.

Although the proportion of the main fibre types is largely inherited, there is some evidence that a small proportion of white fibres might be converted into red fibres by endurance training, and total inactivity may result in a decrease of red muscle fibres. The situation is complicated by the fact that there are at least two types of fast-twitch fibre, one of which has properties intermediate between red and white muscle fibres. This is called a fast-twitch oxidative fibre. It is thought that endurance training results in the conversion of some of the extreme type of white fibre (called fast-twitch glycolytic fibre) into the intermediate type, enabling speed to be sustained for longer periods.

There appears to be a relation between fibre type and body shape, at least in men: slim men tend to have a higher proportion of red muscle fibres than obese men. Red muscle fibres burn up more fat than white fibres. Therefore, if fibre type is largely inherited, it may explain why some people are genetically predisposed to become fat whilst others are predisposed to slimness. Since white fibres fatigue more quickly than red fibres, it may also explain why some obese people find it more difficult to take exercise.

muscle glycogen loading: *See* carbohydrate loading.

muscle group
All the muscles that cause movement at a particular joint when the muscles shorten (i.e. contract concentrically). Thus, all elbow flexors cause the arm to bend. Some muscles which can cause different types of movements belong to more than one muscle group.

muscle growth
Muscles get bigger mainly by an increase in the size of individual muscle fibres (hypertrophy). However, there is a growing body of evidence to suggest that growth may also result from an increase in the number of fibres (hyperplasia). Animal experiments have shown that regular, intense resistance exercises can cause fibres to split longitudinally. This fibre splitting is also thought to occur during high-resistance weight training in humans, but it has not been demonstrated conclusively. *See also* **pumping-up**.

muscle hernia: *See* fascial hernia.

muscle poops: *See* fascial hernia.

muscle pull: *See* muscle strain.

muscle pumping: *See* pumping-up.

muscle soreness
The muscles of exercisers often become sore. There are two main types of muscle soreness: acute muscle soreness and delayed onset muscle soreness.

Acute muscle soreness develops during and immediately after exercise. It is thought to be due to an inadequate blood flow to active muscle, resulting in the accumulation of metabolic waste products such as lactic acid.

Delayed onset muscle soreness (DOMS) develops one or two days after the completion of exercise. The discomfort associated with DOMS may be due to torn muscle fibres or muscle spasms but is most likely to be due to disruption of the connective tissue. DOMS is usually accompanied by increased levels of hydroxyproline in the urine.

Hydroxyproline is a chemical similar to an amino acid and is found only in connective tissue. Its presence in the urine is, therefore, an indication of tissue damage.

DOMS typically affects those who only exercise occasionally or who perform strenuous exercises to which they are unaccustomed. It is greatest following activities that use mainly eccentric contractions in which the muscle lengthens (such as running downhill). Treatment consists of rest and nonsteroidal anti-inflammatory drugs (NSAIDS), such as aspirin or ibuprofen, to relieve the pain. The degree of muscle soreness is correlated to the amount of tissue damage. Therefore, the greater the muscle soreness after an activity, the longer the recovery time required. Slight discomfort may require only a few extra days rest, but severe pain that makes walking difficult may require a month or more of reduced training. Of course, if symptoms persist, medical advice should be sought.

muscle strain (muscle pull)
An injury in which a muscle is damaged by being excessively stretched or overworked. It may result from a direct impact that pushes the muscle against an underlying bone. However, many muscle strains in sport are distraction strains, which occur when a muscle accidentally contracts as it is being stretched. They are relatively common in those who attempt to do vigorous exercise without a sufficient warm-up, or in those suffering fatigue and impaired reflexes. The strains may be slight, causing little discomfort and swelling (first degree strain); they may be quite painful but with no muscle tear (second degree strain); or they be very painful and involve a complete tearing of the muscle when the muscle is stretched beyond its tolerance levels (third degree strain, or distraction rupture). Muscle tears most commonly affect muscles that span two joints. For example, contractions of the hamstring cause the knee and hip to move in opposing directions, normally at different times but if both actions occur simultaneously there is a high risk of a muscle tear. *See also* **muscle soreness**.

muscle strength: *See* strength.

muscle tear: *See* muscle strain.

muscle triglyceride
Fat stored in muscle. Fatty acids and glycerol carried to the muscle by the bloodstream are either metabolized (mainly to release its energy), or recombined to make triglycerides, which are stored. Each triglyceride molecule consists of glycerol bound to three fatty acid chains. Recent evidence shows that muscle triglycerides are an important source of energy during prolonged endurance activities, sparing muscle glycogen. Regular aerobic exercise increases the stores of muscle triglycerides.

mycoprotein
A protein produced by fungi. One particular fungus, a mould called *Fusarium graminearum*, has been the source of a new type of protein-rich food that goes under the trade name of Quorn. It was first approved for food use in the UK in 1984. The mould is fermented for about six weeks after which the resultant liquid is filtered off and the mycelium heat treated. Flavours and colourings are added, along with a little egg albumen to bind the protein, to form the edible mycoprotein. It is marketed as a versatile meat substitute. Quorn is low in fat and a good source of zinc and thiamin.

myocardial infarction: *See* heart attack.

myocarditis
Inflammation of the middle, muscular lining of the heart caused by a bacterial or viral infection. The immediate effects of the inflammation can be serious and may lead to heart failure, but full recovery is possible. The risk of contracting myocarditis during a viral infection, such as a cold, increases if you continue strenuous physical exertion. In the past, exercising during a bout of myocarditis was believed to be very dangerous and an important factor in the cause of sudden exercise-related deaths. Recent studies suggest that sudden cardiac death during the presence of viral myocarditis is a rare event. Nevertheless, it would be very foolish for anyone to test the latest opinion by exercising during a fever.

myoglobin

A red iron-containing protein present in muscle. It combines with oxygen to form oxymyoglobin which acts as a small oxygen store of about 10 millilitres per kilogram of muscle. This source of oxygen seems to be particularly important during intermittent bursts of activity. Oxygen is released during activity and the oxymyoglobin restored during recovery periods. Muscle rich in myoglobin is sometimes called red muscle. It has a preponderance of slow-twitch muscle fibres and is adapted to endurance activities.

N

"I really hate exercise for exercise's sake. It is no disgrace if some people prefer their exercise vicariously. There is a tendency with television for people to just sit there with feet up, eating pretzels, and drinking and that is their participation in sport. I don't think that is bad."
Richard Nixon, former President of the United States. Quoted in (1979) *The book of sports quotes.* Omnibus Press.

narcotic

A drug which when swallowed, inhaled, or injected induces stupor, sleep, and insensibility. Most narcotics are derived from opium, the dried latex of the poppy, *Papaver somniferum*. Some narcotics, especially morphine and its derivatives, are used in medicine to control moderate to severe pain. However, most have severe side-effects: for example, high doses can reduce breathing movements to the point of asphyxiation. In addition, narcotic use carries a high risk of physical and psychological dependence.

Narcotics have been used as analgesics (painkillers) in sport, enabling athletes to continue to compete with injuries that otherwise would be incapacitating. There is also evidence that some athletes use them to induce a sense of euphoria and reduce feelings of fatigue. The International Olympic Committee has banned their use. Its list of banned substances includes codeine which, in the UK, is readily available in over-the-counter cough and cold medicines.

The human body produces its own natural narcotics, encephalins and endorphins. These have pain-relieving effects very similar to those of morphine and they also induce a sense of euphoria (*see* **runner's high**).

neck extension exercise

An isometric exercise that strengthens the head and neck extensor muscles (figure 46).
■ Place your hands on the back of your neck. Keep your neck straight and attempt to push your head backwards while resisting the movement with your hands. Hold for a few seconds, then relax.

neck flexion

An isometric exercise that strengthens the neck flexors (figure 46).
■ Place your hands on your forehead. Try to bend your neck forwards while resisting the movement with your hands. Hold for a few seconds, then relax.

neck flexion and extension

A weight-training exercise that strengthens the neck muscles (figure 46).

Figure 46 Neck extension and flexion

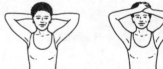

Neck Extension   Neck flexion

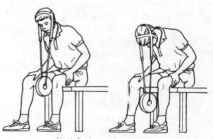

Neck flexion and extension

■ Sit with your hands on thighs and hold your body firm. With weights attached to a neck harness, use your neck muscles to lift and lower the weights slowly.

neck rotation exercise

An exercise that strengthens and stretches the neck rotators, and relieves stiffness. It is important to perform the exercise with the head and neck in good axial alignment.

■ Place the palm of your right hand against your right cheek, with your fingers pointing backwards and your elbow pointing forwards. Try to turn your head towards the right while resisting with your right hand. Hold for 6–10 seconds. Relax and, without straining, turn your head towards the left as far as possible. Hold for about 6 seconds then repeat on the other side.

neck shrugging

A very simple exercise for stretching the upper body, particularly the neck muscles.

■ Stand upright and relaxed with your hands on your hips. Turn your head slowly to one side, hold, and then turn it to the other side whilst shrugging your shoulders. After these sideways movements, slowly lower your head onto your chest. Hold for a few seconds, then, again slowly, raise your head so that your chin is in the air.

During the exercise, you should feel the neck muscles being stretched, but be careful not to overstretch them.

neck stretches

Two simple exercises for neck muscles.

■ To warm up the rotator muscles, gently and slowly turn your head to one side until you can feel a resistance; hold for 10 seconds, then turn to the opposite side and repeat. Do not force the movements; keep them slow and smooth. To warm up the lateral flexors, place your left arm behind your back and grasp it around the wrist with your right hand. Tilt your head to the left and gently pull your left arm. Hold for about 10 seconds and repeat on the other side.

This exercise also warms up the trapezius muscle, the large triangular muscle in the upper back.

negative calories

There is a theory that the process of eating some foods, such as celery, uses more energy than the food contains. Such foods are said to have negative calories. It is true that these foods have few calories (mainly because of their high water content), and that there is an energy cost to chewing and digestion. However, the amounts of energy involved are very small and have no significant effect on weight control or loss.

negative-change goal

A lifestyle goal that emphasizes *not* doing something. Psychologists generally recommend replacing negative-change goals with positive ones. Negative-change goals are common in dieting. For example, overweight people often try *not* to eat fattening things such as cheese snacks (negative-change goal). They are more likely to lose weight if they try to eat fruit at snack times (positive-change goal).

negative-resistance training

Weight training in which muscles contract eccentrically. That is, the muscles lengthen while still under tension. Lowering a barbell, bending down, running downhill, are all examples of negative-resistance training. Many bodybuilders use this type of training because it is reputed to increase muscle size more quickly than other types. They usually recruit training partners to lift the weights in position so that they can concentrate on lowering the weights. *See also* **muscle contraction**.

negative sit-up test

A simple test of abdominal strength.

■ Sit down with your knees bent, hands on the top of your head, and feet flat on the floor. Slowly lower yourself backwards halfway to the floor. Time how long you can hold the position in reasonable comfort: 25 seconds or more is excellent; 15–24 seconds, good; 5–14 seconds, fair; less than 5 seconds, poor.

neohesperidine

A sweetener derived from orange peel used, for example, in some Belgian beers and chewing gum. It has a liquorice flavour which gives it a lingering aftertaste.

nephrolithiasis: *See* kidney stones.

netball
Netball is an energetic game requiring high speed changes in direction and good ball handling skills. It is played mainly by women, among whom it is the most popular sport in Australia, but it is also played recreationally by men. Competitive players require high levels of agility, endurance, and speed, and moderate levels of strength and flexibility. Training often includes running and agility practice (e.g. doing shuttle sprints, dodging around a series of cones). The quick changes of direction, and landing from jumps, impose considerable strain on the feet and legs. Players should wear shoes specially designed to meet these demands. In particular, the shoe should provide good cushioning of the ball of the foot.

neutral fat: *See* fat.

niacin (nicotinamide; nicotinic acid; vitamin B₃)
A water-soluble nutrient belonging to the vitamin B complex. Like other B vitamins, niacin plays an important role in carbohydrate metabolism. It is also indispensable for fat and protein metabolism, and inhibits cholesterol synthesis.

The link between niacin (specifically nicotinic acid) and cholesterol reduction was first made by Dr R. Altschul in 1955, but it was brought to public attention in 1990 by Robert Kowalski in his book entitled *The 8-week cholesterol cure*. As a result, some people have taken excessive amounts of niacin in the belief that it will protect against high blood cholesterol levels. This practice is potentially dangerous. High doses (greater than 500 mg per day), or slow-release preparations of niacin which elevate blood concentrations for a long time, can lead to irreversible liver damage. Large doses of niacin can also decrease fat mobilization and the ability to do physical work.

Although the precise amount varies depending on energy expenditure, approximately 20 milligrams of niacin are needed per day. The body stores very little. It can synthesize niacin from the amino acid tryptophan. This synthesis may be enough to meet the daily requirement, but niacin can also be obtained from foods such as meat, fish, brown rice, beans, and yeast extract (the richest source, with as much as 67 mg per 100 g). Deficiency can result in a disease called pellagra, early symptoms of which include muscular weakness, general fatigue, loss of appetite, indigestion, and minor skin complaints. Pellagra is unlikely to occur in individuals who eat a balanced diet.

nicotinamide: *See* niacin.

nicotine
A drug that acts as a stimulant on the central nervous system. *See also* **smoking**.

nicotinic acid: *See* niacin.

Nieder press
An advanced weight-training exercise named after Bill Nieder, a famous American shot-putter, who used it to improve his upper body strength.
■ Hold the barbell at the shoulders. Vigorously thrust the barbell directly forwards by extending your arms, then immediately return the barbell to your shoulders. You may have to lean back a little to maintain balance as you thrust the barbell forwards.

nitrates
Nitrogen-containing ions (electrically charged atoms) that occur naturally in soils. Soil nitrates are essential for plant growth and levels are increased by artificial fertilizers. Unfortunately, about half the nitrate leaches out into the groundwater and, after a delay of up to 30 years, this nitrate can find its way into public water supplies. After drinking the water, the nitrate may be converted to nitrite by bacteria in the mouth. Once absorbed into the bloodstream, the nitrites can combine with haemoglobin to form a blue pigment, methaemoglobin. The presence of methaemoglobin in the blood reduces its ability to carry oxygen. This can be particularly serious in babies, causing the life threatening 'blue

baby syndrome'. In the UK, nitrate levels in drinking water are monitored. The public are advised (e.g. to give babies bottled water, low in nitrates) when safe levels are exceeded. Nitrate and nitrites are present in small amounts in living animal and plant tissue. Their concentration is significantly higher in preserved cured meats (e.g. bacon and hot dogs) in which they are used to prevent bacterial infections. Nitrates and nitrites have been found to promote cancers of the oesophagus and stomach in laboratory animals, possibly by being converted to carcinogenic nitrosamines. However, the evidence that nitrates cause human cancer is weak and inconclusive. Nevertheless, if nitrates are carcinogenic in humans, vitamin C may offer some protection by inhibiting the conversion of nitrates or nitrites to nitrosamines.

nitrites: *See* nitrates.

nitrosamine
A compound (e.g. dimethylnitrosamine) formed by the combination of amines and nitrates or nitrites. This conversion can occur in an acid environment such as the stomach. Nitrosamines have been found to be carcinogenic in laboratory animals. *See also* nitrates.

non-insulin-dependent diabetes: *See* diabetes.

non-haem iron
Iron not contained within the red blood pigment haemoglobin, myoglobin, and cytochromes. Non-haem iron, commonly referred to as inorganic iron, makes up all the iron in eggs, plants, and dairy products, and up to 60 per cent of the iron in animal tissue. It is not as good a dietary source of iron as that contained within haemoglobin because it is not so readily absorbed. However, vitamin C increases the absorption of non-haem iron considerably. *See also* iron.

non-starch polysaccharide
A term used by nutritionists in the UK for the most easily measured and most precisely defined form of non-digestible food. The term is used in dietary guidelines in preference to dietary fibre, which is an ill-defined term and includes a range of different chemical components, with different effects on the body. The numerical value of non-starch polysaccharide is always lower than that of dietary fibre (by about two-thirds). *See also* **fibre**.

non-steroidal anti-inflammatory drug (NSAID)
A drug, such as aspirin, that reduces the swelling and pain associated with an injury, but which is not related to the steroid group of drugs.

'no pain, no gain'
A phrase which encapsulates the idea that an exerciser must work hard and feel discomfort in order to improve physical fitness. In moderation, this exhortation might be a useful motivation since, for any training benefit to occur, the effort exerted during exercise must be greater than that used during normal, daily activities (*see* **overload principle**). However, the concept is sometimes taken to extremes, and a person may be encouraged to exercise beyond normal limits of tolerance, producing new injuries or aggravating pre-existing ones. A wise exerciser will listen to his or her body, and learn to distinguish between the symptoms indicating harmful overtraining and those which are the natural result of beneficial exertion. *See also* **stretch stress**.

noradrenaline (norepinephrine)
A stimulant drug banned by the International Olympic Committee. It is a hormone secreted by the adrenal gland, and a neurotransmitter, secreted by nerve endings.

norepinephrine: *See* noradrenaline.

normal active range: *See* range of movement.

NOS: *See* eating disorder not otherwise specified.

NSAID: *See* non-steroidal anti-inflammatory drug.

nutrient
A substance present in food and used by the body to promote normal growth,

maintenance, and repair. The major nutrients needed to maintain health are carbohydrates, fats, proteins, minerals, vitamins, and water. Roughage (fibre), although not assimilated into the body and therefore not a nutrient, is also regarded as an essential component of a balanced diet.

nutrient density

The measurement of the amount of carbohydrates, fats, proteins, minerals, and vitamins per 100 kilocalories of a food. A distinction is usually made between energy nutrients (carbohydrates and fats) and the other essential nutrients. Therefore, nutrient density is sometimes expressed as amount of vitamins and minerals (and sometimes proteins) per unit of energy. Foods high in energy often contain a low density of most of the other essential nutrients (*see* **junk food**). Those who follow a low calorie diet should try to consume foods with a high nutrient density.

Nutron diet

A food intolerance diet devised by Dr Patrick Kingsley and Ian Stoakes. Before taking the diet, you have a blood test to find out if you are intolerant to any of about 100 common foods. After the blood test you are given a personal diet plan. The main tenet of the diet is that people can become overweight because of excess water retention associated with the food intolerance. If foods to which an overweight person is intolerant are eliminated, then fluid is no longer retained and weight is lost. Although 15 000 doctors in the UK are willing to carry out blood tests for people who wish to take the Nutron diet, the theory of food intolerance as described by Dr Kingsley is not accepted by the medical profession as a whole. You might lose weight on this diet but it may not be because of the reasons given by Patrick Kingsley and Ian Stoakes. The diet restricts the choice of foods and you are advised to cut out alcohol for a month. This will probably reduce overall energy (calorie) intake.

O

"I'm fat, but I'm thin inside. Has it ever struck you that there's a thin man inside every fat man . . ."

George Orwell, in (1939) *Coming up for air.*

obesity

Obesity is due to the excessive storage of fat in the body, particularly under the skin and around certain internal organs. In 1985, 34 million Americans were obese. Of British adults surveyed in 1991, 13 per cent of men and 15 per cent of women were obese; double the percentage of people who were obese in 1981. A 1995 survey indicates that these figures are continuing to rise. Obesity can be caused by diseases, such as certain cancers, gall-bladder diseases, and hormonal imbalances, but these causes are rare. Many obese people suggest that their condition is due to underactive thyroid glands, but this accounts for less than one in a thousand cases. Most obesity results from eating too much and not exercising enough. This results in a positive energy balance, more energy is consumed than expended. For every 3500 Calories consumed above requirements, approximately one pound of fat is stored in the body.

Obesity is difficult to define quantitatively without knowing how much fat is normal for a given person. Nevertheless, it is generally agreed that the proportion of fat in the body should not exceed 20–25 per cent in men and 28–30 per cent in women. Many medical authorities use body mass as an indicator (*see* **body mass index**); people with a body mass index exceeding 30 are considered obese. However, obesity is not the same as being overweight. A very muscular person may be heavy but still have a very low fat content. Heavy body-builders often have less than 10 per cent body fat. There are two main types of obesity: childhood onset obesity and adult onset obesity.

Childhood onset obesity may develop

because of hormonal imbalances or some other illness, but it is usually caused by overeating when young. This results in the production of an abnormally high number of adipocytes, cells specialized for fat storage. Adults who were obese as children tend to retain a high number of adipocytes, even if they are thin and have a low fat diet. The high number of adipocytes means that a large storage space is always available for fat. Thus adults who suffered childhood onset obesity are generally predisposed to obesity.

Adult onset obesity occurs when a person becomes obese for the first time after reaching adulthood. He or she usually has a normal number of adipocytes but each one is enlarged with fat. Slimming leads to the fat cells returning to normal size. Adults who have suffered adult onset obesity usually find it much easier to control their weight than adults who were obese as children.

Obesity is a major health hazard. Obese people are predisposed to a number of diseases, including diabetes, high blood pressure, and cardiovascular diseases. Some medical experts suggest that life expectancy decreases by approximately 1 per cent for each pound of excess fat carried by an individual between the ages of 45 and 50.

obesity gene

Forty-five years ago a genetic defect was identified in mice which leads them to become morbidly obese. The gene concerned was called 'ob'. When functioning correctly, it instructs fat cells to secrete a hormone as they become inflated with fat. The hormone depresses appetite and increases metabolism. Mice with defective genes become obese. In 1994, scientists unravelled the genetic sequence of the ob gene. Since then the gene has been cloned and a genetically engineered ob protein manufactured. Fat mice have been made thin by daily injections of the protein. Humans are believed to have a gene similar to the ob gene of mice. The gene is for a protein hormone that somehow controls appetite on a long-term basis. Although lack of this gene explains obesity in mutant mice, there is no evidence that injections of the protein hormone will help treat human obesity.

A third of adults in the US are 20 per cent or more overweight. Huge amounts of money are spent on dieting and treatments for obesity. Biotechnology and pharmaceutical companies have been quick to realize the commercial possibilities of anti-fat drugs for human use. One biotechnology company (Amgen) is planning clinical trials of the ob protein on humans in 1996. If these prove to be both safe and effective, they will have an injectable 'cure' for fatness that could reap enormous rewards. However, those suffering from obesity should guard against premature optimism. There is an enormous leap from something that works on obese mice to something that works on people. It has been estimated that less than 25 per cent of human obesity is due to genetic problems; most is probably due to inactivity and eating high-fat food.

OBLA: *See* **lactic acid.**

octacosanol
An alcohol found in wheatgerm oil. It is taken by athletes as a performance enhancer in the belief that it improves endurance. There is no unequivocal, scientific evidence to support this belief.

oesophagitis
Inflammation of the oesophagus usually caused by regurgitating acidic contents of the stomach. Regurgitation may occur if the sphincter muscle between the oesophagus and stomach cannot close tightly enough, or if there is a hiatus hernia in which the top of the stomach protrudes into the thoracic cavity. The oesophagus has little protection against stomach acids which irritate and inflame

its lining, causing pain behind the breastbone similar to that associated with some heart conditions. The pain is usually relieved by taking antacids. Sufferers should reduce their intake of fatty foods, refrain from smoking, and moderate their alcohol intake. However, effective treatment requires first identifying and then dealing with the underlying cause.

oestrogen
A steroid, sex hormone produced by the ovary, the placenta and, in small amounts, by the male testis and adrenal cortex. Oestrogen causes the development of secondary sexual characteristics (e.g. breasts) in adolescent girls, and is involved in repairing the uterine wall after menstruation. Oestrogen also plays a role in calcium uptake and balance. Lack of oestrogen in post-menopausal women results in demineralization of bones, a major cause of fractures in the elderly (*see* **osteoporosis**). Oestrogen hormone replacement therapy for postmenopausal women is effective in slowing down osteoporosis.

Synthetic oestrogens are major constituents of many contraceptive pills. Excessively high levels can cause nausea, vomiting, irregular vaginal bleeding in women, and feminization (development of female secondary sexual characteristics) in men. They may also be linked to certain cancers and an increased risk of deep vein thromboses. This is why oestrogen levels have been reduced or eliminated in most modern contraceptive pills.

There are alarming reports of high levels of oestrogen, or chemicals with very similar effects, in lakes and rivers used as sources of drinking water, and in hormone-rich dairy products. These chemicals may cause male alligators to develop tiny, useless penises, and fish to become sterile. Some scientists believe that they are responsible for the increased incidence of testicular, breast, and womb cancers, and the reduction of human male fertility.

In the mid 1980s, new oestrogen-like chemicals were discovered in human urine. The chemicals were derived from plants so they were called phytoestrogens. Soya bean products and some other tropical legumes are particularly rich sources. Phytoestrogens are so similar to oestrogens that they bind on to the same receptor sites but do not cause the same responses. Although research is in its early stages, it has been tentatively suggested that phytoestrogens may reduce the risk of breast cancer by preventing true oestrogens from attaching onto cells, diluting their impact, and protecting the body against too much exposure.

omega-3 fatty acids

A group of unsaturated fatty acids found in some fish oils and linseed oil. Omega–3 fatty acids may change the chemistry of blood, reducing the risk of heart disease. Consumption of foods with high levels of these fatty acids may be 'cardioprotective' because they help to lower blood cholesterol and prevent arteries from being clogged with cholesterol-rich plaques. It has been suggested that one oily-fish meal a week provides the same protection as three or more. Fish oil capsules containing omega-3 fatty acids are now on the market, but according to the American Medical Association, the capsules may not be as effective as eating fish and other oily seafood. It is possible that the fatty acids only work effectively with other components in fish that are absent from the capsules. Moreover, there is insufficient clinical research data to determine the proper dosage of the fish oils. *See also* **cholesterol**.

omnikinetic resistance machine

A machine with hydraulic cylinders offering a resistance that takes account of variations in the strength of the user. Resistance varies throughout the range of movement. It is high at the strongest points and low at the weakest points. The machines can offer resistance in both directions of a movement so that, for example, after pushing your arm up, you have to actively pull against a resistance to bring the arm down again. Training on such machines is sometimes called hydrafitness training. A typical workout lasts about 30 minutes and uses up to 400 calories. *See also* **variable resistance exercise**.

one food diets

One food diets may be based on grapefruit, egg, poultry, melon, banana, steak, beer, yogurt, rice, or some other food. Dieters are allowed to eat as much as they like of their chosen food, but other foods are either prohibited or severely restricted. The diet is usually supplemented with multi-vitamins and dieters are advised to drink plenty of fluid. The diets appear to be designed to reduce food intake by being boring. They generally do no harm (and no good) because they are so boring that dieters usually give up after a few days. Nevertheless, one food diets are potentially dangerous if taken for a long time. Despite supplementation, it is virtually impossible to obtain a proper balance of nutrients from one food.

onset of blood lactate accumulation: *See* **lactic acid**.

opiate

Any drug containing or derived from opium, the dried latex from unripe seeds of the oriental poppy, *Papaver somniferum*. Opiates include codeine and morphine. They are all banned by the International Olympic Committee because of their addictive and potentially harmful properties. *See also* **narcotic**.

opium: *See* **opiate**.

organic food

A term that has acquired the meaning of foods grown under natural conditions (without the use of inorganic fertilizers, pesticides, or herbicides; and either not processed, or processed without the use of additives). The term, when used on food labels, has no legal meaning. In some states of North America, it is used to indicate food grown in places where no pesticides are used, or that no chemicals are added to the feed and water given to the animals. According to the *Manual of nutrition*, a Ministry of Fisheries and Agriculture (UK) booklet, 'There is little difference between organic and non-organic produce in terms of nutritional value, which is largely determined by the species of plant or animal'. Advocates of organic food would dispute this statement.

orienteering

Orienteering was invented by a Swede, Major Ernst Killander, in 1918. Sometimes called 'cunning running', it combines the physical skills of cross-country running or skiing with the mental skills of route finding. Competitors set off at timed intervals and find their way around a course, using a map and compass, via a number of checkpoints. It is an excellent aerobic activity for the whole family and caters for a wide range of abilities. At the recreational level, mothers and fathers can be seen at local events carrying their infants in backpacks. However, orienteering can be extremely competitive. World championships have been staged since 1966. These demand very high levels of stamina and map reading. Elite orienteers are usually outstanding distance runners. Training and competing regularly over rough terrain tends to reduce flexibility and muscle strength, and reduce maximum running speed. Hence, elite orienteers often incorporate circuit training and interval running into their training schedules.

In recent years, orienteering has gained notoriety because of a number of sudden deaths among young participants. In 1993, Sweden withdrew its ski orienteers from an international meeting following the deaths of seven young athletes from sudden heart failure. The Swedish federation also banned intensive training for both foot and ski orienteering because of evidence that vigorous exercise during a respiratory infection can cause death. Doctors at Uppsala hospital conducted an investigation which suggested that a bacterium called TWAR (Taiwan Acute Respiratory Infection) or a related microorganism was responsible; it causes inflammation of the heart, disrupting normal heartbeat.

orotic acid

A water-soluble substance often found with the B complex vitamins. It was once known as vitamin B_{13}, but it is no longer regarded as a vitamin because it can be synthesized by the body. It plays a role in the metabolism of DNA and RNA, but no symptoms of deficiency have been reported.

orthostatic hypotension: *See* postural hypotension.

orthostatic proteinuria: *See* postural proteinuria.

orthotics

Custom-built devices, such as moulded insoles, which fit in a shoe to make foot motion more efficient, to reduce the risk of foot injury, or to correct certain anatomical imbalances that may lead to pain in the back, hips, knees, and feet.

Some international runners, cyclists, and skiers use orthotics to improve their performance. Many long-distance runners use soft inlays to reduce mechanical shock on the ball of the foot; semi-rigid orthotics are often used to relieve plantar fasciitis (inflammation of connective tissue on the sole of the foot). The use of orthotics to correct anatomical abnormalities of the bones or joints, is controversial. Misuse can result in a worsening of the condition, for example, if the orthotic device is not constructed correctly or not adjusted in response to any growth changes in the anatomical structure.

Osgood-Schlatter's disease

A relatively common overuse injury caused by chronic, repetitive stress to the attachment of the patellar tendon (the tendon between the knee bone and shin bone) on the bony outgrowth at the top of the shin bone. The injury commonly occurs in children who take part in sports such as skating, gymnastics, and football. These sports require a lot of knee bending and jumping and expose the bony outgrowth to great tensile stress. This may damage the cartilaginous growth zone (epiphyseal plate), causing it to separate from the surrounding bone. The condition usually heals spontaneously after rest, but it may lead to permanent damage if the sufferer does not rest; activity may have to be restricted for several months. Occasionally surgical treatment is required.

osteitis pubis: *See* groin pain.

osteoarthritis

Osteoarthritis is a degenerative disease of the cartilage overlying bone within a joint. It may progress into the bone itself, causing pain and stiffness. Although osteoarthritis affects some children, it is more common in the elderly. It results in more than 50 000 hip and knee replacements each year in the UK. Its development is associated with obesity, low bone density, abnormalities in the structure of the joint, and repeated mechanical stress. However, a comparison of the incidence of osteoarthritis in pairs of identical twins and non-identical twins, indicates that between 39–65 per cent of the disease is genetically determined.

The relationship between exercise and osteoarthritis is complex. In some cases, the wear and tear incurred during exercise may accelerate degeneration. This is particularly likely if people are genetically predisposed to osteoarthritis, or are already suffering from a joint defect and take part in activities, such as running, which impose high impact forces on the joints. However, there is no scientific evidence that people who are not genetically predisposed to the disease and who have normal joints are at risk of osteoarthritis because they exercise. On the contrary, many experts claim that exercise provides some protection against the development of osteoarthritis by helping to reduce body weight, improve muscle tone and strength, and increase flexibility. In addition, exercise stimulates the secretion of synovial fluid which lubricates and nourishes the joints. Non-weight-bearing exercise, especially swimming, is often promoted as treatment for mild forms of osteoarthritis. However, those suffering from joint disorders should avoid exercise which puts great stress on the joints.

Osteoarthritis can be kept under control for many years by proper treatment which usually includes the use of analgesics.

osteophytes: *See* **footballer's ankle.**

osteoporosis (brittle bone disease)

A group of diseases characterized by a reduction in bone mass due to bone reabsorption outpacing bone deposition. The disease is usually associated with loss of weight. Other symptoms include feelings of lassitude, bone pains, and acute back pain. However, the most harmful effect of the disease is that bone becomes porous, brittle, and inclined to fracture. Over 250 000 Americans, most of them elderly, fall and break their hips each year, resulting in a $10 billion medical bill. Worldwide, the disease affects 1.7 million people each year. The number is expected to grow to over 6 million a year by 2050. A quarter of these people are expected to die within six months because of complications, usually linked to hip fractures.

Osteoporosis is an age-related disease, primarily affecting post-menopausal women, although it can occur much earlier in life (figure 47). There is always

Figure 47 Osteoporosis. Images such as these have been used by the National Osteoporosis Society (UK) to heighten awareness and to encourage women to take preventative measures

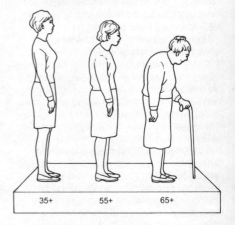

35+   55+   65+

some degree of bone weakening with age, but insufficient exercise and a low calcium diet (especially in early life) may exacerbate this. Excessive exercising and weight-loss dieting are also linked with development of the disease. Development of the disease may be determined to some extent by a single gene. A gene affecting Vitamin D metabolism has been found in Australians which may be responsible for more than 75 per cent of the genetic variation in their bone density. If this gene occurs in a broader population, it may not be long before genetic screening can be used to identify those who are predisposed to the disease, so that preventative measures can be taken.

Physical exercise reduces the risk of osteoporosis. Moderate weight-bearing exercises, such as leisurely cycling, dancing, walking, and tennis, stimulate the deposition of calcium, strengthen bones, and reduce the risk of osteoporosis. However, young people benefit most from exercise; strong and healthy bones are more easily established in adolescents and young adults. A modest amount of jumping (as little as 50 jumps a day) can increase the density of hips in pre-menopausal women by as much as 3 per cent. Although exercise may offer some protection against acquiring the disease, those already suffering from osteoporosis should avoid contact sports and exercise that put undue stress on bones and joints. In particular, flexion exercises of the spine (e.g. sit ups) should be avoided because of the risk of vertebral fractures. Swimming is an especially good exercise for those with the disease.

Slightly overweight post-menopausal women are less likely to suffer from brittle bones than slim women. Possible reasons are that fat acts as a protective cushion; bones of plump women may be heavier and stronger; and the extra fat of plumper women enables them to produce more oestrogen which offers some protection against demineralization of bones.

A diet that includes a good intake of calcium-rich food (e.g. milk, yogurt, and cheese) may help prevent and minimize problems associated with this disease. It appears that it is particularly important for pre-menopausal women to have adequate calcium intakes so that they can achieve maximum peak bone densities. At present, the UK Reference Nutrient Intake is thought by The National Osteoporosis Society (UK) to be too low. They recommend the following calcium intakes:

- children 7–12 years   800 mg per day
- teenagers/adults   1000 mg per day
- women over 45
  (not on HRT)   1500 mg per day
- women over 45
  (on HRT)   1000 mg per day
- pregnant and
  lactating teenagers   1500 mg per day

- pregnant and
  lactating adults   1200 mg per day
- men over 45 years   1500 mg per day

Some doctors believe that the best way to prevent osteoporosis in post-menopausal women is hormone replacement therapy (see **menopause**), but this treatment is not suitable for all women. *See also* **amenorrhoea** and **parathyroid hormone**.

os trigonum

A small bone behind the ankle. It is present in only about 7 per cent of the population. The bone develops as an extension of the ankle bone and then becomes detached. It usually causes no problems except during exercises, such as repeated, energetic bounding movements, common in ballet and gymnastics. The bone can then become squeezed between the ankle bone and the shin bone, causing pain and damaging the surrounding tissue. Surgical removal may then be necessary.

over distance training

Training over a distance greater than the competitive distance, but slower than race pace. Over distance training is believed to improve fat metabolism, enabling a competitor to use fat stores more efficiently during competition.

overload principle

A fundamental training principle which states that fitness improves only when workloads are greater than those normally encountered. The workload can be quantified in terms of training intensity (rate of doing work) or training volume (the total amount of work done). The principle applies to all aspects of fitness including strength, speed, and endurance of muscle contractions. It also applies to improvements in flexibility and the strength of bones, joints, and ligaments.

The overload principle is most easily demonstrated in weight training; the best results occur when a muscle performs at the maximal limits of its strength and endurance. *See also* **progression**.

overpronation: *See* pronation.

overreaching

A form of overtraining resulting from doing too much on one or two days.

Training fatigue occurs but this can be reversed by a slightly longer than normal period of rest. Overreaching is sometimes planned as part of a training programme. As long as it is followed by sufficient rest, it can stimulate the body to adapt to increased training loads. However, overreaching is often unplanned, and results in poor performance and feelings of frustration. Exercisers usually respond to these feelings by training even harder in order to improve. Unfortunately, the effects may be opposite to those intended. Without sufficient rest, overreaching can quickly degenerate into a chronic overtraining syndrome, difficult to reverse.

overstrain

An acute condition resulting from doing too much exercise on one occasion. Long distance runners, cross-country skiers, and others whose activities require excessively high energy outputs, often suffer from overstrain. *See also* **overreaching** and **overtraining**.

overtraining

Overtraining is a major concern to coaches and competitors. It is defined by experts at the British Olympic Medical Centre as prolonged fatigue and underperformance following a period of heavy training or competition lasting at least two weeks. It often occurs because of the false belief that, since training is a good thing, harder training must be better. In fact, the opposite is true. Beyond a certain optimum level of training, further increases in training intensity lead to poorer performances. More good athletes fail because they do too much training than too little. Overtraining is a particular problem for elite competitors, especially endurance athletes, who feel compelled to train up to their physiological limits to succeed. The signs and symptoms associated with overtraining are well documented by sports physicians. They include:

- intestinal disturbances
- decreased libido
- a persistent drop in quality or quantity of sleep
- persistent fatigue and loss of vigour
- decreased appetite

- rapid or persistent loss of body weight
- increased basal metabolic rate
- increased incidence of infections (e.g. mouth ulcers)
- slow healing of wounds and injuries
- increased resting pulse rate.

Some endurance athletes have very consistent resting pulse rates (usually less than 50 beats per minute) and if they experience increases of even two beats per minute they become concerned. However, overtraining can occur without a rise in resting heart rate.

Overtraining may also cause complex hormonal changes with a disturbance in the secretion of stress hormones (e.g. adrenaline) and a decrease in testosterone (male sex hormone) levels. If you respond to the occurrence of overtraining symptoms immediately by taking some rest, you can avoid its worse effects. However, if you ignore the symptoms and continue to train hard, you are likely to suffer from chronic overtraining. To recover completely from this, you may need to take weeks or months of rest.

overuse injury

An injury resulting from an imbalance between training and recovery. The mechanical stresses imposed by training damages tissues (especially muscles, tendons, and ligaments) at a rate faster than they can be repaired during the rest period. Internal factors contributing to overuse injuries include age, malalignments of joints, muscle imbalances, and inflexibility; external factors include errors in technique, poor equipment, poor environment, and overtraining. Overuse injuries range from those which cause mild pain during the activity only, to those which severely limit performance and produce chronic, unremitting pain. Overuse injuries are common in aerobic activities involving repetitive movements over a long period of time. Certain sites, such as the tendons of the shoulders, wrists, hips, knees, and ankles are particularly susceptible to overuse injuries. The injuries are usually quite easy to treat in the early stages with a combination of relative rest, ice, stretching, and progressive resistance exercises. If, however, a person continues to train with an overuse injury, it may become much more difficult to treat; anti-inflammatories and other more intrusive treatments, including surgery, may be needed to resolve the condition.

overweight
There is no universally agreed definition, but most people are considered overweight if they are 15–20 per cent greater than their ideal weight as determined by standard tables. These tables usually take into account age, height, build, and sex. Excess weight can put great strains on the body, particularly the joints in the legs and back. Although there is a connection between overweight and obesity, not all overweight people are obese. Muscle has a higher density than fat, so highly muscular people may be overweight but not obese. Conversely, a sedentary person with normal body weight could have a small muscle mass, large fat stores, and be suffering from obesity. *See also* **body mass index**.

oxalic acid
A naturally occurring chemical found in vegetables such as beetroot, spinach, and rhubarb. Oxalic acid also occurs in relatively high concentrations in tea, chocolate, and other cocoa products. It combines with calcium and magnesium in the gut to form insoluble salts which impede the absorption of these essential minerals. High concentrations of oxalic acid are toxic, which is why we do not eat rhubarb leaves (they contain very much more oxalic acid than the stems). Oxalic acid is also produced in the human body. About 5 per cent of the population suffer from recurrent kidney stones as a result of internal oxalic acid production.

oxygen
An odourless, colourless gas that makes up about one-fifth of the atmosphere. It is essential for survival. A person completely starved of oxygen would die after only a few minutes. Artificial supplies have been used to improve athletic performance and to aid recovery after exertion. However, routine administration of supplemental oxygen for brief periods before, during, or after exercise has minimal benefits, unless the normal oxygen supply to the tissues is in some way restricted. Supplemental oxygen will benefit people exercising at high altitudes and those suffering from a medical condition (e.g. a disease of the heart, lungs, or blood) that reduces the ability to absorb and transport oxygen. The greatest benefits to a healthy person are gained when oxygen is continuously supplied during exercise, but this has little practical use because of the problems of administering the gas to an active exerciser. Oxygen inhaled under high pressure may be an effective therapy for some sports injuries (*see* **hyperbaric oxygen therapy**), but it should be administered only under medical supervision because of the danger of poisoning (*see* **oxygen poisoning**).

oxygen cost
The amount of oxygen used by body tissues during an activity. It is related to the energy demands of the activity and (to a much lesser extent) whether the energy source is carbohydrate, protein, or fat. *See also* **calorimetry**.

oxygen debt
The name given to the volume of extra oxygen consumed after exercise. This is most obvious immediately after short bursts of intense activity when a person breathing heavily is said to be 'paying off the oxygen debt'. The term implies that the oxygen has been borrowed from a store during activity and replaced afterwards. Indeed, some of it is used to re-oxygenate myoglobin, the special red pigment which acts as a small oxygen store in muscle. However, only a small proportion is used for this purpose; most is used to convert lactic acid, produced by anaerobic respiration during exercise, into glucose and glycogen (animal starch), or to break down lactic acid to carbon dioxide and water. Therefore, most exercise physiologists prefer to describe the extra oxygen as recovery oxygen or excess postexercise oxygen consumption (EPOC), rather than oxygen debt.

oxygen poisoning
Although oxygen is essential for human life, you can be poisoned by breathing pure oxygen under high pressure.

Symptoms include tingling of the fingers and toes, visual disturbances, auditory hallucinations, confusion, muscle twitching, nausea, vertigo, and convulsions.

oxymyoglobin: *See* myoglobin.

ozone

Ozone is a gas containing three atoms of oxygen per molecule. It occurs naturally at about 0.01 parts per million (ppm), but the concentration can be increased by the photochemical action of sunlight on the products of the combustion of fossil fuels. At concentrations greater than 0.1 ppm, ozone is toxic and can be a potent bronchial irritant, making breathing difficult. High ozone levels in cities hosting endurance activities have caused respiratory distress in some participants.

It seems that we cannot win with regard to ozone levels. Although we have too much in our cities, the ozone layer above the poles is being depleted due to chlorofluorocarbons and other pollutants. This atmospheric ozone protects us against harmful ultraviolet light. Its depletion may increase the incidence of skin cancers.

P

PABA (para-aminobezoic acid)

A chemical found with members of the B complex but not a true vitamin in humans. Gut bacteria may be able to synthesize folic acid from it, but there is no evidence that humans can. Some manufacturers of PABA supplements claim that, if taken in conjunction with dimethylaminoethanol (DMAE), PABA stimulates the brain, reducing the risk of mental illnesses associated with ageing; this claim is not scientifically proven.

Although not a nutrient, PABA is one of the most commonly-used ingredients in lotions and creams that are used to prevent sunburn. Its derivatives effectively screen out the ultraviolet rays responsible for sunburn, but do not offer protection against the full spectrum of ultraviolet rays, including those linked with skin cancer.

pain

Scientists do not know exactly how we feel pain, but it involves the stimulation of specialized nerve-endings. Individuals vary in their sensitivity according to their pain threshold (minimum intensity of stimulation which can evoke pain) and pain tolerance (ability to put up with feelings of pain). Some chemical substances released in the body increase sensitivity. These include bradykinins, histamine, potassium, and serotonin, all of which may be released at sites of tissue damage.

Many sedentary people believe that all exercisers have to experience pain if they are to become fitter: this belief is encouraged by the well known training motto: 'No pain, no gain'. Sensible people interpret this as meaning that it takes effort, dedication, and commitment to improve fitness; it does not mean that exercise has to be a masochistic ordeal. On the contrary, if real pain is experienced, an exerciser should stop. Of course, an athlete who is training for top-class competition must be able to tolerate greater discomfort than a recreational athlete, but even an elite athlete must learn to distinguish between real pain and discomfort. Real pain acts as an important warning signal that something is wrong. If the signal is ignored, serious injury may result.

Pain can be relieved by a variety of means including cold therapy (e.g. application of ice), acupuncture, transcutaneous nerve stimulation, and analgesic drugs. Used correctly, these can provide relief and accelerate recovery. However, used incorrectly they can make a bad condition even worse. Many injured athletes unwisely take painkillers to enable them to continue training or competing. This often leads to further damage and the need for stronger painkillers; a vicious cycle ensues which can only be broken by rest. *See also* **muscle soreness**.

pain cycle

A vicious cycle resulting from training when in pain (figure 48). Initially, pain may follow an intensive training session. Instead of taking this as a warning sign of an injury, an exerciser may attempt to train through it, fearing that fitness will

Figure 48 Pain cycle

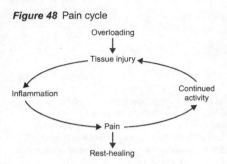

be reduced if training sessions are lost. The pain often disappears during the warm up, creating a false impression that all is well. This encourages the exerciser to continue the training session which may aggravate the injury. Pain may develop again after the training but, unless it is severe, this may not prevent further training. The cycle continues until the exerciser suffers a chronic injury that prevents training, or until the cycle is broken by rest and treatment of the injury. Of course, the earlier the escape from the pain cycle, the less rest is required, and the easier the treatment.

palpitation

Irregular or forceful heartbeats. Palpitations may have a number of causes including excitement, indigestion, alcohol, caffeine, or nicotine in cigarettes. They may also be associated with food intolerance and deficiencies of certain minerals (e.g. magnesium, copper, and potassium), and vitamins (e.g. B_1 and B_6). Many very fit people have slow heart rates and become aware of extra beats at rest. Although unpleasant and worrying, palpitations are not usually caused by heart disease. Moderate exercise often alleviates them. However, if the heart palpitates rapidly at rest, or if palpitations occur suddenly during exercise, medical advice should be sought.

pancreas

A gland that secretes digestive juices into the small intestine, and hormones (insulin and glucagon) into the bloodstream. The pancreatic digestive juices contain enzymes which break down starch, fats, and proteins. If the pancreas becomes inflamed, a condition known as pancreatitis occurs. It is often linked

with a blockage of the bile duct. The inflammation it causes may lead to obstruction of the pancreatic duct and pancreatitis. Heavy drinkers of alcohol often suffer from pancreatitis. Traumatic pancreatitis can also result from an injury to the abdominal region inflicted during a contact sport such as karate. Symptoms include abdominal pain (which often radiates to the back), fever, and vomiting. Traumatic pancreatitis can be dangerous if accompanied by bleeding, and may require surgical correction. Chronic pancreatitis leads to tiredness and loss of weight because of reduced secretion of digestive enzymes.

pancreatitis: *See* pancreas.

pangamic acid ('vitamin B₁₅')

Despite its alternative name, pangamic acid is not a true vitamin; it causes no deficiency disease and has no clearly defined function in the body. Nevertheless, in the form of calcium pangamate and sodium pangamate, it is marketed as one of the 'super-vitamins', essential for those who wish to maximize their physical performance. The marketing claim is based on reports that pangamic acid stimulates oxygen carriage from the blood to active muscles. It has also been suggested that pangamic acid is involved in fat mobilization, formation of anti-stress hormones, and detoxification of poisons and free radicals, but there is little evidence to support the suggestion.

It has been claimed that a one-week course of pangamic acid can improve running endurance on a treadmill by up to 24 per cent. Tim Noakes, an eminent exercise physiologist, personally tested this claim during a marathon race and reported that it was an 'unmitigated failure'.

Some nutritionists believe that, far from being beneficial, some sources of pangamic acid may be potentially poisonous. These sources contain dimethylglycine hydrochloride (DMG) which may be converted by saliva into dimethylnitrosamine, a potent carcinogenic chemical.

pantothenic acid (vitamin B₅)

A water-soluble vitamin, and a member of the B complex. Pantothenic acid is a constituent of coenzyme A which plays an essential part in the intermediate stages of carbohydrate and fat metabolism. Pantothenic acid also plays a role in antibody formation, detoxification of drugs, and the conversion of cholesterol to anti-stress hormones. Some studies indicate that pantothenic acid supplements improve physical fitness, but it is generally agreed that more detailed experimentation is needed to confirm these effects.

Pantothenic acid was discovered because deficiency caused the hair of black rats to turn grey. It was called 'anti-grey hair factor' at one time but there is no evidence that it affects hair colour in humans. Nevertheless, it is used in some hair care preparations as 'pro vitamin B_5'.

Deficiencies do not cause any specific disease in humans but can lead to a condition known as 'burning feet syndrome' when the feet ache, burn, and throb. Other deficiency symptoms include a wide range of mental and physiological disorders, among them headaches, depression, arm and leg cramps, respiratory infections, digestive disorders, and irregularities of heartbeat.

Good sources of pantothenic acid include dried brewer's yeast, pig liver, peas, and other legumes. Pantothenic acid is widespread in foods except fats, oils, and sugar. Healthy people are rarely at risk from deficiencies. The US RDA is 10 mg. There is no RNI in the UK.

para-amino benzoic acid: *See* PABA.

paracetamol
A painkiller which, unlike aspirin, does not increase the tendency to bleed. However, paracetamol acts within the brain and not at the site of tissue damage, so it lacks the power of aspirin to reduce the inflammation associated with many sports injuries. Overdoses can cause liver failure.

parahaemolyticus food poisoning
A form of food poisoning usually caused by eating fish or shellfish contaminated with the bacterium *Vibrio parahaemolyticus*. *See also* **food poisoning**.

paratenon: *See* peritendinitis.

parathormone: *See* parathyroid hormone.

parathyroid glands: *See* parathyroid hormone.

parathyroid hormone:
(parathormone; PTH)
A hormone secreted by the parathyroid glands (four small glands located behind the thyroid). It controls the distribution of calcium and potassium in the body. High levels of PTH cause calcium to be transferred from bones to blood; abnormally low levels result in lowering of blood calcium levels which can lead to tetany (twitching and spasm of muscles). Deficiencies can be compensated for by injections of the hormone.

An overproduction of parathyroid hormone has been linked recently to the development of fragile bones in a group of 14 female long-distance runners. After strenuous workouts they produced abnormally high quantities of parathyroid hormone and abnormally low quantities of another hormone called calcitonin. Calcitonin stimulates bone growth. It is not clear how general is this effect of endurance exercise on females, but it may contribute to the development of osteoporosis (brittle bone disease) in thin athletes.

PAR-Q
The Physical Activity Readiness Questionnaire developed by the British Columbia Ministry of Health and the Multidisciplinary Board on Exercise (MABE). It is designed for self-screening by anyone who is planning to start an exercise programme that includes moderate to strenuous activity, such as aerobics, jogging, cycling, power walking, and swimming (figure 49).

passive exercise
Exercise performed with the assistance of a partner who moves a completely relaxed part of the body. Such exercises are sometimes called passive mobility exercises because they are often performed to increase the range of movement of a joint. The partner gently exerts pressure against a joint to move it into its end position (i.e. the normal limit of its

Figure 49 PAR-Q. Physical Activity Readiness Questionnaire.

Physical Activity Readiness
Questionnaire (PAR-Q)*

NAME OF PARTICIPANT_____

DATE_____

PAR Q & YOU

PAR-Q is designed to help you help yourself. Many health benefits are associated with regular exercise, and completion of PAR-Q is a sensible first step to take if you are planning to increase the amount of physical activity in your life.

For most people, physical activity should not pose any problem or hazard. PAR-Q has been designed to identify the small number of adults for whom physical activity might be inappropriate or those who should have medical advice concerning the type of activity most suitable for them.

Common sense is your best guide in answering these few questions. Please read them carefully and check (✓) the ☐ YES or ☐ NO opposite the question if it applies to you.

YES NO

☐   ☐   1 Has your doctor ever said you have heart trouble?

☐   ☐   2 Do you frequently have pains in your heart and chest?

☐   ☐   3 Do you often feel faint or have spells of severe dizziness?

☐   ☐   4 Has a doctor ever said your blood pressure was too high?

☐   ☐   5 Has your doctor ever told you that you have a bone or joint problem such as arthritis that has been aggravated by exercise, or might be made worse with exercise?

☐   ☐   6 Is there a good physical reason not mentioned here why you should not follow an activity program even if you wanted to?

☐   ☐   7 Are you over the age of 65 and not accustomed to vigorous exercise?

If You Answered ➤

YES to one or more questions

If you have not recently done so, consult with your personal physician by telephone or in person BEFORE increasing your physical activity and/or taking a fitness appraisal. Tell your physician what questions you answered YES to on PAR-Q or present your PAR-Q copy.

programs

After medical evaluation, seek advice from your physician as to your suitability for:
• unrestricted physical activity starting off easily and progressing gradually.
• restricted or supervised activity to meet your specific needs, at least on an initial basis. Check in your community for special programs or services.

NO to all questions

If you answered PAR-Q accurately, you have reasonable assurance of your present suitability for:
• A GRADUATED EXERCISE PROGRAM – a gradual increase in proper exercise promotes good fitness development while minimizing or eliminating discomfort.
• A FITNESS APPRAISAL – the Canadian Standardized Test of Fitness (CSTF)

postpone

If you have a temporary minor illness, such as a common cold.

• Developed by the British Columbia Ministry of Health. Conceptualized and critiqued by the Multidisciplinary Advisory Board on Exercise (MABE).
Reference PAR-Q Validation Report, British Columbia Ministry of Health, May, 1978.
• Produced by the British Columbia Ministry of Health and the Department of National Health & Welfare.

movement). If conducted properly, passive exercises can improve flexibility. They are particularly effective at maintaining mobility when active exercises are not possible, because of, for example, injury. However, there is a danger that an inexperienced and overenthusiastic partner will overextend the joint, and push it beyond its normal range, damaging it. The exercise should stop when pain is felt (*see* **stretch stress**).

patella: *See* kneecap.

patellar tendinitis: *See* jumper's knee.

patellofemoral disorders: *See* knee.

patellofemoral malalignment
A knee disorder with characteristics similar to those of chondromalacia patellae. Both conditions are painful and cause a cracking sound (crepitation) in the knees. However, chondromalacia patellae is due to deterioration of the articular cartilage. Patellofemoral malalignment is due to an abnormal angle of pull of the quadriceps tendon. This tendon passes over the kneecap to attach the quadriceps (the large group of four muscles at the front of the thigh) onto the lower leg. The abnormal angle of pull of the tendons imposes unusual strains on the bones of the knee joint, pulling them out of alignment. Treatment includes rest and the application of heat. Special leg exercises are performed to restore muscle balance and realign the bones of the knee joint. If the condition persists, surgical realignment is sometimes necessary. *See also* **knee**.

pattering
A simple aerobic exercise devised in 1956 by Gordon Richards to train athletes for the Olympic Games. Pattering is similar to running on the spot. The exerciser steps quickly on the spot with the feet moving backwards and forwards but barely leaving the ground. The knees are not lifted, and the arms and legs move in a coordinated manner. Recommended speeds for a slow patter are about 50 steps per 10 seconds; for fast pattering, step as fast as possible. Pattering is tiring and beginners should start slowly doing

only about 5–30 seconds a day (depending on age), gradually extending the session over a period of weeks. No session should exceed 2 minutes.

paunch: *See* pot belly.

peak experience
A rare moment of great happiness and fulfillment, accompanied by loss of fear, inhibition, and insecurity. In sport, peak experiences often occur during personal best performances and are marked by a heightened sense of awareness. The experiences are usually described as being beyond one's control, temporary, and unique, standing apart from normal happenings and experiences. The physiological basis of peak experience has not been analyzed, but it is probably associated with the release of brain chemicals (*see* **endorphins**). *See also* **flow** and **runner's high**.

peaking
In sport, achieving an optimal performance on a specific occasion or for a given period of time. Ideally, peaking should occur on the very day, even the very minute, of an important competition. It requires a thorough knowledge of training and its effects so that a training programme can be tailored to meet the specific requirements of an individual. Peaking for vigorous activities usually requires a short period of high-intensity, low-volume training (so-called peaking training) near the time of competition, but not immediately before it when training should taper down.

Training to peak has to be done sparingly because it is very demanding. It is believed to use up energy (*see* **adaptation energy**), increasing susceptibility to infection and injury. There is a fine dividing line between optimizing performance and underachieving. Most coaches agree that peaking training should continue for only short periods (no more than about 8–12 weeks). Although an optimal performance can occur only once, high-level performances may be maintained for about 6 weeks or so before they begin to fall. If training intensity is lowered during peaking training, the duration can be extended and the high performances maintained for a longer period. However, the peak performance will probably be lower.

pear-shaped obesity: *See* gynoid fat distribution.

pec deck
A weight-training machine designed to allow an exerciser to isolate the pectoral muscles while in a seated position. It is quite effective at improving the strength of the chest muscles, but many trainers regard free weights as the best method.

pecs: *See* pectoral muscles.

pectin
A mixture of relatively soluble, complex carbohydrates found in fibre. Pectin forms a kind of cement in plant cell walls. It is particularly abundant in fruits. The concentrated extracts of fruit pectins contain methyl pectate, used as a setting agent for jams and other foods. Pectin delays stomach emptying, helping to prevent blood sugar swings. It may also help to lower blood cholesterol levels. *See also* **fibre**.

pectoral muscles (pecs)
The chest muscles. The pectoralis major is a large, fan-shaped muscle covering the upper part of the chest and forming the front of the armpit. It draws the arm forward and across the chest, and rotates it inwards. These movements are important in climbing and rowing. The pecs also help to move the rib cage during heavy breathing. The pectoralis minor is also flat, but it is thinner and lies beneath the pectoralis major. It lowers the shoulder, drawing the shoulder blade closer to the chest. These muscles are quite easily strained causing pains in the chest which sufferers often confuse with symptoms of heart disease.

pectoral stretch
A flexibility exercise for the chest muscles.

■ Stand in a doorway with one foot a stride in front of the other. Raise your arms to shoulder height, bend your elbows, and grasp the door frame with your hands. Using your arm muscles, press forward on the door frame as hard as you can. Hold the contraction for a few seconds. Relax and shift your weight forward so that the chest muscles and those at the front of your shoulders are stretched. Hold the stretch for about 6 seconds, then relax.

pellagra
A disease due to a deficiency of niacin, a member of the vitamin B complex. Early signs of pellagra include listlessness, headache, and weight loss. This progresses to a sore tongue, nausea, vomiting, and photosensitive dermatitis, resulting in ulcerated skin. The symptoms are sometimes referred to as the 'four Ds': dermatitis, dementia, diarrhoea, and death.

pelvic floor exercises
Exercises designed specifically to develop the pelvic floor muscles. *See also* **pelvic floor lift** and **stride jumps**.

pelvic floor lift
An exercise, specifically designed for women, to develop the muscles in the perineum or pelvic floor. These muscles are responsible for holding the lower part of the abdominal contents in the pelvic girdle. The perineum weakens after childbirth or through lack of exercise. This weakening is often associated with stress incontinence induced by coughing, jogging, jumping, or similar activities. Pelvic floor lifts reduce the risk of incontinence. The exercise can be done standing, sitting, or lying, but is easiest in a lying position.

■ Lie on your back with knees bent and feet approximately hip distance apart and flat on the floor. Tilt the pelvic floor (hips) upwards while tightening the muscles of the anus, vagina, and urethra, and clenching the buttocks together. Hold the position for 2–3 seconds then relax. Repeat.

pelvic floor muscles
Deep muscles in the floor of the pelvis. Their technical name is pubococcygeal muscles but they are often referred to as the 'love muscles'. They play a particularly important role in women. They are wrapped around the anus, urinary opening, and vagina, cradling them in a hammock-like structure. The muscles are used when emptying the bowels or

urinating, and during sexual intercourse, pregnancy, and childbirth. They also react to coughing, sneezing, laughing, and physical exertion of the abdomen. Weak pelvic floor muscles can cause stress incontinence. *See also* **pelvic floor lift** and **stride jumps**.

pelvic tilt

A simple exercise which can help realign the body, extending the back and pulling the abdominal muscles in (figure 50).

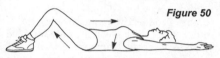

Figure 50

■ Lie on your back with knees bent and feet flat on the floor. Pull in your stomach muscles and press your lower back against the floor. At the same time, tighten the hip and thigh muscles so that the pubic bone is pulled forward and up slightly. Hold, then relax.

pep pills: *See* amphetamines.

pep talk

A talk aimed at heightening arousal. In sport, pep talks are usually given just before a competition or during an interval in play. They are a traditional, almost ritualistic, feature of managerial talks to soccer teams and often include exhortations to try harder. This may help some performers to reach an optimal level of arousal, but can cause others to become over-aroused and anxious, leading to a poor performance.

peptic ulcer

A breach in the lining of the stomach or the first part of the duodenum. The lining is covered by a layer of mucin which protects it against acids and pepsin secreted by the stomach. It is thought that ulcers are caused when the stomach secretes excessive amounts of acid and pepsin (a protein-digesting enzyme) or when the wall of the stomach or duodenum is damaged. Until recently, the disease has been attributed to stress and poor dietary habits which result in over-secretion of acids. Traditionally, treatment of peptic ulcers has been with antacids, drugs that control gastric acid

secretion (these permit the ulcer to heal), and, in severe cases, surgery. But in the last few years research in Australia has suggested that the formation of peptic ulcers is linked with the presence in the stomach of bacteria belonging to the genus *Helicobacter*. Several patients have been treated successfully with a special concoction of antibiotics to eliminate the bacteria; their ulcers have disappeared and there has been no recurrence of the disease. However, the treatment requires large doses of antibiotics and can cause side-effects (e.g. nausea and diarrhoea). This research disproved the previously-held belief that the stomach is too hostile an environment for any bacteria to survive. Whether the bacteria are the direct cause of peptic ulcers is still a subject of debate.

peptide hormones

A class of drugs banned by the International Olympic Committee. They include HCG (*see* **human chorionic gonadotrophin**), EPO (*see* **erythropoietin**), and hGH (*see* **growth hormone**). Other closely related chemicals and those which stimulate the secretion of these hormones are also banned.

perceived exertion

Subjective assessment of the demands of a training session. Gunnar Borg, a Swedish physiologist, devised a set of ratings (called the Borg scale) which numerically grades perceived exertion. His original rating consisted of 15 grades, from very, very light exertion to very, very hard exertion. This has been modified into the New Borg Scale to take into account the fact that exercisers become more sensitive to changes of exertion at higher work rates:

RATINGS OF PERCEIVED EXERTION (RPE) SCALE: THE NEW BORG SCALE

RATING	PERCEPTION OF EFFORT
0	nothing at all
0.5	very, very weak (just noticeable)
1	very weak
2	weak
3	moderate

RATING	PERCEPTION OF EFFORT
4	somewhat strong
5	strong (heavy)
6	
7	very strong
8	
9	
10	very, very strong (almost maximal)
>10 (any number)	maximal

Adapted from Noble, *et al.* (1983) *Medicine and Science in Sports and Exercise*. **15** (2): 523.

The perceived ratings follow changes in heart rate (which is directly related to exercise intensity) quite closely, indicating that perceived exertion is a reasonable indicator of actual exertion. A record of perceived exertion in a training diary can be a very useful means of monitoring exercise intensity and fitness. As fitness improves, a person should be able to exercise at higher ratings of perceived exertion with less fatigue. If a person feels unusually tired after exercising at low ratings of perceived exertion, it probably means that he or she needs a rest.

performance plateau: *See* plateau.

periodization
A training programme which divides training into periods with different objectives. A typical example consists of five periods, each about 4–6 weeks in length:

1 PREPARATION (whole-body conditioning)
2 STRENGTH PERIOD
3 STRENGTH/POWER PERIOD (completion of strength development and major work on power and speed)
4 MAINTENANCE PERIOD (competition period)
5 TRANSITION PERIOD (active rest to enable recovery from competition).

During the first three periods, training gradually changes from non-specific, general conditioning activities of long duration and short intensity, to more specific, special training of high intensity and short duration. The programme is designed so that athletes peak during the maintenance period and this is timed to coincide with major competitions. The precise duration of the periods and the total length of the complete cycle depends on when the athlete wants to peak. Most training programmes adopt a single periodization per year; some adopt a double periodization in one year so that the athlete can peak twice; and others have periodization lasting 2–4 years (for example when preparing for the Olympic Games) or even longer.

periosteum
A glistening-white, double-layered membrane of connective tissue covering the outer surface of bone. It is richly supplied with nerve fibres, lymph vessels, and blood vessels. The periosteum may become inflamed (a painful condition known as periostitis), when the insertion point of a tendon is severely strained, stretched or torn. This overuse injury commonly occurs when exercisers run on hard roads, or when they change technique or equipment. Periostitis is much more common in poorly conditioned exercisers than in fit athletes. *See also* **shin splints**.

periostitis: *See* periosteum.

peritendinitis
Inflammation of the paratenon, the tissue which surrounds and nourishes a tendon. Peritendinitis produces a crackling sensation over the area involved. It is a common overuse injury experienced by overenthusiastic exercisers. If not treated properly, the injury is potentially disabling. It is important for the damaged tissue to heal completely before training is resumed. If an injured person persists in training, there is a danger of the condition becoming chronic; permanent scarring of tissue may develop, increasing the thickness of the paratenon and reducing mobility, in which case surgery may be needed.

peritonitis
Inflammation of the peritoneum, the membrane lining the organs within the abdomen and the wall of the abdominal cavity. Peritonitis is classified as bacterial, chemical, or haemorrhagic, depending on the cause. Bacterial peritonitis can be

caused by perforation of an infected organ, such as the appendix. Chemical peritonitis can be caused by chemicals released from the digestive tract, such as bile or stomach acids. Haemorrhagic peritonitis may be caused by a violent blow to the abdomen causing internal bleeding. Whatever the cause, peritonitis is a grave condition and usually requires surgical treatment and hospitalization.

pernicious anaemia

A progressive decrease in the number, but an increase in the size, of red blood cells resulting from a lack of vitamin B_{12} in the diet or an inability to absorb the vitamin (see **intrinsic factor**). It shares the same symptoms as other forms of anaemia (e.g. breathlessness when exercising and lethargy) but victims of pernicious anaemia also often have a sore tongue, fever, and abdominal pain. Strict vegetarians who do not consume any supplements are at risk of deficiency because there are no plant sources of B_{12}. However, the vitamin does occur in micro-organisms, including yeast.

personality

The sum of an individual's underlying behaviour traits; the relatively stable and enduring attributes of character, temperament, intellect, and physique that make an individual unique. Each trait refers to the way a person behaves in a particular situation. People who always believe they can succeed in a sports competition, for example, have the trait of 'self-confidence'.

Several studies have shown that regular exercise over a period of several years can change personality by increasing vitality; improving patience and humour, and making a person better tempered and more easy-going. They also show that high levels of fitness are often associated with high levels of self-assurance, self-confidence, and emotional stability. These studies refer to ordinary people. They seem to be contradicted by the behaviour of some elite sports people, especially those participating in highly competitive sports such as tennis and football. By their very nature, these sports attract people with aggressive, competitive personalities. However, who

is to say that tennis players and footballers would not be much more aggressive if they did not have their sport as an emotional outlet!

Exercisers may suffer less from anxiety, depression, and tension than non-exercisers. This finding is supported by psychological profiles of elite athletes, who tend to score low on negative mood states and high on vigour (see **Profile Of Mood States**). Many sports psychologists are convinced that vigorous, regular exercise has important social benefits, helping to develop qualities such as dependability, perseverance, and determination. See also **type A behaviour** and **type B behaviour**.

perspiration: See sweating.

phantom

A hypothetical person used as a model for assessing body shape. The unisex phantom is defined by designated body measurements and skin fold measurements, and has an arbitrary stature of 1.7 metres, and a body mass of 64.8 kg.

pH control agents

Food and drink additives which control acidity or alkalinity, and also affect texture and taste. They are often constituents of soft drinks, baked foods, and fruit products. They are added to low-acid canned goods to prevent botulism. pH control agents include citric acid, acetic acid, and some alkalis .

phenylalanine

An essential amino acid contained in many foods, especially meat and dairy products. It is also one of the amino acids in the artificial sweetener, aspartame. Excess phenylalanine is not stored in the body and has to be broken down by a specific enzyme. People lacking this enzyme develop the condition known as phenylketonuria. For this reason, aspartame products carry a warning that they contain phenylalanine.

phenylbutazone (bute)

A non-steroidal anti-inflammatory drug introduced in 1949 to treat arthritis. It is a very powerful painkiller. Unfortunately, it has harmful side-effects and has been implicated in a number of fatalities. Consequently, its use has been restricted. Nevertheless, many physicians still believe that it is a very good drug for treating certain conditions, including ankylosing spondylitis (abnormal rigidity of the backbone, sometimes called 'bamboo spine'). Other physicians think that it is too dangerous for human use although it has been used frequently in a form known as 'bute' for the treatment of soft tissue injuries in horses.

phenylketonuria

A genetic defect resulting in a lack of the enzyme needed to metabolize phenylalanine. Phenylalanine is an essential amino acid used to make proteins, but excessive amounts damage the central nervous system. Phenylketonuria is especially dangerous to infants because it can damage the developing brain and cause severe mental retardation. The disease can be prevented by dietary restriction provided treatment is begun within 60 days of birth. The adverse effects of phenylketonuria are avoided by restricting the amounts of phenylalanine in the diet. Aspartame (an artificial sweetener) may not be suitable for those suffering phenylketonuria because it contains phenylalanine.

phenylpropanolamine (PPA)

A stimulant drug used in many slimming pills. In high doses, PPA has effects similar to amphetamines or 'speed'. In lower doses, it may suppress appetite and aid weight reduction but some users suffer harmful side-effects, including raised blood pressure and irregular heartbeats.

phonophoresis: *See* ultrasound.

phosphagen

An energy-rich phosphate compound. Breakdown of a phosphagen such as creatine phosphate enables ATP (adenosine triphosphate) to be generated very quickly without oxygen. ATP is the only chemical energy which can be used directly by contracting muscles.

phosphagen system
(ATP-PCr system)

The quickest, and most powerful source of energy for muscle movement. The phosphagen system is a form of anaerobic metabolism. It uses creatine phosphate to generate ATP (adenosine triphosphate, the chemical which provides energy for all body processes). Unfortunately, it will support activity for only about 10 seconds, just enough time for top-class runners to complete a 100 metre sprint. Although the phosphagen system produces only a little ATP, it generates energy very quickly. This provides the maximal power needed for short bursts of activity, such as when a sprinter explodes out of the blocks, or when a weight-lifter performs a clean-and-jerk. Creatine phosphate is stored in muscle and its depletion causes fatigue. Dietary supplements which increase creatine phosphate levels in muscles may delay fatigue and improve the explosive power of sprinters and other athletes. *See also* creatine.

phosphatidylcholine: *See* lecithin.

phosphocreatine: *See* phosphagen system.

phospholipids

An organic compound made from a combination of glycerol, two fatty acids, and a phosphate group. Phospholipids are major components of all cell membranes. They are involved in the transport of fat in the blood and lymph, and also take part in many other metabolic reactions throughout the body.

phosphorus

A non-metallic element which is an essential component of the diet. It is a constituent of many vital compounds in the body, including ATP, DNA, and phospholipids (*see* separate entries), but it is found mainly in bones. Vitamin D and calcium regulate the availability of phosphorus for bone formation. Most meats and fish are rich sources of phosphorus; deficiencies lead to rickets and poor growth, but this is rare compared with the effects of calcium and vitamin D deficiency on bone development.

Physical Activity Level (PAL; Physical Activity Index; PAI) and Physical Activity Ratio (PAR)

The energy used for a particular activity can be calculated by multiplying the basal metabolic rate (BMR) by a factor appropriate to that activity. This factor is known as the Physical Activity Ratio (PAR) and is calculated as follows:

PAR = energy cost of an activity per minute/energy cost of BMR per minute

Thus the energy cost of sitting at rest is 1.2; for walking at a normal pace, 4; and for jogging, 7. The sum of the cost of all the activities over a 24-hour period can be used to calculate the daily physical activity, and is expressed as the Physical Activity Level (PAL) or Physical Activity Index (PAI):

PAL = total energy required over 24 hours/ BMR over 24 hours

According to World Heath Organization statistics, the desirable PAL for cardiovascular health is 1.7; the average PAL in the UK is 1.4, with only 13 per cent of women and 22 per cent of men achieving a PAL of 1.7. For those engaged in hard physical activity, the PAL is 2.14. In a group of novice athletes training for the half marathon, the average PAL at the start of training was 1.66, and after 10 weeks of training it was 2.03.

physical fitness

If you are physically fit, you are free from illness, and able to function efficiently and effectively, to enjoy leisure, and to cope with emergencies. Health-related components of physical fitness include body composition, cardiovascular fitness, flexibility, muscular endurance, and muscle strength. Skill-related components include agility, balance, coordination, power, reaction time, and speed.

physical recreation

Physical activity pursued for enjoyment and to refresh health and spirits. Physical recreation is usually more purposeful and planned than play, but tends to be less organized than competitive sport. Nevertheless, some highly competitive sports are pursued as recreation, in which case the main motivation for taking part is to gain refreshment and not to compete. See also **play** and **sport**.

physical work capacity

The maximum amount of work a person can do during a physical activity. It is usually measured as the VO₂ max (see **maximal oxygen consumption**).

physiological limit

The level of physical activity beyond which an individual cannot normally go. In ordinary circumstances individuals do not reach their physiological limit, although it might be approached in the heat of competition when motivation is very high. Often a plateau is reached in training when people believe they have reached their physiological limit.

physiotherapy

The use of physical methods to assist recovery of damaged tissue, especially in muscles and joints. Sports physiotherapists are specially trained to treat sports injuries. Their role is to return an exerciser to full fitness using the safest and quickest methods. Many exercisers consult physiotherapists only when they have a serious injury which is not getting better. However, most, even those with minor injuries, would benefit from early advice and treatment. See also **cryotherapy; heat treatment; massage;** and **electrotherapy**.

phytic acid

A combination of inositol (a substance related to hexose sugars) and phosphorous. In the gut, phytic acid reduces the absorption of some minerals (e.g. calcium, iron, magnesium, and zinc) by forming insoluble salts with the minerals. Relatively high concentrations of phytic acid occur in wholegrain cereals and some other foods rich in fibre.

Calcium was first added to flour because of the suspicion that high levels of phytic acid in bread interfere with calcium absorption and cause rickets. However, the link between rickets and foods rich in phytic acid is far from conclusive and it is not certain to what extent these foods interfere with mineral absorption. There is some evidence that those who regularly eat high fibre diets adapt to the high phytic acid content by secreting an enzyme which can break phytic acid down into inositol and phosphorus.

phytochemical

A member of a wide range of chemicals found in fruits and vegetables that may have beneficial effects on human health. Phytochemicals are biologically very active. They include antioxidants, phyto-oestrogens, and compounds that modify potential toxins and carcinogens. In plants, they are not involved in photosynthesis, respiration, or protein synthesis, but they may function as attractants for pollinating insects or repellants against insect pests. Some phytochemicals are known to have medically important effects. Isoflavanoids from soya beans, for example, may reduce the risk of cancers induced by excessive intakes of synthetic oestrogen (see **oestrogen**). Allicin, a component of garlic, may offer some protection against heart disease. In 1989, the National Cancer Institute started a multimillion dollar project that includes the study of phytochemicals. It is likely that many new phytochemicals will be discovered which have an important effect on human health and disease.

pica

A craving for substances not normally considered to be nutrients. The curious behaviour of some pregnant women who crave for ice (pagophagia) or eat mouthfuls of clay (geophagia) may be caused by a real need for extra minerals, especially iron and zinc. If pica is due to a mineral deficiency, it clears up very quickly after the appropriate mineral supplement is taken.

Pilates

A system of training popular among dancers and other performers. Exercises, designed to strengthen the whole body without strain or injury, are performed lying down on a machine fitted with springs, the tension of which can be varied to suit the user. During Pilates, the emphasis is on relaxed, rhythmic breathing while performing smooth, coordinated movements. The movements, based on yoga and dance exercises, are particularly good at strengthening the stomach, thigh, and buttock muscles. The resistances are relatively low so that the exerciser is more likely to develop a sleek appearance rather than a muscular physique.

The training system has a very low risk of injury because there are virtually no impact forces on the joints and bones. Consequently, it is suitable for people of a wide fitness range, but it is probably not sufficiently vigorous to improve aerobic fitness.

piles: See **haemorrhoids**.

pitcher's elbow: See **thrower's elbow**.

pituitary

An endocrine gland at the base of the brain. It is sometimes called the 'conductor of the endocrine orchestra' because it coordinates the activities of many other endocrine glands. Some of its hormones are banned by the International Olympic Committee (see **growth hormone**).

placebo

An inert, harmless substance which resembles a medicine. Placebos are used in research when new medicines and dietary supplements are tested. They enable a researcher to distinguish between the psychological effects of a treatment and its physiological effects. If a person expects a substance to be of benefit, it often is. This was demonstrated in a classic study of the effects of vitamin C on the frequency of colds. One group of subjects was given a placebo and told it was vitamin C, while another comparable group was given vitamin C and told it was a placebo. Surprisingly, the group taking the placebo reported fewer colds than the group taking vitamin C, illustrating how strong the power of suggestion can be. The placebo effect may be reinforced by overt suggestions; for example, by exaggerated claims of manufacturers that they have produced a new wonder drug. In properly controlled tests of a drug, neither the investigators nor the subjects should know who is taking the drug and who is taking the placebo. The placebo effect is often used by physicians who prescribe an inert, innocuous substance to patients who need the psychological boost of being given something they believe will heal them. This effect is also used by sports trainers. Placebo salves with no pharmacologically active ingredients have been used to relieve muscle fatigue. The placebo effect is also a major consideration when evaluating the effectiveness of a training system. Some of the physiological improvements associated with the training may be brought about by a psychological belief that the system works, independent of what the actual system is (as long as the system itself is not harmful) . There is a suggestion that the placebo effect may be due to the release of chemicals in the brain which have an effect similar to morphine (*see* **endorphins**).

plantar fasciitis
Inflammation of the plantar fascia (the thick band of tissue along the sole of the foot) at its attachment point to the heel bone. Plantar fasciitis is characterized by a gnawing pain or discomfort in the heel that radiates along the sole of the foot. It may be caused by mechanical stress and is common in exercisers who jump or run excessively. It usually responds well to treatment with anti-inflammatory medication, without the need for surgery. However, it can take a long time to resolve, in some cases as long as 4 years.

plastic surgery
Surgery to revise or reconstruct tissue of superficial organs (i.e. those which can be seen easily) in a damaged area. Plastic surgery used solely to improve a person's appearance is more properly called cosmetic surgery.

plateau (arrested progress)
A period during training or the learning of a skill when there is no apparent improvement in performance even though practice continues. This is sometimes called the 'plateau of despond' because it is so discouraging. The condition may be due to staleness or the need of the body to have time to adapt to the demands of training. If staleness is the cause, improvement usually follows

quickly after a short rest or a change in the type of training. If staleness is not the cause and training continues, the plateau invariably passes and is often followed by a period of accelerated improvement. However, there is a risk of overtraining. *See also* **physiological limit**.

play
Spontaneous, childlike physical activity producing immediate pleasure. There is no goal other than sheer enjoyment. Play involves some rules which are freely accepted by participants. Feelings of exhilaration and tension often accompany play, with mirth and relaxation following. Although it appears to be an unnecessary activity with no material purpose, sociologists and psychologists believe that play is a necessary part of physical development, learning, social behaviour, and personality development. Many of the best sports coaches and exercise trainers incorporate play into their regimes to reduce boredom and maintain motivation. Very few people sustain their commitment to exercise unless it has an element of fun.

plumpness
Western society tends to denigrate plump people, regarding them as slobbish, lazy, and inherently unhealthy. There is no doubt that extreme obesity is unhealthy, but people with body fat slightly above average are unlikely to be jeopardizing their health. On the contrary, the general medical consensus is that moderate plumpness, particularly in younger women, has several health advantages. These include a lower risk of suffering osteoporosis and some other postmenopausal disorders. Plumpness in men may carry more risk, especially if the fat is distributed mainly around the waist (*see* **Syndrome X**). Nevertheless, even in men, slight plumpness is unlikely to be harmful.

It is often forgotten that the risks from being underweight can be as great or greater than those from being overweight. As far as health is concerned, there is probably an optimum weight and level of body fat for each individual dependent on a number of factors, including height (*see* **body mass index**) and body build. As a person's weight diverges from this optimum, the risks to health increase. Because of Western society's obsession with slimness, the body weight that most people prefer is probably less than the optimal weight for health.

plyometrics

Exercises, including hops, bounds, and jumps, in which maximum effort is expended while a muscle group is lengthening. During plyometrics, a concentric contraction (shortening) of muscle is immediately followed by an eccentric contraction (lengthening). Plyometrics forms part of the training programmes for most sprinters, jumpers, and throwers because they improve explosive power. However, there is a high risk of injury for those who are not well conditioned.

PMR: *See* progressive muscle relaxation.

PNF: *See* proprioceptive neuromuscular facilitation.

polyunsaturated fat (polyunsaturates)

Fats that have carbon chains with more than one double bond. A polyunsaturated fat has four or more fewer hydrogen atoms than its equivalent saturated fat. Polyunsaturates are classified as cis and trans fatty acids according to the arrangement of the hydrogen atoms closest to the double bond. In the cis form, the two hydrogen atoms are on same side of the double bond; in the trans form, they are on opposite sides of the double bond. In nature, polyunsaturated fatty acids are usually in the cis form, but hydrogenated polyunsaturates (e.g. some margarines) have a greater proportion in the trans form. This has important dietary implications because trans fatty acids have characteristics very similar to saturated fats and are regarded as being more harmful than cis fatty acids. Consequently, although it is recommended that up to 6 per cent of food energy may be obtained from polyunsaturates, no more than 2 per cent of food energy should be obtained from trans fatty acids

Polyunsaturated fatty acids include the essential fatty acids, linoleic acid and alpha-linolenic acid. A number of other polyunsaturated fatty acids occur in high concentrations in fish and vegetable oils and are thought to be particularly beneficial to health (*see* **eicosapentaenoic acid** and **gamma-linolenic-acid**). Nutritionists advise us to make sure that we have sufficient quantities of the essential fatty acids in our diets (in the UK, the Committee on Medical Aspects of Food Policy, recommend that linoleic and alpha-linolenic acid should provide at least 1.0 and 0.2 per cent, respectively, of total dietary energy). At the same time, however, we are also told to make sure that our total fat intake does not exceed 35 per cent of dietary intake. *See also* **unsaturated fat**.

polyunsaturates: *See* polyunsaturated fat.

ponderal index: *See* body size.

pooling

Accumulation of blood in the lower limbs due to gravity. *See also* **postural hypotension**.

postural hypotension (orthostatic hypotension)

A fall in blood pressure that occurs when a person stands up quickly after sitting or lying down. When sitting or lying down, blood accumulates or pools in the lower part of the body. When you stand up there is a temporary shortage of blood to the brain that may cause dizziness for a few seconds. Fit, active people are particularly susceptible to postural hypotension. After a strenuous workout, the blood vessels are usually highly dilated. This encourages pooling. Consequently, if a fit person stands still after exercise he or she may faint due to lack of blood returning to the heart. Lying down allows the heart to receive blood once again and to perfuse the brain. A cooling down procedure, such as walking or mild exercise, prevents pooling.

postural proteinuria (orthostatic proteinuria)

The occurrence of proteins in the urine as a result of prolonged standing or prolonged exercise; it occurs particularly in young adults. Protein in the urine is usually a sign that all is not well with the kidneys, but postural proteinuria is relatively benign and quickly disappears after bed rest.

posture
The position or attitude of a person's body. Static posture is the posture of a person standing, sitting, or lying still; dynamic posture is posture in movement. Correct posture results in the body being aligned so that the centre of gravity passes through the centre of the body and the position is maintained with a minimum of effort. If the body is off-centre, compensatory movements are made. This sets up stresses and strains that can result in aches and pains, particularly in the back. Posture is maintained largely subconsciously, but it can be improved by training. You can improve posture by exercising to improve muscle tone, muscular strength and endurance, and flex-ibility. If you have bad posture, you will need to make a conscious effort to establish correct body positioning.

potassium
An important mineral element in the human body. Optimal levels of potassium in the blood help to strengthen arteries, may reduce the damage to blood vessels associated with ageing, and are essential for the efficient functioning of the heart. Potassium-rich diets may reduce blood pressure and counteract some of the harmful effects of high sodium intakes. Some nutritionists suggest that the addition of one piece of potassium-rich fruit or vegetable per day may reduce the risk of a fatal stroke by 40 per cent.

Although deficiencies are rare, they may result from severe diarrhoea, sweat-ing, or vomiting. Mild deficiencies can lead to muscular weakness, increased heart rates, and nausea. Severe deficiencies may lead to heart failure unless supplements are given.

Potassium is found in many foods (including apricots, meat, fish, and poultry). Fruit and vegetables are especially valuable sources of potassium because they tend be relatively low in sodium. Bananas are an excellent recovery food for replacing potassium lost in sweat and they are very convenient (the original pre-wrapped food!). For these reasons, many professional cyclists eat bananas during races.

Potassium toxicity is rare, but excessively high intakes can lead to muscular weakness and heart complaints, and may accompany kidney disease. The daily potassium requirement is about 2–4 grams (UK recommended level for adults is 3.5 g per day).

pot belly (paunch)
A large, extended abdomen, due to the accumulation of body fluids and fat. It can sometimes be the result of malnutrition (e.g. in children deprived of protein, a pot belly may develop due to the infiltration of fat into the liver; see **kwashiorkor**), but is more often due to overindulgence in food and alcohol, and poor abdominal muscle tone. It is more common in men and is linked with several metabolic disorders. See also **abdominal muscles; android fat distribution;** and **Syndrome X**.

power clean
A weight-training exercise that develops all-round explosive power by strengthening the legs, trunk, and shoulder girdle muscles (figure 51). This is an advanced

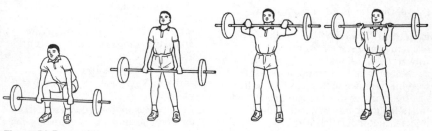

Figure 51 Power clean

lift and is not recommended for young or novice exercisers. You should always wear a weight belt when performing a power lift.

■ Crouch down, feet shoulder width apart. Lean forward to grip the bar firmly with an overhand grasp. Before you start the lift, your back and arms should be straight, hips low, shoulders just forward of the bar, and eyes focused forwards. Use your thighs to initiate the lift and then pull powerfully with your upper body to bring the bar to your shoulders in one movement. Keep the bar close to your body. Bend your knees quickly and force your elbows under the bar to 'catch' it. Hop slightly forward between the extension and catch and bend your knees into a slight squat position to receive the barbell at your shoulders. Do not hook the bar over in an arch at the top of the pull. This will cause the bar to hit your chest, pushing it backwards and imposing an unnecessary strain on your lower back. Lower the bar first onto your thighs and then to the floor.

power lifting
Weight lifting with the emphasis on pure strength rather than technique. The three power lifts (known as the Power Set) used in competition are the Two Hands Dead Lift, Press on Bench, and the Squat.

power sport
A sport, such as weight lifting, that involves short bursts of extremely high levels of activity. Power sports include those such as basketball in which players perform intermittent bursts of activity during a game.

PPA: *See* phenylpropanolamine.

praise
One of the best forms of motivation a coach or trainer can use on athletes and exercisers. To be effective praise must be warranted and not excessive. Unwarranted, excessive praise can be counter-productive because it loses its credibility. Praise should be given either during an activity or immediately following it. It should also be accompanied by information indicating why it is given. If applied properly, praise can encourage athletes and exercisers to persist with their training despite difficulties.

preacher curls
A weight-training exercise in which the elbows are rested on a special bench (called a preacher bench).

■ Use an underhand grip to grasp a barbell. Curl the barbell towards your chest slowly and smoothly and then return it to the start position.

pre-activity meal: *See* pre-competition meal.

pre-competition meal
Many athletes treat the pre-competition meal as a ritual which must be followed to ensure success. A thick steak with all the trimmings, the traditional meal of footballers, may have psychological benefits but is not nutritionally sound. The advice of most sports nutritionists is to avoid protein-rich foods for at least 12 hours before intensive exercise. Protein stimulates the secretion of acids in the stomach which can act as an irritant. It is also the most difficult type of food to digest. Other advice generally given to those about to compete or exercise intensively includes the following.

● EAT SOMETHING ON THE MORNING OF COMPETITION. Liver glycogen stores will have been reduced by 50–60 per cent overnight.

● AVOID SALTY, SPICY, AND GREASY FOODS.

● AVOID VERY SUGARY FOODS. Paradoxically, they may reduce the blood glucose levels (*see* **insulin rebound**), and they may delay fluid absorption, increasing the risk of dehydration.

● LIMIT YOUR INTAKE OF HIGH FIBRE FOODS. Vigorous physical activity stimulates movement of food along the gut. If this is further accelerated by high fibre foods, the results could be uncomfortable or even embarrassing.

● EAT AT LEAST 2–3 HOURS BEFORE COMPETITION. This allows digestion to take place.

● EAT COMPLEX CARBOHYDRATES. Pasta, for example, does not cause wild fluctuations in blood glucose levels

(*see* **glycaemic index**); avoid simple sugars such as honey, sweets, or candies.
- EAT FAMILIAR FOODS. Eat foods you know you can digest easily. A pre-competition meal is not the time to surprise your digestive system with new foods.
- DO NOT OVEREAT. During exercise, blood flow is diverted from the gut to the muscles and the food remains undigested, trapped in the gut. This may lead to constipation and stomach cramps.
- RELAX AFTER YOUR PRE-COMPETITION MEAL. Do not rush around as this will upset digestion.
- DRINK PLENTY OF FLUIDS (*see* **water replacement**).

If the competition lasts a long time, make sure you replace fluid and energy losses. Starchy carbohydrates (e.g. bananas) are a good source of energy and minerals. Many athletes use commercial carbohydrate drinks specially formulated for this purpose (*see* **energy drink**).

pre-exhaustion system: *See* pre-fatigue method.

pre-fatigue method (pre-exhaustion system)
A method used to ensure that, during weight training involving the simultaneous action of two muscles of different strength, both muscles are fully stimulated. Normally, the training would have to stop when the weaker muscle becomes fatigued, long before the stronger one is fully stimulated. To overcome this problem, a preliminary exercise (called an isolation exercise) is performed using only the stronger muscle so that it is 'pre-fatigued'. When the two-muscle exercise is performed immediately afterwards, both muscles will have a similar relative strength and will have to work equally hard during the training. The pre-fatigue method is used, for example, before the incline press which involves the pectorals and the weaker triceps. Either dumbbell flyes or cable crossovers are used as the isolation exercise, pre-fatiguing the pectorals.

pregnancy
Although women with a history of poor health may be prescribed rest at various stages of pregnancy, it is now generally accepted that moderate exercise can be beneficial. The reported benefits include:

- maintenance of physical fitness
- avoidance of excessive weight increase
- decreased risk of problems such as constipation, backache, and varicose veins
- improved sleep
- improved self-image and less risk of postnatal depression
- easier labour.

An exercise programme for pregnant mothers should take into consideration physiological and anatomical changes. The mother's heart, lungs, and other vital organs are working much harder than usual, and hormonal changes make some joints less stable. Pregnancy is not the time to start a fitness programme, but most regular exercisers can continue their normal exercise programme, with their doctor's permission.

Several elite athletes have continued to train and compete successfully during the early stages of pregnancy. Three gold medallists in the 1956 Melbourne Olympics were pregnant when they competed. During the later stages of pregnancy (usually after the 5th month) strenuous physical activity is not recommended.

Exercises which are particularly beneficial during pregnancy should be learned in special, medically-approved antenatal classes. These include exercises to improve posture and general mobility; pelvic floor exercises to maintain the perineal muscles and reduce the risk of stress incontinence in later years; and relaxation exercises, to improve neuromuscular control and the ability to cope with the pain of labour. Many experts advise against excessive stretching because the hormone relaxin is present in the body during pregnancy. Relaxin causes ligaments to relax, particularly those in the pelvis, which needs to widen during birth. Lax ligaments mean that joints can be overstretched easily, causing long-term problems of joint instability. During pregnancy the rectus abdominis (one of the stomach muscles) separates to accommodate an enlarged uterus. Sit-ups, or other strenuous abdominal exercises, can exaggerate the separation and result in an enlarged abdomen after giving birth. The American College of Obstetricians and Gynaecologists' guidelines for exercise during pregnancy state that pregnant mothers should be especially careful to take plenty of fluids before and during exercise to limit the risk of dehydration and assist cooling (maternal body temperature should not exceed 38°C).

During pregnancy, the mother is eating for both herself and her baby. At least in the later stages of pregnancy, she needs to consume more energy than usual, but this does not mean eating twice as much. The average weight gained during pregnancy is about 10–12.5 kg (22–28 lb). There is no merit in putting on less than that, but there are disadvantages in gaining much more. Carrying excess weight is tiring. It can also increase the risk of problems such as backache, diabetes, and varicose veins. On average, pregnancy demands 200 additional Calories daily. In the UK, the Health Education Authority recommend that these extra calories should be taken only during the last three months of pregnancy. It is only then that the energy cost of providing for the baby is high enough to necessitate a greater food intake, but this assumes that activity levels are reduced during pregnancy.

Pregnancy also increases nutrient requirements. It is important that the mother's diet contains sufficient protein, iron, calcium, folate, and vitamins C and D for the formation of the baby's muscles, bones, and teeth, and to make haemoglobin. Most extra nutrients are obtained simply by eating a balanced diet that satisfies the increased energy requirements. However, all women should take folate supplements to reduce the risk of neural defects in their babies (see **folic acid**). Pregnant women are advised not to eat liver or liver products although they are rich in folate, because of the possible harmful effects of their high vitamin A content on the health of the baby. Supplementary iron and vitamins C and D are often recommended, but iron tablets can cause constipation

and other distressing effects in some people. Any supplements should be taken only after consultation with a medically-qualified person or dietitian.

premenstrual tension (PMT)

As many as 90 per cent of women suffer from premenstrual tension (also known as premenstrual stress and premenstrual syndrome). The disruptive emotional and physical symptoms (including appetite changes, irritability, and headaches) that precede menstruation may last up to two weeks or longer. The symptoms vary considerably in intensity from very mild and barely perceptible, to so severe that work and domestic harmony are threatened. Physical changes associated with premenstrual tension are an increase in breast size, increased fluid retention with associated weight gain, abdominal distension, and an increase in skin pigmentation.

There appears to be no single cause of PMT, but it is probably linked to a hormonal imbalance (such as lack of progesterone during the second half of the menstrual cycle). Some experts suggest that nutritional deficiencies can disrupt the body's delicate hormonal balance. These include a lack of gamma-linoleic acid (GLA), vitamins, and minerals (such as zinc, magnesium, and vitamin B_6). There is, however, no conclusive evidence that supplements of these nutrients have any beneficial effects, and there is a risk of toxicity if doses higher than 50 mg per day of vitamin B_6 are taken. Other factors (alcohol, stress, ageing, a diet high in saturated fats, and viral infections) may also precipitate PMT. Sufferers are generally advised to reduce their intake of saturated fats and salty foods, increase their consumption of fruit and green vegetables, and drink plenty of fluids during attacks; even if this has no effect on PMT, the dietary changes should improve overall health.

Some gynaecologists believe that fatigue can cause PMT and recommend that women rest before a period is due. However, moderate exercise significantly reduces the severity of premenstrual symptoms in many women. In addition to improving fitness, regular aerobic training can reduce feelings of depression and anxiety.

prepatellar bursitis: *See* housemaid's knee.

preservatives
Substances added to food and drink to retard spoilage. Some preservatives (such as nitrates and sulphites) inhibit the growth of moulds and bacteria, while others (such as ascorbic acid, BHA, and BHT) stop fats from going rancid too quickly. Due to public concern about the safety of some of the artificial preservatives (e.g. BHT), there is a trend among manufacturers to replace these synthetic preservatives with natural ones (e.g. vitamin E).

press: *See* military press.

press-up
An exercise for developing strength in the arms and shoulders. When performed properly, press-ups can also benefit the back, stomach, and legs.

■ Lie face down, with your arms at about shoulder level and legs stretched out behind you; support your body on the palms of your hands and the balls of your feet. Gently lower your body by bending your arms until your chest touches the ground. Then lift your body by straightening your arms. Repeat. Make sure that you keep your back and legs straight throughout the exercise.

For those who find the full press-up too difficult:

■ Start from a kneeling position with your head held up, arms and back straight, and hands flat on the ground. Lower your body by bending your arms until your chest touches the floor. Return to the starting position by pushing up with your arms.

In both forms of press-up, regular, smooth breathing is maintained by inhaling as the body is lowered and exhaling as it is being pushed up (figure 52).

pressure training
A training system much used in team sports. It consists of deliberately creating intensive conditions for skill practice, much more difficult than those required in the actual game. In tennis, for example, a player may be put under pressure by being made to deal in a particular way

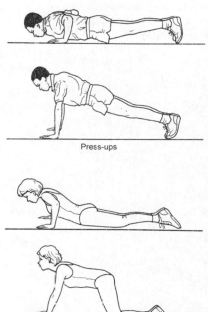

Figure 52 Press-up and kneeling press-up

Press-ups

Kneeling press-ups

with a much more rapid sequence of balls than would normally occur in a real game. Pressure training may improve the speed of executing skilled movements, and help performers retain the skills under the duress of competition. However, if training continues after the skill breaks down, players may have their confidence destroyed and perform less well in competition.

priapism
A persistent, painful erection. Priapism sometimes occurs among cyclists due to pressure on the pudendal nerve (the nerve which serves the genitalia) from a badly-fitted saddle pushing up against the area just behind the testicles. Treatment may include sedation to reduce the erection and the acquisition of a better saddle.

prime mover
A muscle which has the main responsibility for bringing about a particular movement.

principle of progression: *See* progression.

Pritikin diet

A high fibre diet, low in protein and fat, devised by a New York food writer, Nathan Pritikin. It was tested at the Longevity Research Institute, California as part of the treatment for heart patients.

Pritikin believed that we should keep our intake of salt, sugar, fats, and proteins to an absolute minimum. Coffee and tea are avoided, and alcohol greatly restricted. Consequently, the diet consists of 80 per cent unrefined carbohydrates, 10 per cent fats, and 10 per cent proteins. Because the diet consists mainly of vegetable material, you have to eat a large amount of food each day. To supply 700 Calories, about 2 kg (4lb) of food are required. Pritikin also incorporated exercise plans in his weight-control programmes.

The Pritikin diet is generally regarded as nutritious but some people complain that the high fibre intake causes flatulence and makes them feel bloated. Others find the diet too bland and restrictive despite the wide range of recipes suggested in Pritikin's books (e.g. (1982) *The Pritikin permanent weight-loss manual*. Bantam Books). *See also* **F-plan diet**.

probenecid

A drug sometimes misused by athletes to alter the integrity of a urine sample and escape detection by dope tests. Probenecid affects the transport of chemicals across tissue barriers, such as that between the blood and the kidneys. In medicine, this effect is taken advantage of to treat gout by reducing the amount of uric acid in the blood. However, the same effect is misused by athletes to reduce the amount of drugs, such as anabolic steroids, released into the urine, making them much more difficult to detect by conventional dope tests. Because of misuse, probenecid is listed among the banned drugs of the International Olympic Committee. Fortunately, its presence is easily detected in a urine sample.

Profile of Mood States

A test designed to measure certain psychological traits. Profile Of Mood States (POMS) is a popular tool among sport psychologists who have used it to compare the prevailing moods of elite athletes and non-athletes. Six mood states are used in POMS:

- tension
- depression
- anger
- vigour
- fatigue
- confusion.

Subjects are given a score for each trait according to their responses to certain statements which include key words such as unhappy, tense, careless, and cheerful. For each statement, subjects state how they feel at that moment, or how they felt over the previous day, few days, or week, by choosing one of the following responses: not at all; a little; moderately; quite a lot; extremely.

Elite athletes from different sports (including runners, rowers, and wrestlers) tend to score below average for negative states such as tension, depression, fatigue, and confusion; and score well above average on vigour. When presented on a graph, the POMS profile for these elite athletes assumes a characteristic shape that has been called the 'iceberg' profile; the better the athlete, the more pronounced the profile (figure 53).

Figure 53 Profile of Mood States. The 'iceberg' profile characteristic of elite athletes. From Morgan, W.P. (1980) Test of the champions: the iceberg profile. *Psychology Today*. 6 July. 92–108.

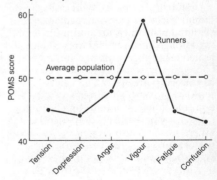

POMS may be used to diagnose over-training because the shape of the profile becomes inverted when an athlete overtrains.

programme setting

If you are to benefit from long-term exercise, you should plan an exercise programme to suit your individual needs. For general fitness, you should exercise for at least 20 minutes, three to four times each week. Swimming, jogging, cycling, and brisk walking are all popular and highly beneficial activities. Each exercise session should consist of warm-up and cool-down exercises which enable you to stretch all parts of your body. Many general fitness exercisers benefit from incorporating at least one strength-training session into their weekly exercise programme. It should include at least one arm and shoulder exercise (e.g. bench press), one trunk exercise (e.g. trunk twist), and one leg exercise (e.g. leg press) with two or three supplementary exercises to strengthen specific muscles. When setting your exercise programme, you should predetermine the exercise intensity and total workload. For strength training this will include planning the number of sets, repetitions, and weights to be used in each session. Be careful to conform to fundamental training principles (see **overload principle**; **progression**; and **specific training principle**) so that you obtain maximum benefits from the exercise.

progression

A major training principle which states that the benefits accrued from training will continue only if training workloads are gradually increased. Workloads should also be higher than usual (see **overload principle**). The minimum level of training which satisfies the overload principle increases as fitness improves. Consequently, workloads have to be increased progressively. This can be achieved by varying the frequency, duration, and intensity of training. Changes in intensity have the greatest effect on fitness, but they also present the greatest risk of sports injuries. Therefore, most coaches and exercise physiologists agree that it is best to vary first the frequency,

keeping the intensity low until the desired number of sessions per week are reached (e.g. three); then to increase duration; and finally to increase intensity when the fitness level is sufficiently high to cope with the demands. The key to successful training is to increase the workload gradually over a long period so that improvements can be maintained and overtraining avoided. Workloads which are too high, and abrupt increases in frequency, duration, or intensity, can provoke overuse injuries.

progressive muscle relaxation (PMR)

A highly-effective relaxation technique used to reduce stress, tension, and worry. Individual muscle groups are tensed for a few seconds and then relaxed in sequence, starting with those in the toes and feet, and progressing up the body to those in the neck and face. All the major muscle groups are contracted. A typical sequence might be: toes, feet, calves, thighs, hips, lower back, stomach, chest, upper back, hands, arms, shoulders, neck, and face. Tensing the muscles really hard produces a correspondingly high level of relaxation in the muscle. It also enables a person to recognize and learn the difference between tense and relaxed muscles. With practice, it is possible to become fully relaxed in a matter of seconds. The technique is used by those who have trouble getting to sleep, and by elite athletes to prevent overarousal and the needless dissipation of nervous energy prior to competition. PMR is best practised in a quiet, comfortable room, free from distraction. To be effective, it should be practised regularly every day. Typically, the complete routine takes about 15 minutes and is performed up to three times a day, with the last session just before going to sleep. Significant benefits are usually gained in a few weeks.

progressive resistance exercise

An exercise in which the workload is increased in predetermined steps. Ideally, the increments are sufficient to stimulate improvements (see **overload principle**) but not great enough to cause damage (see **overtraining** and **overuse injury**). In weight training, progressive resistance exercises are generally based on the repetition maximum (RM). The RM is the maximum load a muscle group can lift for a given number of repetitions, so that a 10-RM is the maximum load that can be lifted 10 times. Typically, in one session several sets of exercises are performed, each at a higher intensity than the preceding one. The following example consists of three sets of repetitions with a short rest of 1–2 minutes between each:

- set 1 at 50 per cent 10-RM
- set 2 at 75 per cent 10-RM
- set 3 at 100 per cent 10-RM.

Between sessions, the 10-RM is re-evaluated to ensure that training conforms with the overload principle. *See also* **progression**.

prolapsed intervertebral disc
(herniated disc; slipped disc)
Displacement of part of the gelatinous interior of an intervertebral disc so that it protrudes through the fibrous outer coat. The exuded disc material may press against adjacent nerves and cause severe pain. So-called slipped discs preclude physical activity but, once the patient has recovered, exercises are often used to strengthen the abdominal and back muscles in order to reduce the risk of a recurrence of the prolapse. *See also* **sciatica**.

pronation
1 Movement of the forearm so that the palm faces downwards. Pronation is the natural position of the forearm when a person is standing in a relaxed position.

2 During running or walking, an inward rolling motion just after the heel strikes the ground and when the weight is shifted to the middle of the foot. It is a natural action which serves as a shock-absorbing and an energy-return mechanism. However, overpronation can become a problem. When the foot rolls too far inwards, the foot arches, ankle, or knee may be damaged. Special shoes, usually with a firmer midsole, have been designed for those who tend to overpronate. *Compare* **supination**.

pronator
A person who exhibits excessive pronation during walking and running.

proprioceptive neuromuscular facilitation
Proprioceptive neuromuscular facilitation (PNF) includes a variety of stretching techniques designed to improve flexibility. Usually an isometric (static) contraction is followed by an isotonic contraction or a passive stretch. An example is described below:

- Tense the muscles at the top of your thigh (quadriceps) by pushing your leg against a resistance produced by your partner. This isometric contraction is followed by your partner passively stretching the hamstring muscles by raising the leg to, or even just beyond, the end point of the normal range.

There is some dispute about the effectiveness of PNF. Many coaches believe it is a good way of improving flexibility if both the subject and partner are well trained in the technique. Unfortunately, if the partner is overzealous there is a high risk of joint and muscle injury.

prostaglandin
One of a group of compounds derived from fatty acids, such as arachidonic acid (a polyunsaturated fatty acid found in low concentrations throughout the body; it can be formed from linoleic acid). Prostaglandins are found in cell membranes. Their effects include stimulating the smooth muscle in the uterus and gut to contract, and regulating blood pressure. They are also involved in the inflammation response after injury. They dilate blood vessels and increase their permeability to fluid and proteins. This results in a rise in temperature and swelling of the affected area. Prostaglandins also increase the sensitivity of nerve endings to pain. Some of the beneficial effects of aspirin, linolenic acid, and omega-3 fatty acids may be due to their action on prostaglandins: aspirin tends to reduce prostaglandin synthesis; linolenic acid and omega-3 fatty acids affect the proportion of the different types of prostaglandins.

protective muscle spasm
A sustained, involuntary muscle contraction, often occurring after muscle injury as a protective mechanism to prevent further movement and damage. Such spasms commonly result in stiffness.

protective protein theory
A theory that regular, vigorous exercise increases the level of fat-carrying, high-density lipoproteins in the blood, reducing the risk of heart disease. *See* **lipoprotein**.

protein
Proteins have been described as the very stuff of life. The word 'protein' is from a Greek word meaning 'of first importance'. This aptly describes the vital part proteins have in the structure and function of every living cell in the body. They comprise between 10–30 per cent of cell mass. They have many varied roles, acting as enzymes, hormones, respiratory pigments (haemoglobin is a protein), and antibodies. The two main contractile elements in muscle cells, actin, and myosin, are proteins.

Chemically, proteins are a group of organic compounds containing carbon, hydrogen, oxygen, and nitrogen. They consist of large molecules, or polymers, containing chains of amino acids linked together by peptide bonds.

Protein consumed in foods is digested in the stomach and small intestine into amino acids which are absorbed into the bloodstream and taken to the liver for initial processing. Some amino acids are transported to muscles and tissues where they are rebuilt into protein. According to the UK Dietary Reference Values, the amount of protein sufficient for most individuals aged 19 or over is 0.75 g per kg per day (about 45 g for the average female and 55.5 g for the average male). Those who are very active, suffering from severe illness, or recovering from surgery need more protein. For example, in a report of an international conference on *Foods, Nutrition and Soccer Performance* held in Zurich in 1994, sports nutritionists stated that soccer players require between 1.4 to 1.7 grams of protein per kilogram body weight. Protein requirements are also relatively high in children,

pregnant women, and nursing mothers. Very active people can meet the body's demands for extra protein by having a well-balanced diet adjusted to their higher energy requirements. Attempts to increase muscle size artificially by consuming excessively high protein diets are thought by most dietitians to be useless. As protein in the diet increases, proportionately less is absorbed from the intestine. Amino acids not needed for growth or repair of body tissues are broken down and excreted as urea, or converted into either glucose (to be used as an energy source) or body fat. One gram of protein yields about 4 Calories. Protein can supply up to 10 per cent of the energy needed to sustain prolonged exercise.

Consumption of excess protein may cause dehydration and constipation, and can lead to obesity. It may also cause deficiencies in vitamin B_6, and a loss of calcium with an increased risk of osteoporosis, but these effects are not fully established. Protein deficiency causes profound weight loss, mental and physical retardation in children, oedema, and anaemia.

Protein-rich foods include meat products, grains, legumes, and vegetables. *See also* **amino acids**.

protein efficiency ratio (PER)
A biological assay of the quality of a particular protein, measured as the gain in weight of an animal per gram of the protein eaten. The ratio is not used so much now, but until 1991 the PER was the legally required way of expressing protein quality for nutrition labelling in the USA.

protein-sparing modified fast (PSMF)
A very low-calorie diet specifically designed for people suffering from severe obesity detrimental to their health. Some very low-calorie diets have inadequate protein, causing body muscles to waste away. The PSMF diet relies on protein as the main energy source, thus sparing body protein and minimizing muscle wasting. The PSMF diet is meant to be used only under medical supervision because it can result in very rapid weight loss, potentially harmful to health. Commercial imitations are available to

ordinary dieters seeking to lose weight quickly. The general use of these diets is unjustified and unsafe.

protein supplement
A food supplement, usually in the form of a powder, containing amino acids. It is claimed, without good scientific evidence, that these accelerate muscle growth and repair, and stimulate fat metabolism for fat reduction. *See also* **amino acid supplements**.

proteinuria
Exercise can produce effects on the human body which, in a sedentary person, may indicate a serious disease. One such effect is proteinuria: the occurrence of abnormally large amounts of protein in the urine. At one time, this was regarded as a very reliable indicator of kidney damage because protein molecules were thought to be too large to pass from blood into the urine unless the kidney was damaged. However, it is now recognized that moderate proteinuria after heavy exertion is common in healthy, young adults. This condition is sometimes called athletic pseudonephritis because the symptoms are similar to those of a very serious kidney disease, glomerular nephritis. Unlike the disease, athletic pseudonephritis is not pathological and is quickly reversed when the exerciser lies down and rests.

prozac
Prozac (fluoxetine) has been hailed as a new miracle cure. It was first marketed in 1988 and is now widely used in the USA as an antidepressant. It has been prescribed for eating disorders and chronic fatigue. Some sports doctors also believe that it may reduce feelings of run down and mental fatigue associated with overtraining. Its use by athletes gained publicity in October 1994 when Alberto Salazar said that it helped him to win the Comrades Marathon in South Africa. This event is generally accepted as one of the most gruelling ultradistance events in the world, and Salazar's form for several years prior to the event had not been good.

In medical parlance, prozac is a selective serotonin reuptake inhibitor (SSRI).

Although we are not sure exactly how it works, it seems to increase the level of serotonin and acts as a relaxant. Therefore, its apparent positive effects on Salazar's endurance were a surprise to some sports scientists. Another SSRI actually reduces endurance capacity. However, it is possible that prozac improves the performance of athletes who have been mentally depressed.

Prozac does not benefit everyone. One psychiatrist said that it is '. . . helpful to some, but wretchedly unhelpful to others'. Side-effects are not experienced by everyone, but they can include nausea, diarrhoea, vomiting, and akathisia (a disorder characterized by extreme restlessness and an inability to sit still).

P/S
A measure of the relative amounts of polyunsaturates in the diet, where P is the amount of polyunsaturated fats and S is the amount of saturated fats. Many dietitians believe we should aim to increase our P/S values by eating more fats of plant origin. Butter, for example, has a P/S value of 0.05, while margarine made only from polyunsaturated vegetable oils has a P/S of 3.15. The World Health Organization recommends a P/S of 1.0 or higher. In the UK, the average P/S is 0.35.

pseudo-allergy: *See* **food intolerance**.

PSMF: *See* **protein-sparing modified fast**.

psyche
An ancient Greek word meaning soul or mind. In addition to psychology and related terms, several sporting expressions are derived from the word 'psyche'. These include 'psyching-up' and being 'psyched-out'.

Psyching-up is a motivational strategy used in sport to increase arousal so that a competitor responds more readily to the demands of competition. It often takes the form of an exhortation from a coach or manager to try harder (*see also* **pep talk**). Sometimes, the exhortation is too stimulating. The competitor becomes over-aroused and even anxious, resulting in a disturbance of mental balance, known as being 'psyched-out'. This usually leads to poorer performances. Psyching-out is also sometimes attempted by competitors who try to make their opponents over-aroused by purposely irritating them. *See also* **catastrophe theory.**

psyched-out: *See* psyche.

psyching-up: *See* psyche.

psychoneuromuscular theory
A theory explaining the positive effects of mental practice during which a person only imagines performing an activity successfully. It is suggested that a vivid, imagined activity produces electrical responses in the muscles and nerves similar to those produced during an actual activity. Slight movements corresponding to those produced during the activity may also occur, but these may be so small that they are barely detectable without sensitive recording equipment. Support for the theory comes from electromyography of skiers using an instrument to measure muscle excitability and electrical activity. The electromyograph patterns in the muscles of skiers who were asked to imagine that they were performing a downhill slalom, closely approximated the pattern recorded when skiers were actually negotiating the slalom.

pteroyl-L-glutamic acid: *See* folic acid.

PTH: *See* parathyroid hormone.

puberty
The period between the first appearance of pubic hair and (in females) the first menstrual flow, or (in males) the first development of active sperm. The age of puberty varies: in females it is usually between 9 and 15 years, and in males between 11 and 14 years. During puberty, young people undergo quite dramatic physical and psychological changes. Regular, well-structured exercise and sport can help them to cope with these changes by providing emotional and physical release. Involvement in sport can also encourage personal responsibility for health and an interest in sound nutrition. In addition to its cardiovascular benefits, regular aerobic exercise may also help to ease menstrual pain in girls.

Despite all these advantages, some types of exercise are dangerous during puberty because bones are still growing and the cartilaginous growth zones (epiphyseal discs) are easily damaged. Consequently, hard anaerobic exercise and training with heavy weights should not take place until two years after the final growth spurt, which may be any time between 10 and 18 years. Excessive aerobic activity, such as long-distance running, can also place intolerable stresses on joints and soft tissues causing permanent damage.

pull up: *See* chin-up.

pulse
The pulse is a rhythmic expansion and recoil of the arteries. It results from a wave of pressure produced by the contraction of the heart. You can feel your pulse in any artery that passes over a bone sufficiently close to the body surface.

Many training programmes prescribe exercise intensities in terms of target heart rates. In healthy individuals, pulse rates are usually identical to heart rates. Most exercisers find it easier to take their pulse rate and generally use that as an indicator of exercise intensity.

The best site for checking the pulse is in the groove directly above the base of the thumb on the underside of the wrist (figure 54). This is called the radial pulse

Figure 54 Taking the radial pulse.

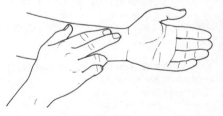

because it is where the radial artery passes alongside the radius. To count the pulse, simply press the fingertips of your middle and index fingers gently but firmly against the radial artery. The pressure should be sufficient to feel the pulse, but not so great that the artery is blocked. It usually takes a few seconds to become aware of the pulse and a few seconds more to become sensitive to its rhythm. Once this is established, an accurate count can be made over a period of 10 or 15 seconds and the pulse rate per minute calculated. (If an exerciser stops to take the pulse for a full minute, the heart rate will have slowed down by the time the minute has elapsed). Sometimes the carotid pulse is taken by pressing the carotid artery which lies along the forward side of the throat, but this pulse can produce inaccurate results. Also, pressure against the artery can affect a sense organ, the carotid sinus (*see* **carotid artery**), which may cause the heart rate to decrease by more than 15 beats per minute.

pulse raiser
An activity that raises the heart rate, increasing blood flow through active muscle, and raises body temperature. *See* **warm-up**.

pumping-up
A body-builder's term to describe the process of increasing the apparent size of muscle by lifting comparatively light weights many times in quick succession. The contraction of muscle compresses veins so that less blood leaves the capillaries than enters through the arteries. The pressure within the capillaries is raised, forcing some of the fluid out into the tissue spaces and increasing the size of the muscles. Shortly after exercise, the pressure is reduced as the excess fluid in the tissue spaces returns to the blood, and the size of the muscle returns to normal.

punch-drunk syndrome (dementia pugilistica; encephalopathy)
A neurological disorder commonly caused by repeated blows to the head in contact sports such as boxing. The victim becomes unsteady when standing, fatu-

ous, euphoric, voluble when speaking, and even aggressive. Memory and intellect may become impaired and, in advanced cases, may lead to chronic headaches and seizures. Punch-drunk syndrome has also been recognized among American footballers, rugby players, and wrestlers.

purging
Removal of food from the alimentary canal by self-induced vomiting, the use of laxatives, enemas, or colonic irrigation. Occasional purging is probably harmless, but chronic purging forms part of the behaviour characteristic of people with bulimia nervosa. The intention then is to reduce the effects of bingeing. In addition to self-induced vomiting and the use of laxatives, bulimics often attempt to purge themselves through diuretics, fasting, and exercising to excess. Purging reduces the feelings of guilt associated with bingeing and also relieves the physical discomfort caused by having an over-full stomach.

push-up: *See* **press-up**.

pyramid system
A weight-training system in which loads are increased successively in each set while the number of repetitions in a set is reduced. Assuming a 2-RM (*see* **repetition maximum**) of 45 kg, a typical session might consist of:

- seven repetitions at 20 kg
- six repetitions at 25 kg
- five repetitions at 30 kg
- four repetitions at 35 kg
- three repetitions at 40 kg
- two repetitions at 45 kg.

pyrexia: *See* **fever**.

pyridoxine: *See* **vitamin B$_6$**.

pyrosis: *See* **heartburn**.

Q

Q-angle (quadriceps angle)

An important indicator of biomechanical function, the Q-angle is the angle formed between the longitudinal axis of the femur, representing the line of pull of the quadriceps muscle, and a line that represents the pull of the patellar tendon. The patellar tendon is a band of strong connective tissue attaching the shin bone to the knee cap. When the quads are relaxed, the Q-angle is normally less than 15 degrees in men and less than 20 degrees in women. An abnormally large Q-angle usually results in a disorder called abnormal quadriceps pull. When the quadriceps muscle contracts, it pulls the kneecap sideways resulting in an overpronation and internal rotation which can lead to knee problems.

quadriceps (quads)

A group of four muscles (rectus femoris, vastus intermedius, vastus lateralis, and vastus medialis) which extend down the front of the thigh. The rectus femoris originates in the pelvis but the others originate from different points on the thigh bone. The four muscles join in a single tendon which crosses the knee cap to insert onto the shin bone. They are usually the most powerful muscles in the body and are the major extensors for straightening the leg. They play a vital role in any activity that involves running, walking, jumping, or even standing. Overextension, for instance when kicking, commonly results in the quads being strained (quadriceps muscle-pull). The leg hurts when touched and feels sore when the quads contract, for example, when going up stairs, hill running or doing squats. Overuse can also lead to a strain in the tendon, causing pain just above

the knee cap. The quads are also actively involved in restraining the leg during downhill movements; the muscles contract eccentrically to resist the pull of gravity. Consequently, excessive downhill running is a common cause of muscle soreness in the quads. *See also* **Q-angle**.

quad stretch

A simple exercise that stretches the quadriceps muscles at the front of the thighs (figure 55). During the exercise you will need to stand on one leg, so hold on to something, such as the back of a chair, to maintain balance.

Figure 55

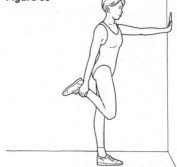

■ Stand upright on your left leg, grasp your right foot around the ankle and slowly move the heel towards your buttocks. Hold the stretched position for about 10 seconds; during the hold, contract your buttocks muscles, drawing them downwards to increase the stretch on the quadriceps muscles. To minimize the risk of injury, try not to allow your back to arch during the exercise, and keep your right knee pointing directly downwards throughout the stretch. This will ensure that the bones and muscles of the leg are correctly aligned. Repeat the stretch on the other leg.

Quetelet index: *See* body mass index.

Quorn: *See* mycoprotein.

R

"For when the One Great Scorer comes
To write against your name,
He marks – not that you won or lost –
But how you played the game."

Grantland Rice, 1880–1954, *Alumnus Foctball*. Quoted in (1979)
The Oxford dictionary of quotations. Oxford University Press, Oxford.

....

radial pulse: *See* pulse.

range of motion: *See* range of
movement.

range of movement
The extent to which a joint can be moved
through the arc of a circle. Range of
movement is determined by a number of
factors, including the shape of the joint's
bony surfaces, the length of its ligaments,
and the elasticity of its connective tissue.
Muscle contractions and gravity are the
main forces which can both cause and
resist joint movements.

There are a number of ways to describe
range of movement. A joint's maximum
passive range of movement is the range
that can be produced by any means (e.g.
manipulation by a partner). For example,
a knee joint which forms an angle of
30 degrees when fully flexed, and 165
degrees when fully extended, has a maximum passive range of 135 degrees. This is
greater than the extent achieved during
normal movements (the normal active
range), or the maximum movement
which an individual can actively perform
(the maximum active range).

The complete range of movement of a
joint is divided into three equal parts: the
inner range, during which the muscle
responsible for the movement is fully
contracted; the outer range, in which the
muscle is becoming fully stretched; and a
middle range between the two extremes.
When the muscle is fully stretched at the
limit of the outer range, it is said to be in
its end position.

An increase in range of movement is

unlikely unless a joint is taken to its end
position during stretching and flexibility
training. In sports like gymnastics, range
of movement is kept as great as possible.
However, joints may become unstable
and weak unless strength training is combined with flexibility training. *See also*
flexibility and **stretching**.

rate–pressure product
An indicator of the oxygen requirements
of the heart. Rate–pressure product is calculated as the product of heart rate and
systolic blood pressure (the maximum
pressure exerted by the blood on vessel
walls).

The heart is a living pump which needs
a good supply of oxygen and nutrients in
order to work. If these supplies are inadequate, heart failure results. During aerobic exercise, heart rate and systolic blood
pressure are the two main factors determining the workload on the heart. If
these factors increase, the heart has to
work harder, and will require more oxygen and nutrients to keep going. The
response of the heart rate and blood pressure to a fixed level of exercise tends to
decrease with regular, vigorous aerobic
exercise. Therefore, a well-trained person
is better able to satisfy the demands of
the heart for oxygen and nutrients during exercise than an untrained person.
For the same reasons, training is also
thought to offer some protection if there
is any disruption of the blood supply to
the heart muscle.

rating of perceived exertion (RPE):
See **perceived exertion**.

Ratzeburg method

A training method devised in the 1950s by the West German coach Karl Adam and used by the rowing club Ratzeburg R.C. The Ratzeburg method is a combination of interval training (to achieve peak aerobic fitness) and weight lifting (to obtain strength endurance). The interval training was based on that used by track athletes, but was performed in boats. Rowers were encouraged to use the same weight-lifting techniques as competition lifters, and were expected to move the barbell swiftly; rest between sets was kept to a minimum. Between 1956 and 1965, members of Ratzeburg R.C. won three European titles, an Olympic title, and a silver medal in the world championship eights.

RDA: *See* Recommended Dietary Allowance.

reaction time

The delay between the presentation of a stimulus (e.g. the sound of a starting pistol) and the initiation of a response. The delay is due to all the events which have to take place before a person is able to respond. Information in the form of nerve impulses has to travel from the sense organ along nerves to the central nervous system (i.e. the brain or spinal cord) where it is processed. Then a message has to be conveyed to the muscles before they respond. It takes about 14–16 hundredths of a second to respond to an acoustic stimulus (excluding the time it takes for the sound to reach the ear), and 16–18 hundredths of a second to respond to optical stimuli. Reaction times can be improved by training, but even well-trained, elite sprinters cannot respond physiologically in less than 10 hundredths of a second without anticipating the signal; in electronically-timed competitions, any starts quicker than this are regarded as false starts.

You may assess the speed of your reactions by doing the ruler drop test (sometimes called the stick test).

■ Get a partner to hold the top of a metre rule with the thumb and index finger. The rule should be held upright between your thumb and fingers, but you must not touch the rule. Your thumb and fingers should be around the 50 cm mark. When your partner drops the rule catch it as quickly as possible between your thumb and fingers. Repeat three times and calculate the average distance the rule dropped before you caught it. Rating: <8 cm, excellent; 8–12 cm, good; 13–20 cm, fair; >20 cm, poor.

rebound hypoglycaemia: *See* insulin rebound.

Recommended Daily Amounts: *See* Recommended Dietary Allowance.

Recommended Daily Intake (RDI): *See* **Recommended Dietary Allowance**.

Recommended Dietary Allowance (RDA)

A set of reference levels for nutrient intakes. In the USA, the RDA is an estimate of the average safe amount of nutrients and energy needed to maintain good health in a person who is already healthy. RDAs are adjusted for men, women, and children, and for different age groups, as well as for pregnant women. The further below the RDA intake is, the greater the risk of deficiency; the further above the RDA, the greater the risk of toxic effects. RDAs were revised in 1989 by a panel of nutrition specialists. RDAs were based on their expert opinion rather than proven fact. RDAs form the basis of Reference Daily Intakes (RDIs). The Nutrition and Labeling Education Act of 1990 mandates that nearly all foods in the USA should have RDIs on their labels.

Until 1991, RDAs were also published in Britain when they were replaced with Dietary Reference Values. There were considerable differences between the British RDAs and those set in the USA. The standards have been used on both sides of the Atlantic by individuals to check the nutritional adequacy of their diets. However, this is not the intended use of RDAs. They were devised as estimates of average safe levels for population groups. *See also* **Dietary Reference Values**.

recommended dietary goals

Many governments have recognized the importance of diet in relation to their nation's health and economic prosperity. Accordingly, some departments responsible for health have provided guidelines about the quantity of specific nutrients people should eat to ensure adequacy and prevent nutrient deficiency (*see* **Recommended Dietary Allowance**). In addition, some government bodies (such as the US Senate Committee on Nutrition and Human Needs) have made more general dietary recommendations aimed at reducing nutrition-related diseases. Most of these recommendations advise adults to:

- MAINTAIN DESIRABLE WEIGHT. Consume the same amount of energy (calories) as you expend to keep in energy balance. (For male adults, this is about 2500 Calories each day, and 2000 Calories for females)

- INCREASE THE CONSUMPTION OF COMPLEX CARBOHYDRATES. The World Health Organization (WHO) recommend that 70 per cent of our total calorie intake should be complex carbohydrates which include fruit and vegetables, pulses, and grains

- DECREASE REFINED SUGAR INTAKE. Added sugar should contribute no more than 10 per cent of energy intake

- REDUCE TOTAL FAT CONSUMPTION. Countries vary in their recommendations. UK guidelines suggest a decrease in the average fat intake from about 40 per cent to 35 per cent. WHO suggest that only 15–30 per cent of food energy should come from fat with a maximum of 10 per cent as saturated fat

- MODERATE PROTEIN INTAKE. This should be about 10–15 per cent of calorie intake

- REDUCE CHOLESTEROL INTAKE. Restrict consumption to less than 300 mg per day

- EAT LOW-FAT SOURCES OF CALCIUM-RICH FOODS. This is especially important for adolescent and premenopausal women to reduce the risk of osteoporosis

- INCREASE FRUIT AND VEGETABLE INTAKE. Leafy green and yellow vegetables are particularly good sources of vitamins, minerals, and antioxidants. The WHO recommend that we eat more than 400 g each day (about five servings a day)

- INCREASE DIETARY FIBRE INTAKE. Adults should eat about 30 g of fibre each day (18 g of non-starch polysaccharide)

- AVOID OVERCONSUMPTION OF SUPPLEMENTS. Supplements are necessary for some people, but most people can obtain adequate nutrients from a varied, balanced diet. Supplement use can lead to toxicity

- DECREASE SALT CONSUMPTION. Sodium intake should be less than 1.6 g per day (equivalent to about 4 g of table salt a day)

- RESTRICT ALCOHOL CONSUMPTION. Consume no more than one ounce of pure alcohol a day (approximately 3 units, equivalent to about two glasses of wine).

Most dietitians emphasize the advantages of eating a variety of natural, unrefined foods to ensure that we obtain sufficient nutrients. They also say that, with some adjustments, almost anyone's diet can meet the dietary recommendations. There is no need to give up your favourite food!

reconstructive surgery: *See* **plastic surgery.**

recovery
The physiological processes that restore the body to its pre-exercise condition after exercise. Recovery includes replenishment of muscle glycogen and phosphagen (the energy stores in the muscles); removal of lactic acid and other metabolites (the waste products of muscle activity); reoxygenation of myoglobin (the special respiratory pigment which provides muscles with an extra source of oxygen); and replacement of protein (needed to repair muscles damaged during exercise). Recovery can be accelerated by ensuring body fluids lost in sweat are replaced with water; by replacing mineral salts lost in sweat (especially sodium and potassium); and by eating enough nutrients (especially foods that can be converted to muscle glycogen) to replace those lost during the exercise. *See also* **rest.**

recovery period
Period following exercise when the body is restored to its pre-exercise condition. In

Reference man and woman

CHARACTERISTICS	MAN	WOMAN
age	20–24	20–24
height	68.5 ins/ 1.74 m	64.5 ins/ 1.64 m
weight	154 lb/ 69.8 kg	125 lb/ 56.7 kg
total fat	23.1 lb/ 10.5 kg (15%)	33.8 lb/ 15.3 kg (27%)
muscle	69 lb/ 31.3 kg (44.8%)	45 lb/ 20.4 kg (36%)
bone	23 lb/ 10.4 kg (14.9%)	15 lb/ 6.8 kg (12%)
remainder	38.9 lb/ 17.6 kg (25.3%)	31.2 lb/ 14.1 kg (25%)

weight training, the recovery period is the rest interval between sets; each set consisting of a number of complete muscle contractions.

rectus femoris: *See* quadriceps.

recumbent leg press: *See* fixed-weight machine.

reference man and woman
A theoretical man and woman, based upon average physical dimensions from detailed measurements of thousands of people.

Reference Nutrient Intake: *See* Dietary Reference Values.

rehabilitation
The process of restoring an injured person to the level of physical fitness enjoyed before the injury. In the past, rehabilitation usually followed the treatment of an injury, but now treatment and rehabilitation tend to take place simultaneously. The aim of rehabilitation is to restore athletes to full fitness safely and in the shortest possible time so that they can train and compete at a standard as high as, or even higher than, before the injury. Speedy rehabilitation is particularly important to ageing athletes because the longer they are unable to train properly, the harder they must work to regain full, competitive fitness. It takes about twice as long for an athlete aged 60 to recover from an injury as someone aged 20. A rehabilitation programme should include all aspects of physical fitness, especially flexibility, strength, endurance, balance, muscle coordination, agility, and skill. In this respect, it is similar to a conditioning programme. However, in every phase of rehabilitation recovery from injury must have prime consideration and additional stress to the injured area must be avoided. If an athlete returns to competition before complete rehabilitation, there is a high risk of recurrence of the injury or development of a new one. *See also* **RICE**.

relative strength: *See* strength.

relative weight
The ratio of a person's weight to the midpoint of the weight range for people of the same height, body build, and sex, based on standard height/weight charts published by insurance companies. Relative weight is often used to assess the extent to which a person is overweight or obese, but it is not a very reliable or accurate estimate. *See also* **body mass index**; **ideal weight**; **obesity**; and **overweight**.

relaxation
Relaxation is characterized by a reduction or complete absence of muscle activity and a controlled, relatively stable level of arousal that is lower than the normal waking state. Relaxation is incompatible with feelings of worry and anxiety. The famous physiologist, William James, stated long ago: 'If muscular contraction is removed from emotion, no emotion is left'.

Relaxation is a skill anyone can learn. It is possible to reduce muscular activity consciously to induce a state of relaxation and obtain optimal levels of arousal (*see* **progressive muscle relaxation**). Programmes of muscular relaxation have been used to control anxiety, and to treat high blood pressure, insomnia, nervous headaches, stomach distress, and menstrual distress. It has also been used to increase tolerance to loud noises and other painful stimuli.

Other relaxation techniques include psychological strategies such as behaviour therapy, biofeedback training, and meditation. A number of tranquillizer drugs are used as relaxants, but most have unpleasant side-effects such as drowsiness and dizziness. In high doses they can cause abnormal movements and actions. Prolonged use of some tranquillizers may lead to dependence.

relaxin
A hormone secreted by the placenta in the terminal stages of pregnancy. It causes a softening of connective tissues (cartilage and tendons), so that the bones at the front of the pelvis can separate, making it easier for the baby to be born. Unfortunately, relaxin also affects the tissue of other joints, loosening them. These changes may persist for several weeks after delivery. Therefore, most physicians advise expectant mothers to avoid vigorous weight-bearing exercises during the later stages of pregnancy and for a few weeks after birth.

renal stones: See kidney stones.

renin
An enzyme released by the kidneys in response to exercise and stress. It helps maintain the correct salt and fluid balance in the body. It reacts with a substance produced by the liver to form angiotensin which increases blood pressure; overproduction of renin can cause hypertension.

rennin
An enzyme produced in the stomach to coagulate milk protein and delay its passage into the small intestine. The delay enables other enzymes to break the protein down into absorbable amino acids. Relatively large amounts of rennin are present in the gastric juice of infants, but it may be absent in adults. A derivative of rennin, rennet, is used in junket- and cheese-making. Some vegetarians (lacto-vegetarians) will eat dairy products but not other animal products. Cheese for these vegetarians is made using edible plant enzymes or genetically-engineered enzymes which have the same action as rennin. In fact, because they are cheaper, genetically-engineered enzymes are gradually replacing rennet in other cheese-making.

repetition maximum (RM)
The maximum load that a muscle group can lift over a given number of repetitions before becoming fatigued. For example, a 10-RM load is the maximum load that can be lifted over 10 repetitions.

repetitions
1 In interval training, the number of work intervals in one set. For example an interval training prescription of 6×200 m would constitute one set of six repetitions of 200 metre runs.

2 In weight training, the number of times an exercise is performed without rest.

repetition training
A form of training, similar to interval training, used by runners, swimmers, cyclists, and other sports people. It differs from interval training in the length of the work interval and the amount of recovery between repetitions. For runners, it consists of running a given distance in a predetermined time with almost complete rest and recovery (usually walking) after each run. The run is usually at, or near, race pace.

repetitive strain injury (RSI)
An injury to soft tissues (especially tendons) caused by repeated use of a muscle or muscle group. RSI is a generic term for a whole group of overuse injuries including carpal tunnel syndrome, tendonitis, and tenosynovitis. These were once thought to be mainly the preserve of overenthusiastic exercisers. In fact, RSIs are so common in some sports that they have acquired a sporting epithet (for examples, see **golfer's elbow** and **tennis elbow**). In recent years there appears to have been an epidemic of RSIs not associated with sport: the British Trades Union Congress estimated that more than 200 000 people per year miss work

because of the condition, and in 1992 the US Bureau of Labour Statistics reported 282 000 confirmed cases of RSI, a 26 per cent increase on the previous year. The increase has been linked to the advent of personal computers. Repetitive speed-typing on computer keyboards may result in pain and stiffness in the hands, wrists and arms. The pain may be so severe that sufferers cannot drive, or carry bags. In the UK, keyboard-induced RSI has been called Work Related Upper Limb Disorder by the Health and Safety Executive. A few physicians deny the existence of RSI and regard it as largely psychosomatic. However, most treat it in the same way as other overuse injuries, with rest, anti-inflammatories, physiotherapy and, in extreme cases, surgery.

replacement drink

A drink specifically designed to replace energy and electrolytes (mineral salts) and to assist recovery after exercise. *See also* **electrolyte drink** and **energy drink**.

resistance

In weight training, the weight moved by, or whose movement is resisted by, a muscular contraction.

resistance exercise

An exercise against an additional resistance. Resistance exercises include running up a hill or on sand, carrying additional weights (*see* **weight training**) during exercise, and moving against an added drag force (*see* **speed chute**).

Pulling against an elastic exercise band is a form of resistance exercise. Bands vary in tension so that the intensity of exercise may be controlled. A band is easily attached to a stable piece of furniture, such as a table leg, and can be used to strengthen or rehabilitate specific muscles.

resistance stage: *See* general adaptation syndrome.

resistant starch

Dietary starch which behaves like fibre because it remains relatively undigested until it reaches the large intestine. Although it may form only a small percentage of the total starch in a food, it can form a large percentage of its total fibre. For example, some white bread contains only 0.7 per cent resistant starch, but this may make up 30 per cent of its fibre. The proportion of resistant starch in a food varies widely with the extent and type of cooking, freshness of the food, and other factors. Some estimates of dietary fibre ignore the contribution of resistant starch and include only non-starch polysaccharides. *See also* **colonic fermentation**.

respiration

The chemical process by which food is converted into a form of energy that can be used by the body. During this internal or cellular respiration, carbohydrates and fats (and proteins in extreme circumstances) are broken down either without oxygen (anaerobic respiration) or with oxygen (aerobic respiration) to form adenosine triphosphate (ATP). ATP is the only chemical which can be used directly as a source of energy by the body.

respiratory acidosis: *See* acidosis.

respiratory quotient (RQ)

The ratio of the volume of carbon dioxide produced to the volume of oxygen consumed during respiration. The RQ can be used to determine which foods are being used as an energy source. During aerobic respiration, respiration of fat gives an RQ of 0.7; respiration of protein gives an RQ of 0.9; and respiration of carbohydrate gives an RQ of 1.0. An RQ of more than 1.0 indicates that anaerobic respiration is taking place.

rest

Rest is often a forgotten or underestimated element of an exercise programme. However, periods of proper rest are essential. Rest gives the body time to adapt to the demands of vigorous exercise. Without it, there is a serious risk of overtraining and overuse injuries. Lack of rest is a major reason for underachieving in competitions. Rest not only enables you to recover physically from the stress of exercise, it also gives you time to recuperate mentally. Sensible exercisers incorporate at least one day of complete rest each week into their exercise programme.

They also avoid training hard on consecutive days. Serious, competitive sports people usually have a long rest period of 6–8 weeks in their yearly schedules.

Bruce Fordyce, the brilliant distance runner and one of the most successful ultramarathon runners ever (he won the Comrades Marathon every year from 1981 to 1990), gave the following training advice: 'During the hard training phase never be afraid to take a day off. If your legs are feeling unduly stiff and sore, rest; if you are at all sluggish, rest; in fact, if in doubt, rest.'

It is worth remembering that when you are older, it takes longer to recover from intense exercise, and that you will require longer rest periods. *See also* **over-training** and **tapering down**.

rest–pause training

A method of weight training that enables a lifter to perform several repetitions with a weight that normally could be used only once. Ten to fifteen seconds rest is taken after each repetition, allowing the blood to flow back into the muscles. This allows the muscles to recover before another maximum effort. Rest–pause training is demanding even for experienced lifters, but is popular among some body-builders.

retinol: *See* vitamin A.

reversibility principle

A basic training principle that there is a gradual loss of training effects when the intensity, duration, or frequency of training is reduced. *See also* **detraining effects**.

Revolutionary Three in One Diet:
See **aromatherapy**.

rheumatoid arthritis

A chronic inflammation affecting the lining and fluid of joints. It causes stiffness and pain. Treatment may include exercise and changes in diet. Exercise is sometimes beneficial, but sufferers should consult their doctor to find out what type of exercise, if any, is best for them. Some are helped by gentle mobility exercise and others by muscle-building.

There is controversy concerning the affect of diet on rheumatoid arthritis.

The Arthritis and Rheumatism Research Council advises those with rheumatoid arthritis to follow a normal, prudent diet and moderate their intake of fats, especially saturated fats. Most doctors endorse the view that a diet low in saturated fat with plenty of fresh fruit and vegetables may help sufferers, if only because this diet is healthy. However, there is less agreement about prescribing specific foods (e.g. fish oil supplements and evening primrose oils) to reduce inflammation and pain. The greatest disagreement surrounds the use of elimination diets to discover which foods aggravate the symptoms of rheumatoid arthritis. Many doctors are sceptical about interpretations. For example, if a sufferer eliminates chocolate and rheumatoid arthritis symptoms disappear, the sufferer will tend to blame the chocolate for the symptoms, but the effects may be merely coincidental. Nevertheless, some doctors claim that up to a third of their patients manage to control rheumatoid arthritis by dietary changes alone. Foods commonly eliminated include red meat, alcohol, dairy produce, and citrus fruits.

riboflavin: *See* vitamin B$_2$.

RICE

An acronym for the first phases of the rehabilitation of an acute musculo-skeletal injury: 'R', rest the injured body part; 'I', apply ice; 'C', apply compression; and 'E', elevate the injured extremity above heart level. This treatment helps to reduce swelling and restrict the spread of bruising, accelerating the healing process. Rest varies from absolute rest to relative rest, depending on the severity of the injury. Ice is never applied directly to the skin. As well as reducing swelling, the ice also acts as a local anaesthetic, decreasing pain. Compression is usually by means of a bandage wrapped tight enough to reduce swelling, but not so tight that blood flow is restricted. Elevation helps to drain excess fluid to the heart. RICE is one of the best forms of immediate treatment for almost any sports-related musculo-skeletal injury and should be continued for as long as pain and swelling persist. However, the ice should not be applied for longer than 15–20 minutes at any one time as it may impair circulation and damage tissues.

rickets
A deficiency disease of children whose bones do not harden and are deformed due to lack of vitamin D.

rider's strain
A strain of the muscles which pull the thighs and knees together. It is a common injury among horseback riders. *See also* **adductor muscles**.

rock-climbing: *See* climbing.

Rockport Fitness Walking Test
A test developed in the United States by cardiologists and exercise physiologists to determine fitness and monitor progress during an exercise programme. The fitness ratings are based on the speed at which you can walk exactly 1.6 km (1 mile) on a flat course, and the effect of the walk on your heart rate (assessed from a 15 second count of pulse rate immediately after the walk is completed). The faster you can complete the walk and the lower the effect of walking on heart rate, the fitter you are (figure 56). You are advised to warm-up for 10–15 minutes before the test, and to wear loose clothing and good shoes suitable for walking.

The test is generally regarded as quite safe and can be used by anyone. However, if you are over 35 years old, or if you have had any signs of heart disease, you should consult a doctor before doing it.

rope jumping
Rope jumping or skipping has long been regarded by boxers and their trainers as an excellent activity for developing aerobic fitness, strength, agility, and coordination. It has also been endorsed by the American Heart Association as a good exercise for cardiorespiratory fitness. However, it can be very strenuous and it is not easy to control exercise intensity. Jumping at 80 skips a minute can require 9 METS (that is, you will use nine times the amount of oxygen used at rest).

There are many kinds of rope jumping, from the very simple to the very difficult.

The basic bounce consists of jumping with both feet just one or two inches above the floor, and landing on the balls of the feet with knees bent slightly. You should keep feet, ankles, and knees together. Have your forearms out at right angles, and turn the rope by making small circles with your hands and wrists. Keep your body upright with your head and eyes up. You should start slowly and maintain a steady rhythm. The rope is of the correct length if, when you stand on its centre, the handles reach from armpit to armpit.

rotation diet
A diet that alternates periods of low calorie intake with periods of moderate intake. This rotation of low and moderate energy intakes is aimed at preventing the body from lowering its metabolic rate as an adaptation to long-term low calorie intakes. In fact, the whole regime, which includes regular daily exercise, is designed to increase metabolic rate. This chop-and-change system also makes the diet less demanding on willpower than a continuous low-diet regime.

The menus appear to provide a healthy balance of protein, low fat, and high fibre complex-carbohydrate foods, with a strong emphasis on fruit and vegetables. However, this diet, like other low calorie diets, is potentially harmful to certain groups of people. The deviser provides an alternative higher-calorie scheme for diabetics, but anyone wishing to follow the diet should consult their dietitian or doctor first.

rotator cuff
Four small muscles which stabilize the shoulder joint. These muscles are the subscapularis, supraspinatus, infraspinatus, and teres minor. They hold the ball-shaped head of the humerus bone (the long bone in the upper arm) in the socket in the scapula. The rotator cuff assists in some shoulder and arm movements. During throwing activities, the muscles undergo rapid eccentric contractions (they are lengthened under tension) as they decelerate the arm. This puts considerable stress on the tendons of the muscles making them susceptible to overuse injuries.

Figure 56 Rockport Fitness Walking Test

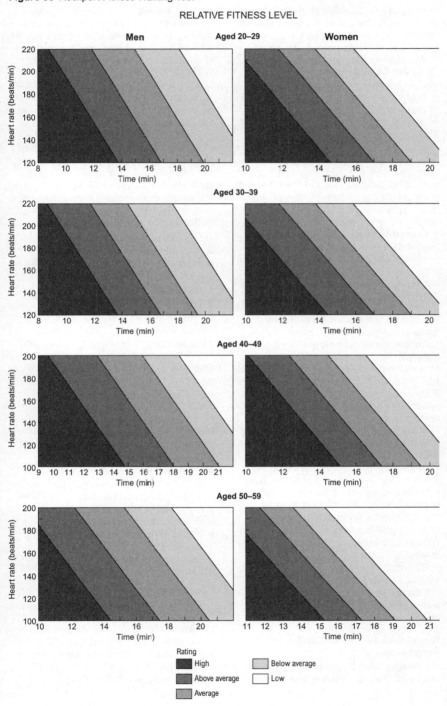

RELATIVE FITNESS LEVEL

rowing

Rowing in a boat with a sliding seat is considered to be one of the best forms of aerobic exercise. It uses muscles in the arms, legs, and torso, providing an all-body workout. This increases bone density in the spine which may offer some protection against osteoporosis.

Rowing is a sport which can be enjoyed at many levels. Even some octogenarians with a modest fitness level row regularly for exercise and pleasure. Many stable types of boats have been developed for non-competitive, recreational rowers. Elite rowers require supreme levels of fitness. World-class rowers have extremely high maximum oxygen consumptions (a measure of aerobic fitness), second only to cross-country skiers.

One attraction of rowing is that the boat supports the body so there is little jarring of the joints and a low risk of stress injuries such as shin splints and sore knees. Nevertheless, because the primary power for rowing comes from the leg muscles linked to the back, injuries to the lower back are relatively common. These injuries are often caused by poor conditioning or poor technique, for example, by overworking the flexible thoracic spine rather than using the combined power of the upper and lower body. To reduce the risk of injury, all rowers should do conditioning training and master the correct techniques. They should also train to develop their aerobic fitness, muscular strength, endurance, and flexibility, so that they can improve their performance and enhance their enjoyment. Training on water usually includes long stretches of rowing at two-thirds maximum effort interspersed with bursts at maximum energy output. Land-based training may involve calisthenics, weight training, running, cycling, and the use of rowing machines.

Despite low injury rates, serious accidents can occur if rowers capsize. All rowers should be able to swim and be fully aware of survival techniques in case of accidents.

Royal Canadian 5BX and XBX Programs

Progressive exercise plans designed by the Royal Canadian Airforce to develop and maintain the physical fitness of their military personnel. The programs have been widely adopted by the public. The basic exercises can be performed without any special equipment and in a confined space.

The 5BX programs are arranged in six charts, each with five exercises. Warming-up is incorporated into the exercises. For example, the first exercise (toe touching for 2 minutes) stretches and loosens the muscles. You start the first exercise easily, and gradually increase vigour and speed. The exercises are graded so that a person increases the number of repetitions of each exercise described on one chart and then progresses to more demanding exercises in the next chart as fitness improves. The exercises in chart one are:

- toe touching: 2 minutes
- partial sit-up (sufficient to see heels): 1 minute
- leg lifts: 1 minute
- push-ups: 1 minute
- stationary running: 6 minutes.

The exercises are completed in about 11 minutes.

The XBX program consists of four charts of 10 exercises, arranged in progressive order of difficulty. As with the 5BX charts, as your fitness improves, you perform more repetitions and then move on to a more difficult chart. The exercises in chart one are, in the order performed:

- toe touching: 30 seconds
- knee raising: 30 seconds
- arm circling: 30 seconds
- partial sit-ups: 30 seconds
- chest and leg raising: 2 minutes
- side leg raising: 1 minute
- push-ups (from a kneeling position): 2 minutes
- leg lifting: 1 minute
- run and hop: 3 minutes.

The 10 exercises are completed in about 12 minutes.

rubber suit

A suit made of material impermeable to water. A sensible use of rubber suits is in water sports, but other rubber and plastic suits are designed and marketed specifically for weight reduction during exercise. These are sometimes called sauna suits. They are worn during exercise to raise body temperature. Perspiration increases and body weight is reduced. However, the weight reduction is almost entirely through water loss and is quickly regained. Such suits can be dangerous because they prevent evaporative cooling of the body. This may cause heat exhaustion, heat stroke, and death even in cold weather if the suits are used during heavy physical exertion.

rugby

Rugby is a fast-flowing contact sport played by men and women. Each position offers its own particular combination of physical challenges. Forwards require great upper body strength combined with powerful legs to drive in the scrum, and backs need great sprinting speed. All players need endurance and good ball-handling skills. High levels of aerobic fitness enable players to maintain their skills at high speed throughout the whole game. Players can improve their endurance through running, cycling, or on rowing machines. They can develop strength by weight training, muscle endurance by circuit training, and powerful sprinting by sprint drills and plyometrics. It is also important that players perform stretching and mobility exercises to compensate for the shortening and tightening of muscles during a game.

Rugby is a hazardous sport. Injuries are frequent and sometimes severe enough to cause death or complete quadriplegia. The most vulnerable age group is that between 15 and 21. Injuries are often related to dangerous or aggressive play. Rule changes have been introduced to reduce the incidence of serious injuries: players must keep their heads and shoulders above hip level; they are not allowed to charge; and penalties are incurred for popping, collapsing, or wheeling the scrum. Poor levels of fitness increase the risk of injuries substantially. It is especially important for members of the scrum to have strong neck muscles.

ruler drop test: *See* reaction time.

run down

In sport and exercise, a decrease in performance caused by:

- factors outside sport which tend to drain the body of physical energy (such as lack of adequate sleep)
- excessive physical exercise (*see* **overtraining**)
- overstraining which may cause exercise-related injuries (*see* **overuse injury**)
- indisposition, due to psychological factors such as worry, or to transient physiological complaints such as fatigue, due to glycogen depletion.

See also **adaptive energy**; **burn out**; **overtraining**; and **stress**.

runner's haematuria: *See* haematuria.

runner's haemolysis: *See* haematuria.

runner's high

A feeling of exhilaration and well being directly associated with vigorous physical activity. Runner's high is thought to be related to the secretions in the brain of endorphins which have narcotic effects similar to those of morphine and related drugs.

runner's knee

An umbrella term for a number of conditions, but usually applied to knee pain resulting from an irritation of the iliotibial band (the tendon on the outside of the thigh which helps to stabilize the knee) when it rubs against the lower end of the thigh bone. This injury has the much more impressive medical name of 'iliotibial band friction syndrome'. It usually occurs in runners who have been running for less than 4 years and who regularly run more than 10 miles (about 16 km) per week. Running on cambered roads and excessive pronation increases the risk of suffering this condition. Treatment includes static stretching exercises of the iliotibial band.

runner's toe: *See* black nail.

rupture

Tearing or bursting apart of an organ or tissue. *See* **hernia**.

S

"You get writers who think that there's some magic formula, and they want to be first to tell the world how to do it. What's the secret? I don't know. But I will tell you one thing. You don't run 26 miles at 5 minutes a mile on good looks and a secret recipe."
Frank Shorter; Olympic Marathon champion, Munich, 1972. Quoted in Noakes, T. (1991)
Lore of Running. Leisure Press, Champaign, Illinois.

saccharin
An artificial sweetener about 300 times as sweet as sucrose but with no calories. Large doses of saccharin cause bladder cancer in laboratory animals, but there is no certain proof that it is carcinogenic in humans. In the USA, foods containing saccharin carry warning labels. Pregnant and lactating women, and children are advised not to use it.

SAD: *See* **seasonal affective disorder.**

Safe Intake: *See* **Dietary Reference Values.**

SAID principle (Specific Adaptations to Imposed Demands principle)
Principle stating that if a person is put under physical stress of varying intensities and duration, the person attempts to overcome the stress by adapting specifically to the imposed demands. *See also* **specific-training principle.**

salicylates
Compounds which are salts of salicylic acid, a drug with bactericidal and fungicidal properties. If salicylic acid is applied to the skin it causes peeling and is used to remove warts and corns. Salicylates can be synthesized but they also occur naturally in many foods and drinks, including dried fruits, some vegetables (e.g. chicory, green peppers, green olives, and radishes), herbs, teas, and some coffees, wines, and beers.
Many salicylates have properties similar to aspirin (acetylsalicylic acid) which is also prepared from salicylic acid. They are administered to reduce swelling and relieve the pain associated with muscle and joint injuries. Overdoses of salicylates and related compounds (including aspirin) can lead to a form of poisoning called salicylism. This is characterized by dizziness, impaired hearing, drowsiness, sweating, and, in extreme cases, delirium and collapse. Even in low doses, salicylates may cause salicylism in some people. Also, hyperactivity in children is sometimes caused by an adverse reaction to salicylates and is treated with a salicylate-free diet.

salicylic acid: *See* **salicylates.**

salicylism: *See* **salicylates.**

salmonellosis
The most common form of food poisoning. It is caused by eating food contaminated with bacteria belonging to the genus *Salmonella.* In the USA, it is estimated that *Salmonella* infects up to 4 million people annually. Symptoms include nausea, vomiting, and abdominal pain. The disease can be fatal in infants, the elderly, and individuals with a weakened immune system.
Most salmonellosis is probably due to poor hygiene in food handling, but some people have attributed the increase in salmonellosis to the use of antibiotics in animal feeds. The antibiotics are administered to improve growth. However, if dosages are not sufficiently high to kill all *Salmonella,* they may enable antibiotic-resistant strains to develop. If the meat is then not handled properly, these super-strains of bacteria could infect humans.

In recent years, another source of *Salmonella* has been raw eggs, which may become infected with bacteria from inside the hen.

salt

A member of a wide range of chemicals formed when one or more hydrogen atoms of an acid has been replaced by a metal. Salts are usually crystalline at normal temperatures and dissolve in water to form positive and negative ions. Salts such as sodium chloride, calcium carbonate, and potassium chloride are common in the body. They play vital roles in physiological functions such as nerve conduction and muscle contractions. The term salt is often used to refer to sodium chloride, the most common type of salt (*see* **table salt**).

salt depletion

The loss of salt from the body, either by sweating, persistent vomiting, or diarrhoea. Salt depletion is common after heavy physical exertion, especially in hot environments. It can lead to muscular weakness and cramps.

salt replacement

The replenishment of salts (especially sodium salts) lost from the body. If they are not replaced there is a risk of suffering from a number of disorders, including cramps. Salt replacement is mainly achieved from the diet. Sports men and sports women rarely need to take salt tablets. Sports drinks sometimes contain salts, but their main value is to accelerate the uptake of water from the small intestine. *See also* **water replacement**.

salt substitute

A flavour enhancer used in the same way as table salt but which does not contain sodium or has a reduced sodium content. People who are sodium-sensitive and have high blood pressure can take substitutes in which potassium and/or ammonium replaces the sodium. This can make the food taste bitter, but potassium may reduce blood pressure.

salt tablet

A tablet containing sodium chloride used to replace the salts lost during sweating.

If the tablets are taken without adequate water, there is a danger of a salt imbalance occurring.

saponins

Soapy chemicals that form colloids (mixtures having properties between those of a solution and a fine suspension) in water and foam when shaken. They occur in foods such as dried beans and peas. Saponins have a bitter taste and are toxic in large amounts. Generally regarded as antinutrients because they interfere with the digestion of some nutrients, some people believe that saponins may help reduce blood cholesterol levels and lower the risk of cardiovascular diseases.

Sargent jump test (vertical jump test)

A test of muscular power, often used in fitness testing. The Sargent jump test consists of measuring the difference between a person's maximum vertical reach before jumping and at the highest point during a jump (figure 57). Typically, the

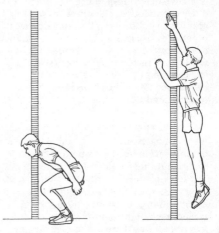

Figure 57

person swings his or her arms downwards and backwards, assumes a crouching position, pauses momentarily to get balance, and then leaps as high as possible, swinging the arms forcefully forwards and upwards. Usually, the fingers are covered in chalk so that a mark can be made on a board to record the heights reached before and after jumping.

RATING	VERTICAL JUMP (CM ABOVE STANDING HEIGHT)	
	MALE	FEMALE
excellent	>60	>55
good	50–60	45–55
average	40–49	35–44
fair	30–39	25–34
poor	<30	<25

saturated fat

A fat or triglyceride having the maximum number of hydrogen atoms attached to the carbon atoms. Because of its chemical structure, molecules of saturated fat can pack tightly together. Consequently, they tend to be solid at room temperature. Consuming large amounts of saturated fats can result in fatty substances such as cholesterol being deposited in the walls of arteries. This may lead to atherosclerosis (narrowing of the arteries) and high blood pressure. Saturated fats come mainly from animal sources (such as beef, butter, whole-milk dairy products, the dark meat of poultry, and poultry skin) as well as some tropical vegetable oils (such as coconut and palm oils). Many governments throughout the world have recommended a decrease in the consumption of saturated fat to reduce the risk of heart disease. *Compare* **unsaturated fat**.

sauna baths

A type of bath originating in Finland. The bather is immersed for a period in hot steam and then subjected to cold water. Some people take a sauna in order to lose weight. Saunas may be invigorating and boost morale, but they result in only a temporary weight reduction due to water loss. When fluids are consumed, weight is regained.

Taking a sauna immediately after strenuous exercise can be dangerous. A 33-year-old Israeli man who had a sauna 15 minutes after a strenuous weight-lifting session, produced an abnormally dark urine. On examination, he was found to be suffering from rhabdomyolitis, a destructive muscle condition usually associated with heat exhaustion. It can cause kidney failure and fluid congestion of heart and lungs. Physicians advise against taking very hot saunas immediately after a hard training session. It is also advisable not to take a sauna immediately after a large meal.

sauna suit: *See* rubber suit.

Scarsdale diet

A weight-loss diet devised by Dr Herman Tarnower in 1979. The dietary regime has two stages which alternate fortnightly. The first stage consists of the medical diet, a strictly prescribed high protein, low carbohydrate, low fat diet. Protein constitutes about 43 per cent of the diet but fats are restricted to about 25 per cent. Sugar, pasta, potatoes, and all bread (except a high protein variety) are excluded and between-meal snacks are restricted to carrots and celery. Tea or coffee can be taken freely, but alcohol is not allowed. The second stage consists of a keep-trim programme. This acts as a relief period from the very strict regime. More foods are allowed and alcohol can be taken in moderation. The diet during the keep-trim programme contains less protein.

Although the Scarsdale diet may result in weight loss, it is potentially harmful. The excessive amounts of protein and low carbohydrate in the medical diet can result in the accumulation of ketones, chemicals that are toxic in high concentrations. These may not be completely eliminated during the keep-trim programme. *See also* **ketogenic diet**.

sciatica

A severe pain radiating down the lower back into the leg. It is caused by inflammation or irritation of the sciatic nerve, the longest and largest nerve in the body. The sciatic nerve supplies the hamstring muscles and runs from the spinal cord to the knee where it divides into two smaller nerves. Onset of sciatica may be sudden; it is often brought on by strain of the lower back or a slipped disc (see **prolapsed intervertebral disc**).

sciatic nerve: *See* sciatica.

scintigraphy

A technique using a radioactive tracer to compile a picture of internal structures.

It is used to diagnose sports injuries such as stress fractures in bones. *See also* **bone scan**.

SCUBA diving

SCUBA is an acronym for Self-Contained Underwater Breathing Apparatus. The sport has become very popular. In the United States alone, there are more than 5 million certified SCUBA divers. It is an extremely pleasurable activity, especially with the development of excellent breathing apparatus and diving suits that retain body heat. The diver can experience the joys of weightlessness and explore unfamiliar, exciting, and beautiful environments. However, SCUBA diving is a high-risk sport. You should do it only after adequate training and a medical examination. Pregnant women and people suffering asthma, epilepsy, and certain other medical conditions should not dive. With adequate supervision, it is an excellent activity for those who are usually wheelchair bound.

scurvy

A disease resulting from a deficiency of vitamin C. Initial signs include bleeding gums. This may be followed by anaemia, red spots in the skin where blood has leaked out of capillaries, degeneration of muscle and cartilage, and weight loss. Most of the symptoms of the disease can be attributed to the breakdown of collagen (a protein that forms an important part of skin). The effects are reversed by treatment with vitamin C supplements. Vitamin intakes as low as 10 mg/day will prevent scurvy.

Although scurvy is rare in Western societies, it still occurs in some infants fed bottled milk, in elderly people who restrict their intake of acidic fruits because of heartburn, and in people addicted to alcohol who do not eat enough food. It may also occur in people who abruptly cease taking megadoses of vitamin C (a condition known as rebound scurvy).

seasonal affective disorder (SAD)

A mood disorder characterized by mild depression and lethargy, apparently triggered by a reduction in the number of daylight hours in autumn and winter. It is often accompanied by intense cravings for sugary foods that might alleviate feelings of depression. SAD sufferers usually lose their cravings when exposed to special, bright artificial lighting for one or two hours each day.

second wind

A phenomenon characterized by a sudden transition from an ill-defined feeling of distress and breathlessness during the early stages of prolonged exercise, to a more comfortable, less stressful feeling later in the exercise. There is some debate about the physiological reality of second wind, but it may be due to an increase in lactic acid at the beginning of the exercise followed by recovery as a steady state is established. It may also be related to a delay before the correct type and number of muscle fibres are recruited and oxygen-rich blood is diverted to the active muscles.

secretin

The first substance to be identified as a hormone. It is secreted by the lining of the small intestine in response to acid chyle (partly-digested food) passing into the duodenum from the stomach. Secretin promotes the flow of bile and pancreatic juices into the intestine, and inhibits the secretion of gastric juices. The pancreatic juices contain bicarbonates which help neutralize the acids in chyme.

segmenting (framing)

A psychological technique that helps an athlete to maintain concentration during endurance activities. The activity is broken down into manageable segments and realistic goals set for each one. A marathon runner, for example, may break down a race into kilometre segments and concentrate on maintaining a given pace determined separately for each kilometre, instead of aiming to achieve an overall time for the marathon.

selenium

A trace element found in meat, seafood, and cereals. Selenium acts as an antioxidant and is a constituent of some enzymes. Its functions are closely related to those of vitamin E. Selenium and vitamin E often work with each other. In the UK, the adult Reference Nutrient Intake (RNI) is 60 micrograms per day for women and 75 micrograms for men. Supplements are not recommended because high levels of selenium can be toxic. The upper limit of safe intake is 6 micrograms of selenium per kilogram body weight per day (about 400–450 micrograms for most adults).

self-concept (self-image)

A person's perception of himself or herself. It is often defined by self-description, for example, 'I am a father, athlete . . .' and so on. It is thought to have three components:

- the ideal self (the person you would like to be)
- the public self (the image you think other people have of you)
- the real self (what you really think about yourself).

Sometimes a conflict between the real self and the other components results in anxiety. In sport, this can be detrimental to performance and there are a number of psychological training methods to improve self-concept. In addition, to maintain good mental health, the public and ideal self should be compatible with the real self. *See also* **body image**.

self-confidence

A person's belief that he or she can succeed. Self-confidence is usually specific to particular tasks, but some people seem to display it in a wide range of activities. In sport, it has long been thought of as an important determinant of performance. It tends to be self-generating: confident athletes set themselves difficult training goals and persevere until they have achieved them. This generates feelings of competence which reinforce their confidence. Sport psychologists refer to situation-specific self-confidence as self-efficacy. According to one theory (Bandura's self-efficacy theory), self-efficacy is enhanced by four main factors: successful performances; vicarious experience; verbal persuasion (including praise and encouragement); and arousal (*see* **catastrophe theory**).

In training, you can enhance your self-confidence in the following ways:

- SET APPROPRIATE GOALS. Break down long-term goals into short-term, attainable goals so as to maximize feelings of success
- VICARIOUS EXPERIENCE OF SUCCESS. Imagine yourself performing the target activities perfectly to maximize the vicarious experience of success (*see also* **visualization**)
- VERBAL ENCOURAGEMENT. Use positive self-talk, by verbally encouraging yourself (e.g. with phrases such as 'This is a great session; I'm doing really well today . . .') to reinforce feelings of self-confidence.

self-efficacy: *See* **self-confidence**.

self-esteem

Positive self-esteem is viewing yourself as a competent and worthy person, and feeling good about yourself. Regular aerobic exercise can enhance self-esteem.

Lack of self-esteem is often associated with being overweight; this is reinforced by the media which portray thinness as essential for success, health, and wealth. Low self-esteem can result in not caring about how one looks, and not bothering to eat well or exercise. Excessive eating and drinking may be pursued as a means of escape from feelings of worthlessness. Many people, particularly women, seek sweet foods, especially chocolates, when they are feeling low. These so-called 'comfort' foods may alter mood by changing brain chemistry. For example, carbohydrate-rich foods increase the concentrations of an amino acid, tryptophan, within the brain. The tryptophan is a building block of serotonin, a neurotransmitter which relieves depression and reduces irritability. Self-esteem can be enhanced by thinking positively: by focusing on successes rather than failures and concentrating on your good points rather than on what you think of as bad points.

self-image: *See* **self-concept**.

self-starvation syndrome: *See* **anorexia nervosa**.

self-talk: *See* **self-confidence**.

semi-vegetarian

A person who has a diet of mainly plant and fungal products supplemented with some animal products. *See also* **vegetarian**.

serotonin (entramine; 5-hydroxytryptamine)

Serotonin is a chemical derived from the amino acid tryptophan. It plays a key part in a number of reactions in the brain and other tissues. In the blood, it acts as a vasoconstrictor, narrowing blood vessels, and is involved in the inflammation response. In the brain, serotonin is a neurotransmitter, affecting the activity of nerve cells. Brain concentrations are affected by diet in quite a complex way depending on the ability of tryptophan to cross the barrier between blood and the brain. Generally, carbohydrate-rich diets increase tryptophan levels, accelerating serotonin production. Some protein-rich diets (those containing the amino acids tyrosine, phenylalanine, leucine, isoleucine, and valine) compete with tryptophan to get across the blood–brain barrier, depress tryptophan uptake into the brain, and reduce serotonin levels.

Changes in serotonin levels can alter mood: increases have a calming effect, relieving depression, insomnia, and irritability; decreases are associated with wakefulness and greater sensitivity to pain. There is also a link between high serotonin levels and the early onset of fatigue: elevated levels induce lethargy and reduce the desire to exercise. Attempts have been made by some sports scientists to see if reducing serotonin levels can improve physical performance, but the results so far are inconclusive. *See also* **branched chain amino acids**.

SERP: *See* **Sport Emotional Reaction Profile**.

serratus anterior: *See* **boxer's muscle**.

set

In weight training, a given number of repetitions. In interval training, a set is a single group of work and relief intervals (*see* **interval training**).

set point theory

A theory suggesting that body weight is kept relatively constant by internal control mechanisms similar to those of a thermostat. According to the theory, each adult has a range of body weights that act as a norm or set point; changes in body weight trigger mechanisms to bring the weight back to this set point.

Some researchers believe that the set point is psychological. An individual establishes a perceived set point weight based on personal and cultural preferences. These preferences may be influenced by the person's appearance, body weight measurements, clothing size, health, and so on. Deviations of weight result in changes of physical activity and eating habits that return the weight back to the set point. Other researchers believe that the set point is physiological, but there are a number of different mechanisms proposed. One proposal is that the set point depends on the activity of the hypothalamus, a hormone-secreting gland at the base of the brain; another proposal is that a hormone is secreted by adipose tissue. In either case, it is suggested that deviations of weight result in a physiological corrective mechanism (e.g. change in basal metabolic rate) being switched on. Although dieting does not appear to affect the set point, exercise may lower it, making it easier to lose weight. *See also* **obesity gene**.

set system

A system of weight-training in which the trainee performs an exercise for a given number of repetitions (the set), rests, and then does another set. Popular variations of the set system include supersets and the super multiple set system.

In supersets, one particular muscle group is exercised for a given number of repetitions, followed immediately by a set of exercises which use the antagonist (opposite) muscle group. For example, one superset may consist of a set of arm curls to exercise the flexor muscles (especially the biceps), followed by a set of arm extensions to exercise the extensor muscles (especially the triceps).

In super multiple set systems, the exerciser completes all the sets for a given muscle group before doing the same number of sets using the antagonist muscle group.

sex and exercise

Heart rates of 180 beats per minute have been recorded during sexual intercourse. This compares with values of between 180 and 220 for athletes in top class condition during competition. It is perhaps not surprising, therefore, that many couples who engage in a regular programme of aerobic exercise report an increase in both the frequency and quality of their lovemaking. However, it should be noted that those with partners who overtrain complain that so much energy can be expended in the gym, or on the track or the playing field, that there is little energy left for anything else. Many sports coaches and managers ban their charges from having sexual intercourse immediately before competition on the assumption that it saps the strength. In answer to this, one leading sports doctor has written that '... from a scientific point of view it is probably fair to say that sex will interfere with sports performance only if both are attempted simultaneously' and an American baseball coach stated: 'It's not the sex but the staying up all night looking for it, that fatigues athletes.'

sex differences

The performance of women in athletics events is improving at a faster rate than men's, but women have to train much harder than men to achieve the same standard of performance in most activities. This is mainly due to biological differences between men and women. Compared to a man of the same age and size, an average woman has:

- less muscle and about 10 per cent more body fat
- a smaller heart volume with 10 per cent less cardiac output (volume of blood pumped with each heart beat)
- a wider pelvis, which decreases the efficiency of the lower leg
- a 10 per cent lower lung capacity
- a shorter Achilles tendon.

In addition, the monthly changes that accompany the female menstrual cycle impose psychological and physiological stresses with which males do not have to cope. *See also* **gender**.

shallow-water blackout: *See* oxygen poisoning.

shaping

A process in which a long-term goal is broken down into a series of gradual steps or intermediate goals, starting with a simple, easily performed task and gradually progressing to more complex and difficult ones. A person who wishes to become fit enough to take part in cross-country skiing, might spend the first two or three months establishing the habit of regular exercise, followed by a period of conditioning to gain general fitness, and finally a period of training to acquire the specific skill of skiing for long periods over variable terrain.

Sheldon's constitutional theory: *See* somatotype.

shigellosis

A form of food poisoning caused by bacteria of the genus *Shigella*. Symptoms include nausea, vomiting, dysentery, and abdominal cramps.

shin fracture

A fracture of the tibia (shin bone); the large bone at the front of the lower leg. The shin bone is very susceptible to fractures as a result of impact during a soccer tackle. An estimated 2500 soccer players are treated by the National Health Service in Britain for shin bone fractures, costing a total of £7.7 million in statutory sick pay.

shin splints

A term used loosely to describe an overuse injury characterized by a dull aching pain brought on by exercise. The pain is felt on either the inside or outside of the shin bone (tibia). Shin splints are commonly caused by repetitive loading of the front of the lower leg. This often results from overtraining (particularly at the start of a season's training), running on hard surfaces in poor shoes, or poor running technique.

The term 'shin splints' is applied to several conditions in which either soft tissues or bones are damaged. These conditions include stress fractures of the tibia or fibula, inflammation of the tendons on the outer side of the ankle (peroneal tendinitis), increased pressure within muscle compartments (*see* **anterior compartment syndrome**), or inflammation of the membrane covering the tibia (medial tibial stress syndrome). Some physicians apply the term only to medial tibial stress syndrome. In all cases of shin splints, the irritation and pain spreads, and continues throughout activity. The symptoms stop only when activity ceases but the leg usually remains tender to the touch.

Treatment depends on the cause, but usually includes quite a long period of rest, indirect application of ice, anti-inflammatory medication, and special stretching exercises. To avoid shin splints:

- wear training shoes that provide adequate protection
- seek coaching advice to ensure that your running technique is correct
- keep training intensities within tolerable limits
- stop training and seek advice if your shins become sore.

See also **periosteum**.

shin stretcher

A stretching exercise (figure 58) that improves the flexibility of muscles at the front of the lower leg and the iliopsoas (a composite of two muscles at the front of the thigh). It also helps to relieve muscle soreness in the shins.

Figure 58

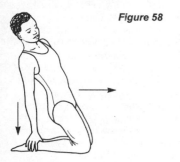

■ Kneel on the floor. Turn to the right and press down on your right ankle with your right hand. Slowly move your pelvis forwards. Hold the stretch for 6 seconds, relax, then repeat on the opposite side.

shock

A general term for a life-threatening state associated with circulatory collapse. It is brought about by a drop in blood pressure to a level too low to maintain an adequate blood supply to tissues. Someone in shock has cold moist skin, a weak rapid pulse, irregular breathing, dilated pupils, and is distressed, thirsty, and restless. Shock may be induced by many causes. Some, such as dehydration, bleeding and severe injury, may be incurred during exercise; others, such as allergic reactions, may be diet related (*see* **anaphylactic shock**).

shock exercises

Specialized form of exercise that involves jumping from an object several feet above the ground. Immediately on landing, the jumper rebounds upwards. The idea behind shock jumping is to stimulate the stretch-shortening cycle in muscles and to improve power output from the legs. When jumpers land, their muscles are stretched before contracting for the rebound. The combined action of stretching and shortening exerts greater power than can be exerted by shortening alone. The enhanced power output is thought to be due to the elastic behaviour of muscles and tendons immediately after they have been stretched. *See also* **plyometrics**.

short leg

Condition in which one leg is either functionally or anatomically shorter than other. In anatomical short leg, the actual lengths of the legs are different. In functional short leg, the legs are the same length, but because of some defect in gait (e.g. overpronation), one leg acts as if it is shorter than the other. Both conditions impose abnormal stresses on the body during walking and running which may lead to lower back pain and joint disorders.

short wave diathermy: *See* diathermy.

shoulder lifts

A simple exercise for the shoulder muscles, commonly used in warm-up and cool-down routines.

■ Stand upright, feet slightly apart, hands by your side and back straight. Slowly lift your shoulders as high as possible (try to touch

Figure 59 Shoulder shrugs

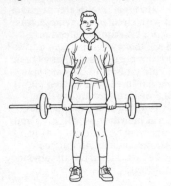 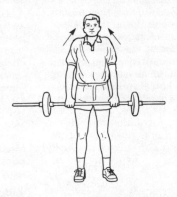

your ears). Hold for a few seconds then gently lower the shoulders. Relax and repeat about five times, remembering to maintain a steady rhythm of breathing in when you lift your shoulders and out when you lower them.

shoulder shrugs
A weight-training exercise that strengthens the muscles of the shoulders (figure 59).
■ Stand upright. With your arms straight, grasp a barbell so that your palms face towards your body and the barbell is resting against your thighs. Keeping your arms and legs straight and feet about shoulder width apart, slowly lift your shoulders as high as you can towards your ears. Then roll the shoulders smoothly backwards, down and forwards. Repeat as many times as is comfortable.

shuttle test
A test of aerobic fitness performed by running to and fro between two lines 20 metres apart. The run is made at a pace usually set by a repeating 'beep' sound (hence the alternative name, beep test). The pace is increased at 1 minute intervals and the test continued until the subject is exhausted. Aerobic fitness is based on the highest pace reached and the number of lengths of the course completed.

sickle cell disease
An hereditary blood disease characterized by abnormal red blood cells. In the full version, sickle cell anaemia, a large percentage of blood cells are sickle-shaped and unable to carry oxygen efficiently. They are removed from circulation, causing anaemia. In the mild version, sickle cell trait, a smaller percentage of blood is abnormal. The disease is endemic in Africa where the trait confers some resistance to malaria. Black people of African origin are more likely to have the disease than whites: about 8 per cent of black Americans have the trait, but less than 0.01 per cent of whites. The trait sometimes produces mild anaemia, particularly when oxygen partial pressures are low (e.g. at altitude), but it usually causes no adverse symptoms. Those with the trait can lead a normal life and participate in sport, even at the highest level. However, extreme conditions (such as maximal exercise in hot weather or at altitude before full acclimatization) can precipitate a life-threatening syndrome called fulminant exertional rhabdomyolysis. Blood cells in limbs become sickle-shaped, leading to kidney failure, collapse, and even death. Dr E. Randy Eichner, Professor of Medicine at the University of Oklahoma and a specialist in anaemia, stated that 'To avoid this syndrome, all athletes – with or without sickle cell trait – should train wisely, stay hydrated, rest when sick, heed environmental stress and early symptoms, and never charge recklessly into heroic exercise.' (In Mellion, M.B. (1993) *Sports medicine secrets*. Hanley and Belfus.)

side bends
A simple upper-body stretching exercise which often forms part of a warm-up routine.

■ Stand upright with your feet slightly apart. Keep your shoulders pulled back and always face straight ahead; maintain this posture throughout the exercise. With one arm, reach down the side of one leg while raising the other arm up the opposite side towards the ear. When you feel a tension in your muscles, hold the position for a few seconds and repeat in the other direction.

side leg raises

A simple exercise to develop abductor muscles on the outer hip and thigh.

■ Lie on your right side. Keeping your legs straight and facing forwards, raise your left leg a few centimetres. Hold the raised position for a few seconds then slowly return to the starting position. Repeat on the other side. Take care to avoid rolling forwards or backwards, and, during the raise, ensure your hips continue to face forwards.

side twist

A stretching exercise to improve the mobility of the trunk and lower back.

■ Stand upright, feet slightly apart. Extend your arms sideways at shoulder height then slowly twist to your right as far as possible. Hold, then twist to your left. Repeat.

simple carbohydrate

A sugar; a monosaccharide (e.g. glucose and fructose); or disaccharide (e.g. maltose and lactose).

single sugar: *See* monosaccharide.

sit-and-reach test

A test of flexibility in which a person sits on the floor and, while keeping the legs straight, bends forward as far as possible.

Figure 60

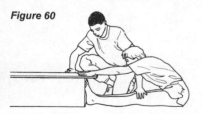

■ Place a box securely on the floor against which your feet can be pressed. Place a ruler on the top of the box so that it extends

15 cm over the end of the box, with the zero end extending towards you. Reach forwards as far as you can go and hold. The distance reached by your finger tips beyond the zero mark on the ruler is a measure of your flexibility. You should perform the test slowly to minimize the risk of imposing too much stress on your back; avoid bouncing movements.

Rating: >30 cm, excellent; 20–30 cm, good; 10–19 cm, average; <10 cm, poor.

sitting tucks

An exercise to strengthen the abdominal and leg muscles (figure 61).

Figure 61

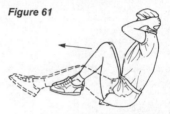

■ Sit so that your back and feet are off the floor. Place your hands on top of your head (not behind your neck). Keeping your back and feet off the floor, alternately bend your legs and bring your knees towards your chest, and then extend your feet away from your body. Repeat.

sit-up

An exercise to improve the strength and endurance of stomach muscles. There are many variations, some of which do more harm than good. Harmful versions include those which put too much strain on the neck and lower back (for example by quickly bringing the chest almost to the knees). Sit-ups are a great exercise, but only when performed correctly.

■ Begin by lying on your back with legs slightly bent at 45 degrees, and with your feet flat on the floor. Rest your hands on your thighs and move them towards the knees during the sit-up. (Your hand position is important because it affects the exercise intensity; this is the safest and easiest position for beginners.) Throughout the whole exercise, press your lower back against the floor; keep your neck and shoulders relaxed and your chin off your chest. Use your stomach muscles to slowly lift your shoulders off the floor, exhaling as you do so. Hold the inclined position for 2–3 seconds, then slowly return to the start position, breathing in as you do so; do not allow your head to touch the floor. Start with no more than 10 repetitions in one set, gradually increasing the workout to three to five sets of 15 repetitions.

Sit-ups are sometimes used as a test of strength and muscular endurance of the abdominal (stomach) muscles. This should be done only if you are in good condition and do not suffer from back problems.

| RATING | NUMBER OF SIT-UPS IN 30 SECONDS | |
	MALE	FEMALE
excellent	>30	>25
good	26–30	21–25
average	20–25	15–20
fair	15–19	10–14
poor	<15	<10

skeletal muscle

Muscle attached to bone and, in some areas, skin. Contraction of the muscle moves parts of the skeleton. Skeletal muscle is sometimes called voluntary muscle because its actions are usually under conscious control. It is also called striated muscle because it contains fibres that appear under the microscope to have alternating dark and light bands. The muscle fibres may be of two main types: fast twitch fibres, adapted to produce quick, powerful movements; and slow twitch fibres, adapted to slower, endurance type movements. *See also* **muscle** and **muscle fibre types**.

skeleton

The rigid framework of the body made of bone and cartilage. It maintains body shape, supports soft tissues, and acts as a system of levers facilitating locomotion. In addition, some parts of the skeleton manufacture red blood cells and store materials, such as some minerals. There are about 200 bones in the body making up more than 20 per cent of the body mass.

skier's thumb

A rupture of a major ligament in the thumb, adjacent to the web between the thumb and forefinger. Skier's thumb often occurs when a skier falls on an outstretched arm, and the ski-pole forces the thumb upwards and outwards. It is also common among over-aggressive ice hockey players when they throw off their gloves and attempt a thumb hold on an opponent's jersey. The opponent, trying to jerk free, damages the ligament. The injury is sometimes called gamekeeper's thumb, presumably because of the frequency with which gamekeepers buttonhole poachers who, understandably, are in a hurry to get away.

skiing

Skiing can be divided into cross-country skiing and alpine skiing. Cross-country skiing (or Nordic skiing) is a low-impact, aerobic activity that conditions the whole body. It is becoming increasingly popular. There are believed to be over 7 million enthusiasts participating in this sport in the United States. Although it is one of the most physically demanding activities (a cross-country skier has the highest recorded aerobic capacity at 80 ml/kg/min), it can be enjoyed even if you have a relatively low skill level. It does not require exorbitant lift fees, and it has a relatively low injury rate (cross-country skiing has an injury rate about 10 times less than alpine skiing). Unlike alpine or downhill skiers who use gravity, cross-country skiers propel themselves about 80–90 per cent of the time, and use muscles in the arms, legs, and trunk in about equal measure. This muscle activity demands a great deal of energy. It has been estimated that cross-country skiing continuously for 150 minutes burns up more than 3000 Calories.

Skiing uses more muscles than running and is less stressful on the legs. During the propulsive phase, skiing produces impact forces of about 1.5 times body weight; running produces forces of up to 3.5 times body weight during the driving phase. This reduces the incidence of overuse injuries common in running. Thanks to a number of manufacturers, you can now obtain the exercise benefits of cross-country skiing without leaving the convenience of your own home. Several home-fitness exercise machines are designed to simulate the demands of cross-country skiing.

Alpine or downhill skiing is a popular family sport shared by people of all ages and athletic abilities. It has less benefits for aerobic fitness than cross-country-skiing because activity is usually in short bursts, but it is good for strengthening muscles particularly those in the upper leg. Alpine skiing is also a tough sport, particularly demanding on the legs. Recreational skiers often succumb to injuries of knee ligaments and ankle tendons because of lack of fitness or poor technique. Many of these injuries could be avoided if people conditioned themselves before embarking on a skiing holiday. Weight-training exercises to strengthen the muscles in the thighs and around the knees, and stretching exercises to improve overall joint mobility, reduce the risk of injury after an awkward fall. Simple activities, such as climbing stairs, brisk walking, jogging, and gentle running, help to develop overall stamina so that you can enjoy a day out on the piste. It is also important to warm-up immediately prior to skiing.

ski jump

A whole-body exercise often used in warm-up routines.

■ Stand upright with your arms stretched over your head, hands slightly clenched, and feet firmly fixed on the ground. Slowly bend your knees and swing your arms smoothly forwards and downwards in an action resembling the start of a ski jump. Continue swinging your arms back behind you, close to your buttocks; at the same time, continue to bend downwards and reach forward with your trunk, remembering not to arch your back. Hold only briefly before swinging your arms forwards and upwards as you return to the upright position, stretching upwards to your full extent, this time briefly going onto your toes if necessary. Immediately drive down again, and try to maintain a steady rhythm of down-and-back, forwards-and-up as you repeat the movements three or four times.

skill

In sport, a special ability acquired through training. Skill acquisition involves learning to execute movements with the minimum effort to achieve predetermined effects. It is a complex process demanding high levels of sensory perception, integration within the central nervous system, and coordination of different muscle groups. There are many different kinds of skill. They form a continuum from fine motor skills, requiring delicate muscular control (used in activities such as putting and rifle shooting), to gross motor skills, requiring coordination of many muscle groups (used in activities such as running). Some are open skills, performed in an unpredictable situation (such as a football match), with outside factors dictating how and when the skill is performed. Others are closed skills, involving movements which can be planned in advance and usually performed in a stable, mainly predictable situation; examples include performing a handstand, serving in tennis, teeing off at golf, and diving from a platform.

skin

The first line of defence against disease and physical damage, the skin is a complex organ containing different types of tissue.

The surface layer consists of dead, keratin-containing cells which swell in response to moisture and are shed daily. Given time, this layer thickens and hardens in response to friction. If friction is excessive, burns, blisters, and corns can develop. One aim of training is to harden the skin gradually so that it can withstand the forces experienced during activity. This is particularly important in martial arts which use parts of the body to inflict blows.

Beneath the outer layer, lie the living cells of the epidermis, protecting the body from injury and invasion from parasites. This layer also helps to prevent dehydration. Epidermal cells are continually dividing to replace dead cells lost from the surface. Since these cells have such a short lifespan, signs of nutritional deficiency develop quickly and skin condition is a good reflection of inner health. Clear, moist, glowing skin usually indicates that a person is healthy and well nourished.

The middle layer of the skin, the dermis or corium, contains cells with a black pigment, melanin. Melanin shields the underlying layers from the potentially damaging effects of ultraviolet radiation. Also in the dermis, sensory receptors and nerves inform the body of changes in body temperature. They enable a person to respond, sometimes defensively, to pressure, touch, and pain. The dermis is well supplied with blood vessel and sweat glands. These, combined with the action of erectile hairs, form part of the temperature-regulating system in the body. Sebaceous glands associated with the hair secrete oils which keep the skin moist and contribute to waterproofing. The dermis is the region in which wrinkles originate.

The deepest layer in the skin is the subcutaneous layer containing the stores of fat which many people spend much effort and time trying to reduce.

A well-balanced diet with plenty of fluid intake, regular aerobic exercise, and moderate exposure to sunlight can help to maintain a healthy skin. Nutrient deficiencies may cause dryness, roughness, wrinkling, and slow healing of wounds. Particularly important dietary components are the essential fatty acids and vitamins, particularly A, C, E, niacin, and riboflavin, but in developed countries deficiencies of these nutrients are very rare. *See also* **chafing; eczema;** and **sun-protection factor.**

skinfold measurements (fatfold test)

A measurement of a fold of body tissue that includes a double layer of skin and underlying fatty tissue, but no muscle. Usually the measurements are taken with special calipers by holding a fold of tissue with the left thumb and index finger at specific sites on the body (figure 62). Such measurements (for instance on the back of the arm, below the scapula, and on the calf) are used to estimate the amount of fat in the body. They may also be used to monitor fat losses. Skinfold measurements should decrease as total body fat is lost.

skin patches: *See* slimming patch.

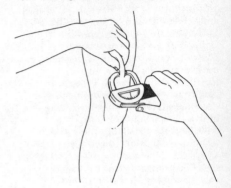

Figure 62 Skinfold measurements: measuring the thickness of the skin on the top of the thigh to estimate body fat

sleep

We spend about one-third of our lives sleeping, but exactly why we need sleep is the subject of much dispute. Traditional views emphasize sleep's restorative value; another view emphasizes the advantages of a period of immobility, for example, in conserving energy. Lack of sleep is associated with lower reaction times, reduced muscular coordination, and poor vigilance. It can also produce distinct alterations in personality.

Although the average person sleeps between 7–8 hours a night, there is no single standard number of hours of sleep that can be applied to everyone. Each person has to determine his or her own optimum. Exercise often restores normal sleep patterns to people who suffer sleeping disorders, and those who exercise vigorously generally need more sleep than sedentary people. *See also* **insomnia.**

slide training

A low-impact, aerobic exercise that strengthens the hips, knees, and ankles. Slide training is performed on a smooth plastic board with bumpers at either end to allow the exerciser to push off and slide. By swinging the arms and pushing with the legs, the exerciser can create a variety of sliding movements similar to those produced by a speed skater. A cloth over each training shoe makes sliding easier. It is a good exercise for promoting cardiovascular fitness, especially when incorporated into circuit training. Some running coaches have advocated slide training because it is especially effective at working the buttock muscles that help to stabilize the body during running, so it improves running economy. Slide training should be avoided by those suffering groin strain, lower back, or knee problems.

slimming patch

A 3 cm-square patch which is claimed by its US manufacturers to make weight loss easy. The patch is worn on hairless skin all day, but removed at night. According to the manufacturers, it contains extracts of a brown seaweed containing iodine which is absorbed into the bloodstream. Iodine is used by the body in the thyroid gland to make thyroxine, a hormone which increases metabolism. The manufacturers of the patch suggest that the absorption of additional iodine from the patch enables the production of extra thyroxine to burn off excess fat. Users are told that the patch will enable them to lose weight without any change in their lifestyle, but they are advised to drink at least eight glasses of water a day and follow a reasonably balanced diet. Loss of weight may be due to following this advice rather than to changes in metabolic rate. Some manufacturers have claimed that wearing the patches results in significant weight loss, particularly in those who are significantly overweight. These claims could not be substantiated to the satisfaction of the Food and Drug Administration and the patches were withdrawn from the US market in 1988, but they are still available in other countries. Tom Sanders, professor of nutrition at King's College, London, UK, is quoted in *The Times* newspaper (14 June 1994) as saying: 'The only way to lose weight with one is to stick it over your mouth.'

slimming pills

Pills containing drugs to help weight reduction. They include appetite suppressants such as the stimulants diethylpropion and fenfluramine; thyroid extract tablets which increase metabolic rate but can be dangerous; diuretics which reduce body fluid content but have little effect on fat content; and starch blockers which are claimed to stop starch digestion but are not effective. Slimming pills should only be taken when prescribed by a medical practitioner. *See also* **amphetamines** and **fibre supplements**.

slipped disc

A misnomer. Discs are firmly wedged between vertebrae and cannot slip (*see* **prolapsed intervertebral disc**).

slow-twitch fibre: *See* **muscle fibre types**.

small intestine: *See* **alimentary canal**.

smoking

Many smokers claim that their habit helps them to relax , but there is no doubt that smoking is harmful to health and has a detrimental effect on athletic performance. Tobacco smoking is a major, preventable factor leading to death. Almost 20 per cent of deaths in the USA have been attributed to diseases associated with inhaling the products of combustion from the tobacco plant, *Nicotiana tobacum*. These products include nicotine, carbon monoxide, and tars.

The psychological and addictive effects of smoking cigarettes are attributed to nicotine, a drug that stimulates the central nervous system and enhances arousal. Nicotine affects blood pressure and heart rate directly, increasing the risk to smokers of coronary heart disease. It also affects hormone production. For example, cigarette smoking lowers blood oestrogen levels and therefore reduces bone mineralization. When inhaled, the carbon monoxide passes into the bloodstream where it combines with haemoglobin, reducing the ability of blood to transport oxygen. Among heavy, chronic smokers the reduction may be as much as 10 per cent, reducing their ability to take part in strenuous exercise, and accounting for the breathlessness experienced by most smokers. Tars inhaled during smoking are microscopic, organic substances which can stick onto cells in the lungs. Some tars release free radicals that may be carcinogenic and increase the risk of lung cancer. The high production of free radicals in smokers may explain why they break down vitamin C faster than non-smokers (vitamin C is one of the antioxidants that mops up free radicals). It is estimated that the vitamin C requirements of smokers may be twice as much as non-smokers. In the UK, the RNI for adult non-smokers is 40 mg but smokers require more vitamin C (possibly as much as an extra 80 mg); in the USA, the RDAs are 60 mg for non-smokers and 100 mg for smokers.

Smoking is highly addictive. Smokers who try to give up may suffer withdrawal symptoms including a persistent craving for tobacco, irritability, poor concentration, and weight gain. The weight gain is popularly attributed to eating more to compensate for the lack of oral gratification provided by smoking. However, the gain may also be due to metabolic changes because nicotine increases metabolic rate, particularly during exercise. It is sensible for ex-smokers to moderate the effects of weight gain by increasing their aerobic activity. They should also control their feeding habits carefully. For example, snacks should consist of nutritious, low calorie foods such as raw vegetables and fruit.

smooth muscle: *See* muscle.

snack

A light, quick meal eaten between, or instead of, a main meal. Snacks have a bad reputation, but the wise use of nutritious snacks can improve the health and vitality of physically active people who lead a hectic lifestyle. Wholesome snacks that may boost energy, take the edge off appetite, and provide useful nutrients include dry cereal, fruits, nuts, seeds, and some vegetables which can be eaten raw, such as carrots. Not snacking can be detrimental since there is a danger of getting too hungry, developing a craving for sweet foods, and overeating at the earliest opportunity. However, the above comments should not be taken as a licence to over-indulge: it goes without saying that the consumption of large numbers of doughnuts (referred to by one nutritionist as 'grease bombs') and chocolate biscuits is not conducive to good health.

snow-blindness

Temporary blindness caused by the ultraviolet radiation in sunlight reflected from snow burning the outer, surface layers of the eye. The cornea and conjunctiva are inflamed and painful. The sufferer becomes very tearful and experiences great discomfort when exposed to strong light. Snow-blindness can be prevented by wearing special ski-goggles to prevent ultraviolet radiation damaging the eye.

soccer

Soccer is played worldwide by young and old, male and female, amateur and professional. The game makes many and varied physical demands on players. Top-class soccer players require very high levels of fitness. During a 90-minute match, their average work rate is about 70 per cent maximum and they burn an extra 1000–1500 Calories. They may cover more than 10 kilometres and have to sprint and jump many times with little chance to recover between bursts of maximum effort. So, in addition to their ball skills, they need to develop sprinting speed, endurance, muscular strength, and muscular power. Training usually involves a mixture of running, weight training, and circuit training, as well as ball work (passing, shooting, ball control, and heading). Flexibility is one aspect of fitness which is often neglected, especially by recreational players. Repeated sprinting, jumping, and kicking tends to tighten muscles in the lower back and legs. Without appropriate flexibility training players are likely to strain or pull muscles and tendons. The most common sites of injury are the calf muscles, Achilles tendons, and hamstrings. Before a match, each player should warm-up by jogging for 5–10 minutes. This should be followed by some flexibility and mobility exercises (especially for the hamstrings and the adductor muscles in the groin), three or four sprints over distances of about 25 metres, and then specific ball skills, such as dribbling and passing.

soccer toe: *See* black nail.

SOD: *See* superoxide dismutase.

sodium

A metallic element which is an important constituent of the human body.

Sodium plays a major role in water balance.

Sodium is one of the major components of table salt. An investigation, called the Intersalt Study, of 10 000 people from 32 countries, found that there was a very strong correlation between a high sodium consumption and high blood pressure, especially in sodium-sensitive people. The results can be interpreted in a number of ways, but most dietitians agree that high sodium intakes can be harmful. Sodium can also increase the risk of oedema (swelling, particularly in joints, caused by an accumulation of fluids). The current average sodium intake of adults in the UK is 3.2 g per day. The government recommends that this should be decreased to 1.6 g. One simple way of reducing sodium intake is not to add table salt to food.

Sodium deficiency is rare, but it can occur if losses from heavy sweating are not replaced. A deficiency leads to nausea and muscular cramps. *See also* **table salt**.

sodium bicarbonate

A salt of sodium that neutralizes acids. Sodium bicarbonate is taken to treat stomach disorders, acidosis, and sodium deficiency. It is used as a raising agent in food (baking powder).

Sodium bicarbonate is also used in tablet form as an ergogenic aid in a process called bicarbonate loading. The extra bicarbonate is taken to increase the blood's alkalinity and buffering capacity so that more lactic acid can be neutralized. This would delay the onset of fatigue. There are conflicting views about its effectiveness, but ingesting at least 300 mg of bicarbonate per kilogram body weight 2–3 hours before exercise may delay fatigue and increase performance in bouts of maximal effort activity lasting more than 1 minute and less than 7 minutes. Bicarbonate loading has improved the performance of average 800 metre runners by several seconds, but it may not have such a marked effect on well-trained, elite athletes. In addition, bicarbonate loading causes unpleasant side-effects in some people, the most common being gastrointestinal distress (e.g. cramping, bloating, and diarrhoea). Improvements in performance can be achieved with less risk by appropriate training. In general, bicarbonate loading should not be given serious consideration by athletes.

soft tissue injury

An injury, such as a sprain, strain, or pull, involving soft tissues (connective tissues which have not hardened into bone or cartilage). Soft tissues include skin, muscles, tendons, ligaments, and the tough connective tissue, called fascia, which lines them.

soft workouts

Any exercise that produces low-impact forces, minimizing the stress imposed on muscles and joints. Low-impact aerobic dance, cycling, and swimming and other water workouts can be used as soft workouts, but brisk walking is probably the most popular form of this exercise.

Regular brisk walking can produce as much cardiovascular benefit as jogging, and walkers tend to suffer far fewer joint and muscle injuries than joggers. Even fit exercisers can benefit from walking, as long as they walk fast enough to reach their target heart rate. Simple ways of increasing the intensity of walking include making vigorous arm movements and carrying light weights, but the best way is by walking uphill.

solanine

A toxic substance found in the skin of green potatoes. In large amounts it interferes with the normal transmission of nerves. Even small amounts cause gastrointestinal distress. Potatoes are stored in the dark to prevent greening and the formation of solanine.

soluble fibre: *See* fibre.

somatotype (body-type)

An individual's characteristic shape and physical appearance, irrespective of size. There are three main somatotypes:

- ENDOMORPH: Characterized by a rounded body shape
- MESOMORPH: Characterized by muscular and stocky physique of medium height
- ECTOMORPH: Characterized by a tall, thin body.

Individuals usually have elements of each type, and their composite somatotype is described in a three-figure rating system. In one system (the Heath-Carter somatotype system) the ratings are based on a number of factors, such as skinfold measurements, age, height, and weight; in another system (Sheldon somatotype classification), the ratings are based on photographs of an individual taken from three different perspectives. In both systems, each rating is from 1 to 7; 1 represents the least amount and 7 the maximum. The first figure represents the degree of endomorphy; the second, mesomorphy; and the third, ectomorphy. Thus, a somatotype of 1–6–2 would indicate no endomorphy, a high degree of mesomorphy, and a little endomorphy.

Certain somatotypes tend to be associated with particular sports. It is not really surprising that distance runners tend towards ectomorphy and wrestlers tend towards mesomorphy. However, although somatotype may contribute to success in specific activities, it is by no means essential. Not all successful distance runners, for example, conform to their expected somatotype. A disadvantageous body shape can be overcome by emphasis on other factors such as skill and dedication.

Sheldon claimed that there is a strong link between somatotype and personality (Sheldon's constitutional theory). He believed that somatotype is inborn, and that it predetermines an individual's character. He suggested that endomorphs tended to be 'viscerotonic' (easy-going, sociable people who take pleasure in eating); mesomorphs tend to be 'somatotonic' (bold and competitive individuals who are risk-taking, adventure-seeking extroverts); and ectomorphs tend to be 'cerebrotonic' (solitary and hyperactive with over-fast reaction times).

Controversy surrounds Sheldon's work. Today, most scientists give little credence to these claims, but Sheldon's constitutional theory was part of mainstream thought in the 1940s and early 1950s. His somatotyping was based on an enormous collection of nude photographs. Thousands of men and women entering certain Ivy League universities were required to pose for photographs sometimes, apparently, against their will. It has been suggested that Sheldon's main purpose was eugenic; that he wanted to establish a planned breeding programme, encouraging individuals with superior physiques to reproduce, while discouraging those with inferior physiques.

spare tyre
Accumulation of fat around the waist. This is more common in men than women and is more of a medical risk than other types of fat distribution. *See also* **android fat distribution** and **waist-hip ratio**.

spasm
A sudden involuntary muscle twitch ranging in severity from the mildly irritating to the very painful. A spasm may be due to a chemical imbalance in muscles; massaging the area often helps to end the spasm.

Specific Adaptations to Imposed Demands principle: *See* SAID principle.

specific-training principle
(specificity principle)
A basic principle of training which states that in order to improve a certain component of physical fitness, a person must train specifically for that component. For example, exercises for strength may do little to improve flexibility, and exercises designed to improve the endurance of arm muscles may do little for leg muscles. The principle applies to muscle groups, movement patterns, and type of contraction.

speed
The ability to execute movements quickly. Speed is a component of physical fitness and refers to distance travelled per unit of time. During running and walking, speed is a product of stride length and stride rate (cadence). Stride length depends partly on flexibility and strength. Stride rate depends on the speed of muscular contractions. *See also* **sprint**.

speed–accuracy trade off
The general principle that the accuracy of a movement tends to decrease when its speed is increased.

speed chute

A small, open parachute attached to the back of a runner. The chute billows out behind a runner during a workout, increasing the resistance against which to run. The manufacturers claim that they improve speed endurance and provide an alternative form of resistance training. There has been little research to test the effectiveness of the chutes. However, studies of sprinters suggest that chute users improve at the same rate as those doing similar training with no chutes. The chutes conferred no special benefits, but they may add variety and fun to resistance training.

speed play: *See* fartlek training.

SPF: *See* sun-protection factor.

spinner's finger

An injury commonly caused by spin bowling in cricket, baseball, and other ball sports. Although the skin in the hand becomes hardened with use, the forces used to impose spin on the ball can cause the skin to crack, leaving open wounds susceptible to infection. If this happens, the skin must be allowed time to heal and harden.

spleen

The most commonly injured organ within the abdomen. The spleen lies just below the 9th and 11th ribs, making it very susceptible to puncture by a fractured rib or a direct blow to the trunk. It can even be ruptured during a non-contact sport as a result of very strenuous activity, especially if it has become enlarged by a viral infection (in athletes, nearly 40 per cent of splenic ruptures are associated with glandular fever caused by a viral infection called infectious mononucleosis). This is one of several important reasons for resting during a fever.

The spleen has a number of functions, including removing worn out red blood cells and dealing with some types of foreign body. In order to carry out these functions, it is very well supplied with blood, making it quite soft and fragile. A rupture often results in torrential internal bleeding which is difficult to stop.

If untreated, this can lead to a serious lowering of blood pressure and death. Sometimes bed rest is sufficient treatment, but often surgical removal is the only viable course of action. Abdominal injuries are often underestimated in sports, especially when young people with enormous reserves of enthusiasm are involved. Consequently, a ruptured spleen may go unnoticed and untreated until the injured person loses so much blood he or she suffers from potentially fatal shock. Abdominal injuries are very difficult to diagnose, but expert medical assistance should always be sought if a person is suffering from persistent abdominal discomfort after a blow or after extreme exertion.

split routine

A system of weight training in which every major muscle of the body is exercised at least once a week. It is particularly popular among body-builders. Typically, the body is divided into two groups of body parts: one group consisting of arms, legs, and midsection; and the other consisting of neck, shoulders, chest, and back. Each group is exercised on alternate days and the exerciser trains 6 days a week.

spondylolithesis: *See* spondylolysis.

spondylolysis

A defect in the spine that causes acute pain on one side of the lower back. The pain is made worse by twisting and bending movements. Spondylolysis was once thought to be congenital. However, although some people are genetically predisposed to the condition, it is now believed to be a stress fracture of a vertebra (one of the bones that form the spinal column) caused by repeated hyperextensions of the lower back (i.e. bending backwards, a movement commonly performed during weight-training exercises). There is a high incidence of spondylolysis in young female gymnasts who perform front and back walk-overs, vaults, flings, and dismounts. Spondylolysis is often linked with another back injury, spondylolisthesis: the slippage of one vertebra on another (usually the fifth lumbar vertebra on the first sacral vertebra). Spondylisthesis reduces flexibility and usually results in tightening of the hamstrings. Physiotherapy, including abdominal strengthening exercises and hamstring stretches, is often sufficient for mild conditions. Surgical treatment may be necessary if, for example, there is more than 50 per cent vertebral slippage.

sport

The term 'sport' is often used loosely to embrace highly organized activities (such as golf, tennis, football, and karate) and recreational activities such as walking and fishing. However, sports scientists tend to restrict the term to highly-structured, goal-directed physical activities governed by rules.

Many people believe that there can be no true sport without the idea of fair play. Participation usually demands a high level of commitment and takes the form of a struggle either with oneself or through competition with others, but it also has some of the elements of play. Sport involves either vigorous physical exertion or the performance of relatively complex skills. Participants are often motivated by a combination of intrinsic satisfaction from the activity itself and external rewards earned through participation.

Sport Emotional Reaction Profile (SERP)

A number of psychological tools have been devised to measure traits that may be important in determining athletic performance. One of these tools is called SERP (sport emotional reaction profile). It was devised by Thomas Tutko and Umberto Tosi who regarded the following traits as important:

- DESIRE. An indication of the ability to set realistic goals: low levels of desire suggest lack of motivation; levels which are too high indicate that unrealistic goals are being set
- ASSERTIVENESS. A measure of an individual's determination to succeed. Low assertiveness suggests that an athlete will be intimidated by others; high levels indicate a tendency towards aggressiveness

- SENSITIVITY. An indication of the amount of pleasure gained from success. A person with high sensitivity may be easily discouraged by lack of success. Low levels suggest resilience
- TENSION CONTROL. The ability to cope with anxiety. Low tension control generally results in poor performance; high tension control is rarely a problem
- CONFIDENCE. Belief in one's own ability. Both low confidence and over-confidence can be a problem and usually result in poor performance
- PERSONAL ACCOUNTABILITY. Ability to cope with failures and mistakes. A person with low personal accountability generally blames others for a lack of success; those with very high levels may blame themselves too much if they make even a small mistake
- SELF-DISCIPLINE. The ability to persevere. Those with low levels of self-discipline give up easily and are generally not persistent trainers.

Each trait is scored on a scale from 5 to 30. To determine the scores, athletes are given 42 statements, such as 'I have nerves of steel during competition', to which they may respond, 'almost always' (about 90 per cent of the time); 'often' (about 75 per cent of the time); 'sometimes' (about 50 per cent of the time); seldom (about 25 per cent of the time); and 'almost never' (about 10 per cent of the time).

SERP is not readily applicable to non-athletes and some sports psychologists doubt its reliability as a research tool. However, it may be useful for self-assessment if the questions are answered honestly. Individual athletes can compare their SERP with a 'normal' profile so that problem areas can be revealed and corrected by psychological training techniques. *See also* **Profile Of Moods States**.

sporting behaviour

Behaviour exhibited by someone who respects and abides by the rules of a sport, and responds fairly, generously, and with good humour whether winning or losing. Sporting behaviour is demonstrated by a competitor who chooses an ethically correct strategy in preference to a success strategy involving 'winning at all costs'.

sport psychologist

A professionally-trained person who observes, describes, and explains the various psychological factors that influence various aspects of participation and performance in sport and physical activity. Sport psychologists support sports people with behavioural problems but they also help athletes to acquire psychological skills so that they can cope with the unusual demands of competition. Sport psychologists are concerned with both enhancing performance and improving the quality of the sport experience.

sports clothes: *See* clothing.

sports injury

Sports injuries are often similar to those sustained in the home or at work. However, there are some so commonly associated with sport that they have acquired special sporting epithets, such as runner's knee, swimmer's shoulder, and tennis elbow. In addition, an injured sports person may need different treatment from an inactive person: fitness prior to injury may subtly change the symptoms; the need to regain peak fitness may necessitate a different rehabilitation programme.

The risk of injury depends on the sport being pursued, as the following table shows:

INJURY RATE PER 100 000 PARTICIPANTS OF VARIOUS SPORTS

basketball	188.0
football	167.0
aquatic activities	46.0
lacrosse	39.5
wrestling	26.0
sledding	24.6
dancing	18.8
martial arts	16.9

From Birrer, R.B., Halbrook, S.P. (1988) Martial arts and injuries. *Am J Sports Med.* **16**:408–10. In: Mellion, M.B. (1993) *Sports medicine secrets.* Hanley and Belfus, xxx Philadelphia.

It may surprise readers to see the low incidence of injury associated with martial arts, but the table shows the number, not the seriousness. Sports injuries tend to be more severe in contact sports.

Professor Greg McLatchie Director of the National Sports Medicine Institute at St. Bartholomew's Hospital, London, UK, conducted a survey of the sites of sports injuries in 1600 patients:

SITE	PERCENTAGE OF INJURIES
lower legs	32.6
upper limbs	30.7
head	17.7
knees	10.4
trunk	6.4
upper leg	2.2

Sports-related injuries are caused by three main groups of factors:

1 direct trauma (i.e. physical contact)
2 overuse (*see* separate entry)
3 environmental factors (those associated with extremes of weather, immersion in water, altitude etc.).

The risk of injury in seemingly innocuous activities such as aerobic dance and jogging, depends very much on environment. These activities subject the body to high impact forces as the foot strikes the ground. Therefore, the type of surface and the degree of protection offered by footwear are important. In addition, high impact sports tend to produce more overuse injuries than low impact sports such as swimming.

Sports injuries are more likely when there is a combination of factors in operation: for example, a rugby player is more likely to incur a knee injury when floored by a lateral tackle if it is a cold day, the pitch is frost-hardened, and the player's knee has already been weakened by overtraining or overplaying.

Many sports injuries are unnecessary and can be avoided by:

● ensuring that you are fit for your activity
● wearing the correct equipment
● being aware of environmental hazards such as slippery surfaces
● always warming-up and cooling down
● allowing your body enough time to adapt to higher levels of activity.

Most sports injuries involve strains, tears, and ruptures of muscle fibres, and are not life-threatening. Your chances of a speedy and complete recovery from these injuries improve if you receive quick, correct treatment. Most muscle injuries, such as bruises and strains, respond well to rest, ice, compression, and elevation (see **RICE**). Heat should never be applied to an injured muscle in the first 48 hours of injury.

A variety of unpleasant and even fatal conditions, including multiple sclerosis, osteomyelitis (bone inflammation), and bone cancer may first appear as an apparent sports injury. For this reason, if for no other, sports injuries should be taken seriously and medical advice should be sought if symptoms persist.

sports medicine
A branch of medicine dealing with the prevention, protection, and correction of sports injuries, and the preparation of an individual for physical activity in its full range of intensity. It includes the study of the effects of different levels of exercise, training, and sport on healthy and ill people.

Originally, the main objective of sports medicine was the welfare of competitive athletes but it now encompasses treatment of anyone engaged in sport and exercise. It is becoming an increasingly important branch of medicine. More general practitioners are being trained in sports medicine than ever before. The training gives them a better understanding of the physical, physiological, and psychological demands of exercise. This helps them to diagnose sports injuries more effectively, and to prescribe the most suitable forms of exercise to improve the health of patients, for example those recovering from heart disease.

Some practitioners trained in sports medicine are employed by sports teams to help athletes improve their performance. Usually, this is by the legitimate and ethical application of their special knowledge. However, sometimes it involves the unethical use of ergogenic aids (artificial performance boosters such as drugs) which transgress the rules of sports governing bodies.

sports science
Any discipline using scientific methods to study sports phenomena. Sports scientists extend our knowledge and understanding of sport by studying the effects of training and competition on performers, and the interactions between performers, their coaches, and spectators. They rely on objective methods (rather than biased judgement and vague impressions) to explain and predict sports phenomena.

spot-reducing: See spot theory of fat reduction.

spotter
A weight-training partner who hands weights to a weight-lifter, controls the weights during lifts, and takes the weights when the lifts are completed. Spotters are essential to reduce the risk of accidents; even the most experienced lifters can get tired.

spot theory of fat reduction
(spot-reducing)
The idea that specific exercises or diets can reduce the amount of fat in a particular area of the body without affecting the amount in other parts. For example, many people intuitively believe that if they have too much fat around the waist, abdominal exercises will reduce the fatty tissue in that area.

Several writers have capitalized on this idea and have promoted spot-reducing diets. One of the most famous is The Hip and Thigh Diet devised by Rosemary Conley. She claims that her very low fat diet (no food with more than 12 per cent fat) and exercise programme can help you lose weight preferentially from the hips and thighs. Although her programme is one of the most commercially successful ever devised (her book has sold more than 2 million copies worldwide), experts do not believe that this or any other diet and exercise programme can help you shed fat from some parts of your body but not others. The idea was disproved several years ago when researchers studied tennis players who played more than 6 hours a week. They expected the arm used to hold the racquet to be more muscular and less fatty than the other arm. Although the racquet-holding arm was more muscular, the amount of fat was the same in both arms.

Other studies confirm that it is not possible to manipulate diet or use exercise to lose fat from specific parts of the body. Fat is lost through the creation of an energy deficit which results in some fat being withdrawn from all the fat stores.

sprain

An injury caused when a joint is moved beyond its normal range of movement, but is not partly or wholly dislocated. Sprains usually arise from a sudden forceful movement that damages a joint capsule and the ligaments that tie together the bones in the joint. Damage to the joint tissue results in pain, swelling, and some loss of function.

Sprains range from small tears to serious ruptures. The severity is graded by degree: with a first degree sprain, there is little damage; with a second degree sprain, partial tearing of the ligament occurs; and with a third degree sprain, there is complete disruption of the ligament.

The primary treatment for a sprain is rest, indirect application of ice, compression with a bandage, and elevation of the damaged joint (see **RICE**). Secondary treatment may include administration of non-steroidal anti-inflammatory drugs (e.g. aspirin or ibuprofen), physical therapy (e.g. ultrasound or heat treatment), and stretching exercises specific for each type of sprain. Sometimes supportive braces or other devices are useful and, in extreme cases (such as a third degree sprain of the anterior cruciate ligament in the knee) surgery may be necessary. Individuals with excessive flexibility are more prone to sprains because the connective tissue surrounding the joint has been stretched and does not contribute so effectively to joint stability. Exercise addicts are also susceptible because they tend to overtrain. They are also reluctant to stop training when injured and do not give the sprain a chance to heal. It is unwise to continue training with a sprain, even with taping or bandaging, because there is a high risk of the sprain growing worse

and becoming more resistant to treatment.

spreads

A general term for butter, soft margarines, and low fat spreads which may not be called margarine (the composition of which is legally defined). Margarines were first developed as a cheap alternative to butter. They were made mainly from hydrogenated plant oils. The addition of hydrogen transforms the oils into solid, saturated fats. They were cheap but difficult to spread after refrigeration and not very tasty. Responding to the demand for a more spreadable and tasty margarine, manufacturers produced soft margarines with a higher content of polyunsaturated fats. These spreads have gained in popularity as people have learned that unsaturated fats are healthier that saturated ones. Some spreads have been developed with the additional advantage to weight-conscious consumers of being low in calories. This is achieved by increasing the water content of the spread or by using fat replacers. Care should be taken when buying spreads because some low calorie varieties have a relatively high percentage of saturated fats.

sprint

A movement over a short distance at top speed in one continuous effort. The best training for sprinting is to run, cycle, swim, or canoe repetitively as fast as possible over short distances. This helps to develop fast-twitch muscle fibres (see **muscle fibre types**) and the enzymes which enable them to contract quickly. However, the training has to be specific. The muscles used for sprint swimming, cycling, or canoeing are not exactly the same as those used for running. Therefore, someone good at sprint cycling may not be any good at sprint running. Although the muscles used differ, all forms of sprinting demand high power outputs. To create quick movements, muscles have to react quickly to instructions from the central nervous system, utilize energy quickly, and go through the mechanics of contraction quickly. Reaction times are sometimes improved by using speed balls (punch balls similar to those used by boxers). The utilization of energy and the mechanics of contraction are often improved by bounding exercises (*see* **plyometrics**), and weight- and flexibility-training specifically designed to improve muscles used in particular forms of sprinting.

sprue: *See* **coeliac disease**.

squash

Squash is a game that requires agility, coordination, and good aerobic fitness. It is generally regarded as one of the most physically demanding sports. Noel Coward said it is 'not exercise – it's flagellation'. A squash game may consist of long rallies and short recovery periods. A match between top-class players can last 90 minutes or more. Repeated bursts of activity within the confined space of a squash court can raise body temperature and elevate the heart rate to dangerously high levels. This can overload the heart of an unfit person. The Squash Rackets Association use the adage 'Get fit to play squash. Don't play squash to get fit', to encourage sensible participation. Most physicians discourage anyone over the age of 50 from taking up squash. The need for caution is emphasized by the table of exercise-related sudden deaths.

Although squash is at the top of the table, Robin Northcote emphasized that there is a very low statistical risk of sudden death from any sport and that the figures do not imply that squash is more dangerous than other sports. Nevertheless, his table does show that a significant number of squash players have probably died unnecessarily.

For those who are fit enough to play squash, it is an excellent game for developing stamina, suppleness, and, to a lesser extent, strength. Even fit squash players are susceptible to pulls, strains, and tears of muscles and tendons, particularly in the lower leg. An adequate warm-up which includes mobility and stretching will reduce the risk of injury. This is particularly important for those over 25 because as you age your muscles and tendons gradually become less elastic. To minimize stress injuries when feet are jarred and dragged on a hard squash court, it is essential to wear shoes that have adequate cushioning in the heels and instep, and adequate reinforcement around the toes. To decrease the risk of eye injury (a squash ball is just the right size to enter the eye socket), squash players should wear smash-resistant eye protectors.

squat

An exercise for conditioning muscles of the legs and buttocks. It can be performed with or without additional weights.

■ Stand erect with feet about shoulder width apart. Keeping your back straight and head up, slowly bend the knees to squat down, and then return to the standing position.

If the knees are bent fully, tremendous mechanical strains are imposed on the joint and can cause irreparable damage. Therefore, the knees are bent only to the half- to two-thirds position. The back is kept straight to reduce the strain on the knees and lower back, and movements should always be slow and controlled.

Squash

EXERCISE-RELATED SUDDEN DEATH IN THE MAINLAND UNITED KINGDOM 1978–87

SPORT/ACTIVITY	NUMBER		MEAN AGE
	MALE	FEMALE	
squash	124	2	44
soccer	53	–	32
swimming	50	6	53
running	38	1	37
badminton	26	–	49
rugby	14	–	30

Table adapted from Northcote, R.J. (1994) Heart and exercise: clinical aspects. In: *Oxford textbook of sports medicine*. p286. Oxford University Press, Oxford.

Squats with additional weights are usually performed with either the barbell resting at the back of the neck (back squat) or across the front of the shoulders and top of the chest (front squat). Both types of squat develop leg, hip, and back strength, but the front squat places more stress on the quadriceps.

There are at least eight other types of squat, each with their own specific advantages and disadvantages. Squats have been called the 'king of all exercises' by some body-builders. If performed properly, squats can greatly strengthen the muscles (especially the quadriceps), bones, tendons, and ligaments in the legs. However, if performed excessively or with poor technique, they can cause a host of stress injuries, including arthritis and torn cartilage of the knee.

squat thrust
An exercise for developing lower-body muscles and aerobic fitness.

■ From a standing position, squat down so that your arms are outside your knees. Support your body with your hands and toes, then thrust both of your legs backwards into the press-up position. Keep your back straight. Move your legs forward so that they come to rest under your arms. Repeat the backwards and forwards movements a number of times, but keep your hands in the same position. Finish the exercise by standing up.

stability: *See* joint stability.

stage training: *See* circuit training.

stamina: *See* endurance.

standing toe-touch test
A commonly-used, indirect test of flexibility.

■ Stand with your hands by your side and your knees straight; lean forward slowly to touch your toes, or, if you can, the floor with your fingertips.

In one test of minimal flexibility, men are expected to be able to touch the floor with their fingertips, and women are expected to be able to touch the floor with the palms of their hands. Many sport's coaches do not like this test because, if performed at speed with bouncing movements, it can put a severe strain on the back.

staphylococcal food poisoning
A form of food poisoning caused by bacteria belonging to the genus *Staphylococcus* (commonly referred to as Staph). The bacteria are present on skin, particularly around boils and pimples. Food is easily contaminated by a food handler with an uncovered skin infection. The bacteria are also spread by coughs and sneezes. They are common in foods that require a lot of handling and multiply rapidly at room temperature. Symptoms are similar to most other forms of food poisoning: nausea, vomiting, abdominal pain, and diarrhoea.

starch
A complex carbohydrate (polysaccharide) made of many glucose units. Uncooked starch is very difficult to digest, but heat opens out starch molecules so that they form a gel-like structure which is more accessible to digestive enzymes. During digestion, enzymes in the gut help to break down the starch into dextrins, and then glucose molecules which are absorbed into the blood. Starch takes much longer to digest than simple sugars, such as sucrose (table sugar). Consequently, starch provides a steady stream of glucose into the bloodstream and is less likely than sucrose to cause blood glucose swings which can provoke the secretion of excess insulin.

High quantities of starch are found in bananas which are still green at their tips (in brown bananas, most of the starch is converted to sugars), breads, corn, oats, pasta, potatoes, rice, and yams. Unrefined forms of these foods also contain other nutrients, especially vitamins, trace minerals, and fibre. They are a much better source of carbohydrates than manufactured, sweet products containing little other than sugar. For example, wholemeal pasta contains high levels of carbohydrate and significant amounts of dietary fibre, minerals, and B complex vitamins. This makes it a favourite pre-race food for many marathon runners: the carbohydrate helps to boost muscle glycogen stores, and the other components help to maintain the health and efficiency of the runner. *See also* **resistant starch**.

starch blockers
Slimming pills said to reduce weight by inhibiting the digestion of starch. They were advertised as a way of eating as much as you like without getting fat. By 1983, millions of starch blockers were sold. They were banned in the USA after researchers found that not only were they ineffective, but they also contained variable amounts of a dangerous toxic substance called lectin.

starch gum: *See* **dextrin**.

starch sugar: *See* **dextrin**.

star jumps: *See* **stride jumps**.

starvation
Total abstinence from food. Starvation for more than one day depletes the body of its glycogen stores. Glycogen is the main source of glucose, an essential fuel for the brain. In order to maintain supplies, the body uses the protein in its own cells to make glucose, resulting in muscle wasting. If starvation continues for a few weeks, the brain adapts and can use the breakdown products of fat as a fuel. Once the fat stores are used, it again resorts to using protein. If this self-destructive process continues, heart muscle is broken down and death is inevitable.

Starvation is sometimes self-inflicted by people who want to lose weight rapidly. This is generally not recommended: it can disturb the body's metabolism and some doctors believe it may lead to eating disorders such as anorexia nervosa. In addition, the muscle lost during starvation is not easily regained, leaving a person physically weaker, less active, and more susceptible to weight gain. *See also* **fasting**.

state anxiety: *See* **anxiety**.

static stretching: *See* **stretching**.

stationary leg change
A mobility exercise that strengthens and improves the flexibility of the leg and hip muscles (figure 63).

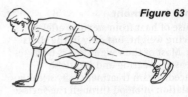

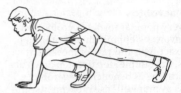

Figure 63

■ Crouch on the floor and rest your weight on your hands and feet. Your left leg should be bent under your chest and your right leg extended behind. Simultaneously bring the right leg up to your chest and extend the left leg backwards. Repeat by swapping the positions of the legs.

steadiness
The ability to maintain the body, or a part of the body, in a fixed position, or the ability to perform a smooth movement without any deviations from the desired course. Steadiness is adversely affected by muscle tremor and usually decreases as the strength of muscle contractions increase. It is an important component of skills requiring very controlled, steady movements (such as pistol marksmanship and snooker). The anxiety caused by competition sometimes results in the loss of steadiness, and a few marksmen and snooker players have resorted to taking drugs, such as beta-blockers, to reduce muscle tension.

steady state exercise
Exercise performed at a level low enough to be maintained for prolonged periods. This type of exercise is mainly aerobic. This means that the amount of oxygen taken in to burn food satisfies energy requirements so there is no oxygen deficit during exercise and no oxygen debt after the exercise.

steam treatment

The use of heat from steam is effective at reducing weight, but only in the short term. Most of the weight loss is from increased sweating and is quickly replaced. Steam treatment may stimulate circulation of blood through the surface tissues and thus invigorate you. It may also help you to relax, for example, before a massage. But on its own it will not help you to lose weight. *See also* **sauna**.

step aerobics

This very popular form of aerobic exercise involves stepping on and off a step. The exact type and rate of movement varies, but simple step-up, step-down aerobics can be as beneficial to aerobic fitness as more intense movements, and less damaging to joints. Step aerobics is linked to more knee injuries than other forms of aerobics. Many of the injuries are due to poor technique and poor tuition in classes that are too large. Stepping rates are usually about 120 per minute and the step is 6–8 inches (about 15–20 cm) high. The higher the step and the higher the rate of stepping, the greater the risk of injury. Therefore, step aerobics should be tailored to individual requirements, and the routine should take into consideration the size and fitness levels of individuals. To minimize risk of injury, steps should be performed gently and carefully. Power stepping (high impact stepping that may involve the use of handweights) is gaining popularity as a more robust form of step aerobics. Although it has a greater effect on strength, it carries a higher risk of injury and does not improve aerobic fitness any more than traditional step aerobics.

stepper

A training machine on which movements similar to running are performed. The exerciser pushes up and down against steps. Resistance is provided by air pressure, so impact forces are low, and there is little risk of stress injuries to bones and joints. Exercise on steppers is good training for active sports such as skiing because it strengthens the quadriceps, hamstrings, and calf muscles in the legs. Resistance is easily varied by changing the air pressure. It is usually set at a low level for developing aerobic fitness, but should be higher to develop muscle endurance. Many steppers are computerized so that stepping frequency, work levels, calories burnt, and duration of exercise can be controlled easily. Some machines have additional gadgets for monitoring pulse rate.

stepping-stone test

A test of dynamic balance in which you leap onto successive spots marked on the floor in an irregular pattern. You try to maintain balance on the landing foot for a few seconds before leaping again. Scoring for the test includes both the time taken and the error rate. *See also* **hexagon test**.

step test

A test of cardiovascular fitness involving a period of stepping on and off a bench or chair and comparing pulse rates before and after the exercise. The quicker the pulse returns to its normal resting rate, the fitter the individual. There are a number of variations. The Harvard step test was devised at Harvard University during the Second World War. In this test, you step on and off a 20 inch (50.8 cm) bench with alternate feet, repeating the sequence at a steady rhythm of 30 times a minute for up to 5 minutes or until exhausted. Your pulse is taken before the exercise and again 1 minute, 2 minutes, and 3 minutes after the exercise. Fitness levels are estimated from the rate at which the pulse returns to its resting level. Although cheap and easy to do, the step test is not very reliable as a medical test of cardiovascular fitness, and has been largely superseded by other exercise tests (*see* **graded exercise test**). However, its beneficial effects on the heart and vascular system have been recognized and incorporated into step aerobics, a very popular type of exercise usually performed to music.

steroid

A fat-soluble organic chemical, formed in the body from cholesterol and fats. Steroids include the male sex hormone, testosterone; the female sex hormone, oestrogen; and the stress hormones secreted by the outer part of the adrenal gland (*see* **corticosteroids**). *See also* **anabolic steroids**.

stevioside
A natural sweetener extracted from a Paraguayan chrysanthemum. It has been used for centuries to sweeten food and drink. Stevioside has the advantage over sugars in not causing tooth decay, but it does have a lingering and bitter aftertaste. *See also* **artificial sweeteners**.

stick test: *See* reaction time.

stiffness
A feeling of restricted mobility often caused by the overuse of a muscle and believed by many to be due to the build up of lactic acid. However, stiffness can also develop when the levels of lactic acid are not high and is probably due to exercise-induced muscle cell damage. *See also* **muscle soreness**.

stimulants
Drugs used as appetite suppressors, weight reducers, and mood enhancers. They have also been misused in sport, particularly in endurance activities, to increase mental alertness, to conceal feelings of exhaustion, and to increase aggressiveness.

Exercisers using stimulants may force their body beyond safe limits. Several sudden deaths have been attributed to stimulants such as amphetamines and cocaine. All stimulants have the potential to increase heart rate and blood pressure with lethal results. In addition, even moderate stimulant use may result in loss of judgement and increase the risk of injury to both the user and others. Stimulants are banned by most sports federations, including the International Olympic Committee.

stitch
A sharp pain usually felt on the right side, immediately below the rib cage. It occurs mainly when exercising upright, for example when running. A stitch often develops during the early stages of exercise and subsides as exercise continues, but the pain may be so severe that it is impossible to continue. Relief can be gained by supporting the abdominal wall, or by lying down with hips raised. The exact cause of a stitch is unknown but it may be due to lack of oxygen to the muscles used in breathing (particularly the diaphragm and intercostals). Factors that increase the likelihood of a stitch include jolting the body, starting an exercise at too high an intensity, eating and drinking before exercise, weakness of the abdominal wall, and lack of training. *See also* **cramp**.

stomach curl
A simple and quick exercise to strengthen the abdominal muscles.
■ Lie on your back, legs bent, and feet flat on the floor. Clasp your hands on top of your head, then slowly and gently raise your legs and move your knees and chin towards each other (do not force your head upwards with your hands). Slowly return to the start position. Most people should be able to do about 10 repetitions.

stomach muscles: *See* abdominal muscles.

stomach stapling
Surgery that seals off and removes parts of the stomach to make it smaller. This extreme procedure is sometimes used to help people suffering from severe obesity when other methods have failed to restrict food consumption. There is little evidence for its long-term effectiveness as a means of weight control.

stomach ulcer: *See* peptic ulcer.

storage fat
Fat deposited under the skin in adipose tissue. It protects internal organs and serves as an energy store. Before it can be used by muscles, it has to be converted into fatty acids (*see* **fat mobilization**).

strain: *See* muscle strain.

strength
The ability to apply a force and overcome a resistance. Strength is an essential part of physical fitness. The term usually refers to maximum, absolute strength, which is the maximum force a person can exert in one effort regardless of body

size or muscle size. A better comparison of people of different body size can be made using relative strength. This is the maximum force an individual can exert in relation to his or her body weight. Other types of strength include dynamic strength and elastic strength.

Dynamic strength is the ability to exert muscle force repeatedly. The muscle contractions involved are isotonic (the muscle shortens and the body or body parts move).

Elastic strength is the ability of muscles to exert forces quickly and to overcome resistance with high speed contractions. Elastic strength requires complex coordination of speed and strength of muscles. It is important in explosive activities such as jumping and sprinting. Sometimes elastic strength is used synonymously with power. It can be improved by special exercises, called plyometrics, which involve bounding movements. There are three main types of muscle contraction: eccentric, in which the muscle increases in length; isometric, in which the muscle maintains a constant length; and isotonic, in which the muscle shortens. A person who has a high level of strength for one type of muscle contraction is not necessarily strong with respect to the other types; training has to be specific.

strength endurance

The ability to resist a force over time or to make repeated muscle contractions against a force. Strength endurance is a measure of the ability of a muscle or muscle group to work continuously. It has a meaning similar to muscle endurance, but with strength endurance there is a greater emphasis on the amount of the force which can be resisted.

strength training

Exercises performed specifically to develop strength. Strength training can be achieved using a wide variety of exercises, including body resistance exercises, exercises with a medicine ball, circuit training, and plyometrics. However most strength training involves progressive resistant exercises using free weights or a weight-training machine. Usually the training programme is based on establishing the repetition maximum (the maximum load that can be lifted for a given number of repetitions) and ensuring that the muscles are systematically overloaded but not overstrained. The main factors which can be varied in strength training are the resistance (the weight being moved or the force resisted); the number of repetitions (the times each exercise or weight-training movement is repeated); the number of sets (each set being a given number of repetitions); and the rest period between the sets. Absolute strength is best gained by increasing the resistance and reducing the number of repetitions. The minimum resistance needed to gain strength is approximately 60 per cent of the maximum resistance that a muscle group can exert. Muscle endurance and elastic strength is best gained by decreasing the resistance, and increasing the number and speed of repetitions.

The following table shows that to develop absolute strength, you should perform high resistance exercises at a low number of repetitions; for endurance, you should perform low resistance exercises at high number of repetitions.

Strength training affects muscles, their nerve supply, and other associated structures. The beneficial effects of strength training include the following:

Strength training

% MAXIMUM RESISTANCE	TRAINING AIM	REPS	SETS	REST (SECS)
90+	absolute strength	1–5	4–8	2–5
75–90	explosive strength	8–10	3–4	1–2
50–75	strength endurance	10–15	3–4	45–90
<50	speed endurance	20+	>4	none

- increase in muscle size and absolute strength
- improved blood supply to the muscles and joints
- toughening of connective tissue in the tendons and ligaments
- increase in bone density and strength
- reduction of the fat content of muscles.

For maximum benefits, strength training should take place at least two or three times a week for 45 minutes each time. Strength training more than three times a week can be damaging and does not allow sufficient time for the muscles to respond to increased demands. It is believed that during a hard training session some of the muscle fibres are split and need time to regrow. It takes several weeks to gain all the benefits of a strength-training programme, the time depending on the person and the muscle groups being exercised.

A strength-training programme should take into account all the basic principles of training: it must be specific, progressive, and provide sufficient overload to stimulate muscle growth. There are a number of different schemes, but they all tend to follow a similar pattern of phases:

- PREPARATION PHASE. General conditioning, including body-weight exercises and light resistance (*see* **circuit training**)
- FOUNDATION PHASE. Continuation of whole-body conditioning, but with an increase in the resistances
- STRENGTH TRANSFER PHASE. Introduction of specific exercises. These will depend on individual aims, but may include absolute strength-gain exercises for those who wish to be weight-lifters, and bounding exercises (*see* **plyometrics**) for potential sprinters, jumpers, and throwers
- SPECIFIC STRENGTH PHASE. Exercises that increase the strength of muscle groups used in a specific activity. A variety of exercises may be performed (e.g. bounding exercises, medicine ball drills, and conventional weight training), but muscles should be worked in the same way as in the activity for which you are training.

The duration of each phase and the choice of exercises will depend on the individual and the activity for which he or she is training. Ideally, during a strength-training session each of the major muscle groups should be used, and, to avoid fatigue, successive exercises should not use the same muscle group.

stress

A psychological condition occurring when individuals feel unable to cope with the demands being made on them. They also believe that this failure will have important consequences. This condition is sometimes called distress, to distinguish it from the positive or pleasant aspects of stressful situations (eustress). Stress is usually associated with feeling a lack of control and involvement in the decisions which affect life and work.

The jobs with the highest strain are those in which there is heavy pressure to perform, where hours and procedures are rigid, there is a threat of redundancy, there is little opportunity to learn new skills, and there is little involvement in decision making. Such jobs tend to be the least prestigious. Workers low in the hierarchy tend to experience the most stress. It is unclear how stress affects health, but one possibility is that it disturbs important systems in the body, such as the hormonal, nervous, or immune system.

Although it may not be possible to change jobs, the effects of stress can be relieved by exercise and a healthy diet. Regular aerobic exercise, consisting of a daily 40-minute brisk walk, can reduce anxiety by as much as 14 per cent. In stressful situations, those who exercise regularly tend to have less muscle tension and lower blood pressure than inactive people.

stress fracture

A microscopic break in a bone caused by repeated loading and unloading. Stress fractures are often slow to develop and are not usually linked to any single injury. They occur when the forces applied repeatedly to a bone exceed its structural strength. According to the fatigue theory, bones are more likely to suffer fractures if they are not adequately supported by surrounding muscles because impact forces are transferred directly to the bones. Consequently, stress fractures tend to be more common in unconditioned exercisers with poor muscle development. Also those with brittle bones, such as older people and females suffering from menstrual irregularities (*see* **amenorrhoea**), are also susceptible to fractures. Stress fractures are characterized by local pain exacerbated by activity but relieved by rest. Most bones can become stress fractured, but more than one-half of all fractures seen in athletes affect the shin bone.

Stress fractures may be difficult to diagnose, except by a bone scan, because they do not always appear on X-rays until well established. *See also* **osteoporosis**.

stress hormone

A hormone secreted in response to stressful or exciting situations. Long-term stress is associated with high levels of cortisol. This is a steroid hormone secreted by the adrenal cortex which has a marked effect on carbohydrate metabolism and acts as an immunosuppressant. In the short term, physiological and psychological arousal results in the secretion of adrenaline into the blood, and noradrenaline into tissues. These hormones evolved so that we could deal rapidly with impending danger. They prepare our bodies for action by improving the blood supply to skeletal muscles and mobilizing energy stores. If stress hormones are too low, muscles have insufficient fuel and oxygen to respond quickly; however, excessive secretion of stress hormones can disturb the balance between fat and carbohydrate metabolism, and damage physical performance.

stress incontinence

The leakage of urine on laughing, coughing, straining, or even walking. It is common in women whose pelvic floor muscles have been weakened during childbirth. Specific postnatal exercises, such as stride jumps, can reduce the risk of stress incontinence.

Female athletes who perform heavy exercises that raise their abdominal pressure (e.g. basketball players, weight-lifters, and javelin throwers) may also suffer stress incontinence. Extreme exertion can reduce the collagen that helps to bind the tissue in the pelvic floor.

Special pelvic floor exercises have been designed to reduce the risk of stress incontinence. One unusual form of exercise uses weights inserted like a tampon into the vagina for 20–30 minutes each day. The pelvic floor muscles are strengthened by the pubococcygeal muscles contracting to keep the weights in place. Sometimes, stress incontinence can be treated by surgery. *See also* **pelvic floor lift**.

stress inoculation training

A form of psychological training devised to overcome the nervousness and anxiety associated with competition. The competitor identifies the factors (stressors) that induce stress and describes the negative thoughts associated with each. Then he or she imagines each stressor in turn, starting with the least worrying. At the same time, the competitor practises physical relaxation techniques and replaces the negative thoughts with positive ones. The training is based on the principle that it is not possible to feel stress and be physically relaxed at the same time.

stretch-and-curl

A relatively easy exercise often used as part of a cool-down routine to reduce muscle tension.

■ Lie flat on your back. Gently stretch out until your arms and legs are fully extended. Slowly raise and bend your arms, trunk, and legs so that you assume a crouched position with your arms wrapped around your knees, the heels of your feet tucked under your buttocks, and your head tucked forwards between your arms. Make yourself into as small a ball as possible. Hold for about 5 seconds then slowly lower yourself back down to the starting position. Repeat the exercise three or four times. The key to this exercise is to move in a relaxed manner, very smoothly and slowly.

stretching

There are two main types of stretching exercises: ballistic stretching and static stretching. Ballistic stretching is performed quickly with bouncing movements. It carries a high risk of muscle tears. In static stretching, the stretched position is reached gently and slowly and is held for a given time (usually 6–60 seconds); there is no movement or bouncing and no extra weight or strain on the muscle.

A programme of static stretching exercises improves flexibility, allowing freer and easier movements. Stretching can also improve posture and a sense of well being. It is particularly useful for older people, because their muscles tend to tighten, particularly those in the backs of the thighs.

Most coaches advocate pre-workout stretching to reduce the risk of muscle injuries. However, stretching can have the opposite effect, especially if it is performed too enthusiastically before you are properly warmed up. If you stretch as part of your warm-up routine, make sure that your muscles are warm before you stretch and perform the stretches gently and slowly. It appears that the best time to stretch is after strenuous activity, during cooling down. This maintains mobility of the joints by loosening muscles which have tightened during the activity. It also reduces the incidence of muscle soreness. It is probably a good idea to include static stretches which are held for only a few seconds (5–10 seconds) towards the end of your warm-up and include longer static stretches (up to 30 seconds) when cooling down.

stretch reflex

The reflex contraction of a muscle when it is stretched. Special sensory receptors (called proprioceptors) in muscle cells constantly monitor the state of muscles. The stretch reflex, by limiting its range of movement, protects a muscle from being overstretched and damaged. However, this protective mechanism can itself be damaging if the muscle is lengthened suddenly, especially when cold. The muscle will automatically and forcibly try to shorten, sometimes rupturing itself. For this reason, sports coaches usually advise exercisers training for flexibility to perform static stretches, or slow, controlled movements.

stretch stress

A feeling experienced when the muscles and connective tissue of a joint are stretched to a point at which some resistance or slight stress is felt but there is no pain. The stretch stress is used to obtain the stretch position when doing flexibility exercises. To gain maximum benefit, this end position is usually held (with no bouncing movements) for 10 or more seconds before the body is returned slowly to its original position. Quick movements are avoided throughout the stretch to minimize the risk of damage.

stride jumps (star jumps)

A simple exercise for toning pelvic floor muscles. It is particularly valuable as a postnatal exercise for women who wish to reduce the risk of stress incontinence. At first, the jumps should be performed when the bladder is empty.

■ Start in a standing position with feet together then jump up, spreading arms and legs out in a wide 'V', and finish with legs together and arms by the side. Usually, 10 repetitions are enough in the early sessions, gradually increasing to about 100 times daily.

stride stretch

A stretching exercise that improves the flexibility of the groin muscles (muscles on the inner surface of the thighs).

■ Stand upright. Assume a stride position with your hands on the floor or on the back of a chair to maintain balance. Lower your buttocks until you feel a stretch. Hold for a few seconds. Return to the starting position. Relax. Repeat with the other leg.

stroke

An interruption of the blood supply to the brain. A blood clot, a head injury, or a burst blood vessel in the brain (an aneurysm) can cause strokes. The main risk factors associated with strokes are high blood pressure, heart diseases, diabetes, smoking, obesity, and physical inactivity.

A stroke results in a portion of the brain being deprived of oxygen often leading to some type of paralysis, but small strokes may occur without symptoms. Large strokes can result in severe paralysis or death. Regular exercise and a healthy, balanced diet lower blood pressure and cholesterol levels, and so can reduce the risk of a stroke

stroke volume
The volume of blood pumped by the left ventricle per heartbeat. A typical value for a relatively inactive man is 75 ml per beat. For a trained man at rest it goes up to 105 ml per beat. *See also* **cardiac output**.

strychnine
An alkaloid drug obtained from the seeds of *Strychnos nux-vomica*. In high doses, strychnine causes severe muscular spasms which can be fatal if respiratory muscles are involved. In low doses it can act as a stimulant, boosting athletic performance. A related chemical was used by the Aztecs to enable them to complete their amazing runs which lasted up to 3 days. In the nineteenth century and the early part of this century, disreputable trainers and coaches sometimes spiked the drinks of their charges with small amounts of strychnine to give them an extra boost during very demanding competitions, such as bare-knuckle fights. In the St. Louis Olympic Games of 1904, the marathon runner, Thomas Hicks, was given strychnine mixed with brandy, in order to inject a bit more pace into his last few kilometres of running.

subluxation: *See* dislocation.

sucrose
A double sugar formed from fructose and glucose. It is a valuable energy source (each 100 grams of sucrose yields about 400 kcal of energy) but it has no other nutritional value and is often referred to as 'empty calories'. Refined sucrose, made from sugar cane and sugar beet, is the table sugar added to foods as a sweetener, flavour enhancer, and preservative. Sucrose also occurs naturally in many vegetables and fruits. *See also* **sugar**.

sudden death
Sudden death during or immediately after exercise is, thankfully, very rare. It has been estimated that one death occurs for every 15 000 to 18 000 exercisers each year. The risk of sudden death during exercise is 4 to 56 times greater than during rest (depending on the activity and age), but regular exercisers are less likely than inactive people to die at rest or during activity. Therefore, regular, vigorous exercise reduces the overall risk of sudden death. Among those under 35 years of age, the usual cause of death is a heart abnormality; of those over 35 who die, about 75 per cent have heart disease. Anyone who suffers from fainting or near-fainting, or has chest pains during activity should consult a doctor before continuing an exercise programme. Myocarditis (an inflammation of the heart) has been implicated in sudden death. However, several sports medicine practitioners question its involvement. Nevertheless, all agree that it is unwise to exercise during any illness which induces fever. *See also* **sudden immersion injury**.

sudden immersion injury
Swimming in very cold water is impossible, even for Olympic champions, because it incapacitates muscles. Sudden entry into freezing water can disturb the activity of the heart and disrupt breathing, resulting in loss of consciousness which may lead to death from drowning, a stroke, or heart attack. Canoeists and participants in other water sports are at obvious risk. Safety procedures for dealing with anyone who falls into the water are vital. Participants should always wear life-jackets and use wet- or dry-suits to retain body heat. Safety procedures should include quick removal, a change into dry clothing, and warm drinks. Alcohol should never be given because it encourages heat loss.

sugar
Sugars are simple carbohydrates. They are sweet, crystalline, and soluble in water. They are classified chemically as monosaccharides and disaccharides. Common monosaccharides are glucose and fructose; common disaccharides are sucrose and lactose. The most common sugar is white table sugar consisting of sucrose.

In the UK, the average person consumes more than 1 kg (2 lb) of sugar each week. Chocolates, biscuits, sweets, and many soft drinks contain very high levels of sugar. Many of these are also high in fat. Highly refined white sugar and its products are often called 'empty calories' because, although they provide energy, they are very low in nutrients such as vitamins and minerals. Unrefined brown sugar, and the sugar in honey, is reputed to have more nutritional value than white sugar, but the difference is insignificant. No sugars contain significant amounts of vitamins and minerals. Sugar is a preservative and flavour enhancer. It is added to many processed foods, such as baked beans and soups.

Sugar has a bad reputation. Table sugar is sometimes referred to as 'pure, white, and deadly'. Obesity, heart disease, and diabetes are just three diseases thought to be linked to high sugar consumption. However, although sugar is not very nutritious, there is little evidence that moderate consumption is harmful. There is much more evidence linking the above three diseases to overeating and lack of exercise. Of course, those people who are particularly carbohydrate-sensitive, or who are already suffering from obesity or diabetes, have to keep sugar consumption within strict limits. Frequent consumption of sucrose can encourage growth of oral bacteria (*see* **tooth decay**) and yeast infections. *See also* **glucose**.

sugar fix
The use of sugar as a quick source of energy, particularly just before or during exercise, to enhance performance. Contrary to popular belief, consuming high quantities of sugar 30–60 minutes before exercise does not boost short-term energy sources. In fact, it may have a negative effect by stimulating the production of insulin thus causing the sugar to be converted to glycogen. This would cause hypoglycaemia, a lowering of blood sugar, which makes a person feel light-headed and interferes with the ability to exercise. Sugar consumed during exercise may improve stamina and is unlikely to lower blood sugar levels because insulin production is inhibited by the exercise. *See also* **energy drink** and **insulin rebound**.

sugar-free food
In the UK, a label used on foods that do not contain table sugar (sucrose).

However, they may contain other sugars such as glucose, fructose, or sugar alcohols (e.g. xylitol, used in 'tooth-friendly' sweets because it deters the growth of bacteria that cause dental caries). Foods containing xylitol are unsuitable for diabetics.

sugar malabsorption
A partial or complete inability to break down disaccharides (double sugars) into monosaccharides. The disaccharides accumulate in the gut and cause diarrhoea. Bacterial decomposition of these sugars in the lower part of the digestive tract results in gas formation and abdominal pain. Vitamins, minerals, and fluid are lost with the diarrhoea. Untreated sugar malabsorption results in fatigue and deterioration in physical performance. Avoiding carbohydrates from which the disaccharides are derived enables normal activity to be resumed. Sugar malabsorption, apart from that due to lactose intolerance, is very rare.

sulphites
Salts containing sulphur and usually derived from sulphur dioxide. They are used as preservatives to prevent oxidation and mould growth in many processed foods and beverages, especially wines. They were formerly used by caterers to maintain the fresh appearance of fruits and vegetables, until it was discovered that some people have an adverse reaction to sulphites. Many asthmatics, children with a history of hyperactivity, and those with liver disorders are particularly sensitive to sulphites or sulphur dioxide. Consequently, their use in raw foods has been banned in the USA. All manufacturers of processed foods must declare the sulphite content in the food label. Although sulphites are a health hazard to only a few people, it is important to be aware that they can destroy thiamin (*see* **vitamin B₁**). Foods containing appreciable quantities of sulphites will not provide this important vitamin. This may be a problem when sulphite is used to blanch chipped potatoes.

sulphur
A non-metallic element that forms part of the essential amino acids, methionine

and cysteine. Sulphur is the third most abundant mineral in the body. Sulphur-containing amino acids are readily available from meat, milk, eggs, and legumes. They form part of a number of proteins and vitamins (e.g. biotin and thiamin), and are particularly abundant in the proteins which form cartilage, tendons, and bones.

sulphur dioxide: *See* sulphites.

sunburn
Skin damage caused by overexposure to the sun's rays, especially ultraviolet rays. There are two main types of ultraviolet light, UVA (wavelengths 320–400 nm) and UVB (wavelengths 290–320 nm). On a dose-to-dose basis, UVB is about 1000 times more harmful than UVA. Exposure to ultraviolet light increases with altitude (4 per cent per 100 metres), increasing the risk of sunburn. Chronic exposure of unprotected skin to sunlight induces premature skin ageing, abnormal pigmentation, and skin cancers. Anyone exercising regularly out of doors has a high risk of sunburn and should use a sunscreen with a high sun-protection factor, which absorbs both UVA and UVB. Acute sunburn is treated with cold compresses and painkillers.

sun-protection factor (SPF)
An indicator on a sunscreen product of the relative degree of protection it provides against sunburn, compared to using no sunscreen. A product with an SPF of 15, for example, allows a person to be exposed to the sun, on average, fifteen times longer than if no sunscreen were applied.

sunstroke
Overheating due to direct exposure of the head and back of the neck to the sun's rays. Symptoms include red skin, a swollen face, buzzing in the ears, dizziness, nausea, increased pulse rate, and rapid breathing. If overheating persists it can become very dangerous (*see* **heatstroke**). Sunstroke is quite common in people exercising outdoors for long periods; tennis players, walkers, and golfers are particularly susceptible. If you suffer from sunstroke, you should stop

exercising, rest in the shade, and loosen your clothing. You should try to keep cool by fanning air over yourself, and apply cool water to your forehead and the back of your neck.

supercompensation: *See* carbohydrate loading.

superoxide dismutase (SOD)
An enzyme that inactivates excess free radicals, preventing them from damaging cell membranes. SOD is taken by some athletes as an ergogenic aid to protect their bodies against the many free radicals produced during vigorous exercise. However, when taken orally this enzyme is digested and made useless.

superset system
A weight-training system (also called supersetting) in which two exercises are performed in order to achieve a balanced development between two opposing muscle groups (known as antagonistic pairs) in the same limb. For example, triceps extensions are performed immediately after a set of biceps curls. The two exercises are alternated until both muscles are worked sufficiently.

supination
1 During running and walking, the outward rolling of the foot in the final stage of the gait cycle. *Compare* **pronation**; *see also* **supinator**.
2 Movement of the forearm so that the palm faces upwards or forwards.

supinator
A runner or walker who rotates the foot outwards during locomotion; the foot makes contact with the ground on the inside edge of the heel, then the foot rolls towards the outer edge of the toes to push off. *Compare* **pronator**.

supplements
Vitamin, mineral, and other food concentrates packaged as tablets, capsules, or liquids. Supplements are big business; in the USA 40 per cent of the population takes some form of food supplement. Those who suffer specific nutrient

deficiencies or who have special dietary requirements may be advised to take food supplements (e.g. expectant mothers, total vegetarians, and those on a low calorie diet). However, most others do not need supplements if they eat a well balanced diet. This applies even to people who are very active, because they usually consume more food and hence more nutrients than sedentary people with smaller appetites. Many people take supplements to compensate for poor dietary habits, or in the belief that the supplement will make them immune to disease or ageing. Some athletes take supplements to improve performance, but this should not be necessary as long as you train well and eat properly.

suppleness
An ability to bend and move easily and gracefully. *See* **flexibility**.

suprascapularis: *See* **rotator cuff**.

supraspinatus: *See* **rotator cuff**.

surfer's ear: *See* **swimmer's ear**.

SWD
Abbreviation for short wave diathermy. *See* **diathermy**.

sweating
It is said that 'pigs sweat, men perspire, but only ladies glow'. Whatever name is given to the process, they all secrete a watery fluid onto their skin to prevent them from overheating during exercise or in hot environments. There are two main types of sweat glands: eccrine glands and apocrine glands.

Eccrine glands are the most common type. They occur all over the body and produce sweat that is a clear fluid containing mainly salt and water. It has small amounts of urea and uroconic acid which may offer the skin some protection against ultraviolet radiation. It also contains small amounts of minerals and water-soluble vitamins that must be replaced if sweating is excessive. Sweating can, for example, cause a significant loss of vitamin B_1 and zinc.

Vigorous physical activity produces heat which must be removed. Otherwise the exerciser will overheat and is in danger of suffering from heat stroke. High body temperatures stimulate the eccrine glands to secrete watery sweat which evaporates from the skin surface, cooling it. The cooled skin subsequently cools blood which has been shunted from the body core to the body surface. One litre of sweat evaporated from the body removes approximately 580 kcal of heat.

A person exercising in the heat may sweat up to 2–3 litres per hour, depending on the conditions. During a World Cup soccer match against Brazil in Mexico, England soccer players lost as much as 5 kg in body weight. Conditions that allow rapid evaporation of sweat include high temperatures, cloud cover, steady breezes, and low humidity. If sweating occurs without sufficient water replacement, overheating and dehydration occur. Sweating also increases during periods of mental and emotional arousal.

The other type of sweat glands are called apocrine glands. They occur under the armpits and around the groin and nipples. They secrete a milky white fluid containing proteins and fatty substances. These substances may be broken down by bacteria to produce a pungent odour which may have a sexual function. *See also* **salt replacement** and **water replacement**.

swimmer's ear (surfer's ear)
An earache that starts as an annoying itch but can develop into a painful infection. It affects swimmers or surfers who neglect to dry their ear canals adequately after long periods in the water. Water trapped in the ear breaks down the lining of the outer canal which becomes infected with bacteria and fungi. Use of cotton-tipped ear swabs increases the risk of infection by removing the protective wax in the ear canal. Swimmers should keep out of the water until the infection has cleared. Ear drops of alcohol and vinegar may clear the infection in its early stages, but persistent infections may need treatment with antibiotics.

swimmer's shoulder
An overuse injury common among swimmers and others, such as throwers, who

make repeated, vigorous movements of the arms. It is characterized by inflammation and intense pain when the arm is lifted upwards and forwards. Soft tissues, mostly the tendons associated with rotator muscles of the shoulder joint, become trapped in the space between the head of the humerus and the shoulder blade. The injury can be prevented by a good upper body conditioning programme, including both strength and flexibility exercises, combined with the development of good technique. Established injuries usually respond to rest, ice, and anti-inflammatories, but surgery may be required in severe cases.

swimming

Many experts believe that swimming is the ideal all-round exercise. People of all ages and levels of fitness can take part. Swimming, especially the front crawl which requires steady, rhythmic movements, helps to develop aerobic fitness, suppleness, and muscular strength. If, however, you are swimming for fitness you will need to do three or four hard sessions a week. The water supports the body so there is little stress or impact on tendons, ligaments, and joints. This does not strengthen bones, but it does make swimming safer than land-based activities for those whose bones are weakened by osteoporosis. It also makes swimming especially suitable for those who suffer from knee or back problems, or who are slightly overweight. Swimming can also be helpful for people with asthma or bronchitis.

Although swimmers are less injury-prone than those involved in high-impact sports which involve running or jumping, they can still suffer overuse injuries. Most injuries affect the shoulder (*see* **swimmer's shoulder**). They are usually caused by either poor technique or lack of muscle balance. Competitive swimmers are particularly prone to overuse injuries so they supplement their swimming with land-based training (especially weight training) to rectify muscle imbalances and strengthen muscles. Injuries can also be reduced by using a variety of strokes that develop different muscles of the body: the front crawl helps develop the arms and chest; backstroke develops

flexibility of the shoulders; breast-stroke develops the upper arms, chest, thighs, and hips; and the butterfly develops the whole upper body.

Although an excellent activity, swimming in cold water may not be a suitable part of a slimming programme because it can stimulate the deposition of fats under the skin to act as an insulating layer.

syncope: *See* **fainting**.

Syndrome X

A set of signs and symptoms associated with the accumulation of fat in the abdomen. This form of fat distribution is common in middle-aged men and is often visible as a pot belly or paunch. Syndrome X is characterized by a number of disorders including gout, impaired glucose metabolism (increasing susceptibility to diabetes), raised blood pressure, and elevated blood cholesterol levels. People with Syndrome X have a high risk of heart disease.

synergist

1 A drug, food additive, or other chemical that interacts with another substance so that their combined effect (known as synergy) is more than the sum of their separate effects. These may be beneficial or harmful. In foods, vitamin E and selenium have overlapping functions, each can replace the other to some extent. When together, they may act as synergists, each increasing the effect of the other as an antioxidant. The term synergist is also applied to health-risk factors. For example, studies in the USA have revealed a synergistic effect of smoking and drinking alcohol on the risk of oral cancer. It was found that moderate drinking increases the risk by 60 per cent; moderate smoking increases the risk by 52 per cent; but moderate drinking combined with moderate smoking increased the risk by 400 per cent.

2 A muscle which aids the action of a prime mover (a muscle which has the main responsibility for a particular movement). The synergist may produce the same movement as the prime mover, or it may stabilize the joints across which the prime mover acts, preventing undesirable movements.

synergy
Coordinated activity of opposing muscle groups (antagonistic pairs, such as the biceps and triceps in the upper arm) that results in smooth, well-controlled movements. *See also* **synergist**.

"I do not believe that diet has much to do with athletic performance. 'You are what you eat' is much less true than 'you are what you do'. . . . I don't think there is anything you can eat which can make you run faster, but I will accept that a diet which is consistently deficient in certain vitamins and minerals will limit your performance."
Bruce Tulloh, distance runner (European 5000 metre champion, 1962) and coach.
Peak Performance. **54**. Stonheart Leisure Magazines, London.

table salt

Common salt used to flavour food and as a preservative. Table salt consists mainly of sodium chloride, but may also contain other chemicals such as anti-caking agents (e.g. magnesium carbonate and sodium hexacyanoferrate II).

Many table salts are also iodized (they have iodine added). Iodization was first carried out in the USA in the 1920s to combat goitre (an abnormal enlargement of the thyroid gland). However, except in the northernmost States where the levels of iodine in the soil are abnormally low, most people can obtain sufficient iodine from a normal balanced diet without using iodized salt.

For several years doctors have expressed concern about the overconsumption of salt because of its high sodium content (approximately 40 per cent). A high dietary intake of sodium salts is associated with high blood pressure and heart disease. Some patients suffering hypertension can reduce their blood pressure by taking a low-salt diet. The WHO recommends that total salt consumption should be around 5 g per person per day. Current intakes in the UK are around 8–10 g of salt each day. In the USA warnings about the hazards of salt consumption have resulted in a remarkable response: although still exceeding 5 g per day, the intake of salty products has decreased by more than 30 per cent and the food industry is processing many more foods with low salt levels.

tachycardia

A rapid, resting heartbeat 20–30 beats above normal. Drinking coffee or tea, and excitement can induce tachycardia, or it may indicate a disorder, such as an impending infection or heart disease. Many sports people monitor their resting pulse rate regularly and find that it keeps relatively constant from day to day. A small elevation (even of 3–5 beats per minute) is often an early indication of overtraining. If wise, they reduce their training load until the resting pulse returns to normal. Those who ignore the warning often succumb to a viral infection or some other disorder.

tae kwon do: *See* **martial arts**.

t'ai chi

A gentle, non-violent form of exercise partly derived from Chinese martial arts and Taoism (a Chinese philosophical system). It consists of 108 complex, slow-motion movements that encourage mental and physical harmony. T'ai chi is unlikely to place sufficient demands on your body to improve cardiovascular fitness, nor is it likely to help you lose weight. However, it may help to improve posture, making you appear taller, slimmer, and more poised.

tannins

Soluble, astringent substances found in some plants, including tea and coffee. Tannins are added to a variety of processed foods, including ice-cream and caramel. They are also used as clearing agents to precipitate proteins in wines and beer.

Tannins are sometimes called 'anti-nutrients' because they may reduce the absorption of some minerals. Drinking more than two cups of tea or coffee without milk a day can rob the body of significant amounts of calcium and iron, and may contribute to the development of osteoporosis (brittle bone disease) and anaemia. These adverse effects can be reduced by drinking tea and coffee between rather than during meals, and the addition of milk or lemon juice neutralizes the effects of tannins on iron absorption. Eating foods rich in vitamin C helps to counteract the effects of tannins on iron absorption.

tapering down

A gradual reduction in training load in the period leading up to competition. Tapering is particularly important for those preparing for endurance events. It gives the body an opportunity to recover fully from months of heavy training and to adapt to increased demands. There are many examples of athletes who performed exceptionally well after they were forced to rest against their wishes. One of the most famous was Emil Zatopek who was training very intensively for the 1950 European Games when he became ill and had to stay in hospital for two weeks. He came out just 2 days before he was due to compete in the 10 000 metres. He won the race convincingly by more than one lap. He went on to complete the 'double' by winning the 5000 metres. Zatopek's performances demonstrated the benefits of tapering so clearly that their effects are sometimes called the 'Zatopek phenomenon'. Despite the well-recorded benefits, many top class athletes do not have the confidence to taper and feel uncomfortable having a period of relative rest before a major competition. However, those who do not taper often underperform and are susceptible to injuries.

There does not seem to be any formula for establishing the optimum tapering period, but many coaches advocate 10–14 days of reduced training load (not complete rest) prior to competition. Duncan MacDougall of the University of Ontario, Canada, found that when middle-distance runners cut their training mileage by 90 per cent, their performances unexpectedly improved as long as they trained at race pace. Swimmers are usually advised not to reduce their training frequency by more than 50 per cent. Swimming is a skill sport and long periods out of the water may result in loss of neuromuscular coordination.

taping

Strapping or taping is the use of tapes and bandages to support a weakened body part without limiting its function. A taped joint should retain its normal range of movement but as the tapes are usually inelastic, they prevent movements beyond the normal range which might stress the weakened area and aggravate an injury. Some coaches and trainers tape uninjured joints as a precautionary measure to improve stability and decrease the risk of injury during strenuous activity. Others never tape uninjured joints. They argue that an immobilized joint cannot take its share of the load and therefore overloads other joints, increasing the risk of injury. They often add that a person injured badly enough to require taping, should not exercise.

tempolauf

A type of training for runners, cyclists, and swimmers which emphasizes high-intensity effort equalling or approaching that required in a race. The aim is to accustom the athlete to the tempo or pace of the race. Tempolauf may take the form of a single time trial or a small number of repetitions with sufficient rest between each to allow recovery to be almost complete.

tendinitis

Inflammation of a tendon which usually becomes swollen, red, and tender to the touch. *See also* **tendon injuries**.

tendinosis

A degeneration of a tendon due to ageing, the accumulation of small ruptures, or both. *See also* **tendon injuries**.

tendon

A white band of tough, rope-like connective tissue which attaches a muscle to a bone or cartilage. Tendons transmit the forces exerted by muscle contraction to move parts of the skeleton. They can tolerate being pulled vigorously by muscles but are less resistant to compression and twisting forces. Each tendon moves up and down within a sheath containing a small amount of fluid to reduce friction. Inflammation of the sheath (paratendinitis) restricts movement of the tendon and can be quite painful.

tendon injuries
Tendons can be ruptured by a single over-enthusiastic movement. Such acute injuries are quite dramatic and usually leave the sufferer unable to move the affected joint. In these cases, surgery may be needed to secure the tendon to its bone. However, most tendon injuries develop insidiously through chronic overuse during activities that produce high compression forces (e.g. road running) or twisting forces (e.g. golf and tennis). One theory suggests that tendons repeatedly subjected to relatively large loads suffer microscopic ruptures. Individual loads are tolerated, but if they are repeated often enough the tendon starts to break down (metal fatigues in a similar way).

Treatment of tendon injuries varies depending on their severity. Rest is the first and most important treatment. Ice and analgesics are often applied to reduce any swelling and pain. Ultrasound, acupuncture, and laser therapy are a few of the many treatments employed by physiotherapists. Stretching exercises are usually an important part of a rehabilitation programme because lack of flexibility of a muscle–tendon unit is a major contributory factor to injury. Unfortunately, tendons have a poor blood supply and are generally slow to heal.

tennis
A top-class tennis match may last over 2 hours and players require high levels of aerobic fitness. A player's average heart rate reaches 60–70 per cent of its maximum level and a burst of maximum activity occurs each time a player contests a point. A point lasts about 12–15 seconds and there may be more than 500 points contested during a match. So,

tennis can be a very demanding sport but it can also be played at many levels of intensity, making it very popular. As long as you can find someone at about the same level to play with, you can play tennis at your own pace.

Doubles is less strenuous than singles (during a doubles match, average heart rate is only about 40 per cent maximum). This makes tennis an activity which can be enjoyed by people of all ages and levels of fitness. Playing tennis involves bending, twisting, stretching, leaping, and running. These movements keep the shoulders, arms, and legs supple and strong, and help to develop good posture and balance. It also improves aerobic fitness. The movements, however, tend to lead to injuries in the shoulder, lower back, and knee, especially if there are muscular weaknesses and imbalances (*see* **tennis elbow**). Injuries are more common in those who are in poor physical condition and those who do not warm-up ade-quately. Rehabilitation from upper-body injuries may include windmill exercises (*see* **windmills**) and 'anchored racquet' exercises in which an elastic band is attached to the racquet to provide controlled resistance for normal stroke movements.

Flexibility and mobility exercises are essential for players of all standards so that they can be adequately prepared for dynamic activity during a game. It is also important to do exercises using both sides of the body to counteract the one-sided development of body musculature. A condition nicknamed 'King Kong' arm is common in players who do not take this advice. The dominant arm becomes overdeveloped because of the asymmetrical increase in size of the dominant shoulder girdle. This affects body posture and may result in stresses and strains causing injuries in other parts of the body. Tennis involves a considerable amount of side-to-side movement. To minimize injuries, tennis shoes should have a strong heel cup and heel counter. Also, the forefoot should be made of sturdy material to cope with the dragging of the trail leg during low ground shots.

tennis elbow
Tennis elbow is an overuse injury of the tendon that attaches one of the finger

and wrist extensor muscles (the extensor carpi radialis brevis) onto the lower part of the humerus. The injury is characterized by pain on the lateral (outer) side of the elbow. The pain may extend from the shoulder to the wrist.

Tennis elbow is associated with any activity in which the wrist is constantly bending while the hand is gripping an object (e.g. canoeing, baseball, fencing, racquet sports, tenpin bowling, and fly fishing). Repeated throwing may also put undue stress on the tendon, especially if the arm and wrist are twisted in an effort to impose spin on a ball. Overuse, poor mechanics, and insufficient conditioning of muscles are contributory factors. In racquet sports, poor backhand technique, inappropriate grip size, and tight racquet strings may overload the tendon. As with other soft-tissue injuries, primary treatment includes rest, ice, and analgesics. *Compare* **golfer's elbow**; *see also* **tendon injuries**.

tennis leg

An injury characterized by a sharp pain in the upper calf described as feeling like 'a shot in the leg'. It is caused by a rupture of one of the tendons of the gastrocnemius muscle at the back of the calf. The injury may result from a sudden extension of the knee when the ankle is dorsiflexed (i.e. the foot is pulled towards the shin), or by a sudden dorsiflexion when the knee is extended. Tennis leg occurs most frequently among middle-aged exercisers who already have some degeneration of the tendon. It is common in all racquet sports and basketball.

tennis toe: *See* black nail.

tenpin bowling: *See* bowling.

TENS: *See* transcutaneous electrical nerve stimulation.

testosterone

The main male sex hormone. Testosterone is secreted by the testes throughout life, but there is some decline with age. To offset this decline and in the hope of retaining youthful virility, some older men take testosterone preparations (in the past, extra testosterone was sometimes obtained by eating testes of monkeys). Surprisingly, testosterone is also secreted in small amounts from the adrenal glands in women. This secretion increases after exercise but decreases with overtraining. Rapid weight loss may also lead to lower testosterone levels. High testosterone levels in females may interfere with some actions of female sex hormones, disrupting the menstrual cycle but reducing premenstrual stress. Low testosterone levels in males may reduce sexual desire. Low levels may also reduce a person's energy capacity by affecting the body's ability to store energy in the form of creatine phosphate and glycogen.

Testosterone has both androgenic (masculinizing) and anabolic (tissue-building) effects. It acts as an androgen by promoting the development of male secondary sexual characteristics. Its anabolic effects include stimulating muscle growth and reducing muscle degradation during training. Both help to improve muscle strength. Most users of synthetic testosterone do not wish to have the masculinizing effects. Therefore, synthetic analogues of testosterone are designed to emphasize the anabolic properties while minimizing the androgenic properties. These preparations can be harmful and have been linked to liver disease, tumour growth, breast development in men, and suppression of normal female hormones. Consequently, the use of testosterone and related drugs has been banned by the International Olympic Committee on the principle that athletes should not be allowed to sacrifice their health to obtain a competitive advantage. However, testosterone supplements do have their valid medical uses. For example, they are administered to some anorexics to help them build muscle mass and aid their recovery. *See also* **anabolic steroids**.

tetanus

In exercise physiology, tetanus refers to a sustained contraction of a muscle block, but most people associate the term with a dreadful disease, lockjaw. A bacterium, *Clostridium tetani*, is responsible for the disease. It can be found anywhere, but is most common on ground contaminated by animal faeces, such as sports fields used by farm animals. Tetanus is regarded as the most serious type of sports-related infection. The infective organisms usually enter the body through a laceration. In recent years, two Scottish rugby players and one soccer player developed tetanus from lacerations acquired during play. Only one player survived. The others died by exhaustion and asphyxiation. Even when not fatal, the disease is very unpleasant. The bacterium releases a toxin which causes simultaneous contraction of all the muscles, making the body go as rigid as a board. Treatment is usually prolonged and painful. Tetanus is preventable by active immunization. Anyone who exercises out of doors is foolish not to take advantage of this protection. Some sports, including orienteering, insist on participants taking measures to reduce the risk of this fearsome condition.

tetany
Spasm and twitching of a muscle which may be due to lack of calcium. It usually affects the hands and feet.

texturizers
Substances such as gums and starch added to food to improve its consistency and to achieve a desired texture.

thaumatin
A sweetener 2000 times sweeter than table sugar. Thaumatin is a natural product extracted from the fruit of the West African plant *Thaumatococcus danielli*. Thaumatin contains many amino acids, some of which give it a lingering aftertaste that limits its human use to products such as medicines. It is also used to enhance the flavour of pet foods. *See also* **artificial sweeteners**.

thermic effect of food: *See* diet induced thermogenesis.

thermogenesis
The production of heat energy. Chemical reactions in the body generate heat, increasing with higher levels of activity. Getting rid of the heat can be a problem when exercising intensely, especially in warm, humid environments. In cold environments, extra heat may be generated

by shivering ('shivering thermogenesis') or by metabolism of special fat cells ('non-shivering thermogenesis'; *see* **brown fat**). *See also* **diet induced thermogenesis**.

thiamin: *See* **vitamin B₁**.

thinness-demand sport
An activity that emphasizes or requires a small body size, thin shape, or low weight. Thinness-demand sports include gymnastics, diving, dance, and figure skating, which base their scoring on appearance and form. Long-distance running is also included because those who have thin, lean bodies often have a high power to body weight ratio which gives them a distinct advantage. Sports which have strict weight classes, such as boxing, wrestling, and horse-racing, often require the participants to lose weight. There is some evidence, albeit inconclusive, that participants in thinness-demand sports have a greater tendency to suffer from eating disorders. It has been estimated, for example, that 75 per cent of college gymnasts in the USA use potentially harmful weight-control methods. *See also* **anorexia** and **making weight**.

thirst
An uncomfortable feeling of dryness in the mouth and throat accompanied by a desire to drink. The stimulus for thirst is an abnormally high concentration of sodium in the blood. This usually occurs after significant amounts of body fluid are lost. Unfortunately, thirst is not a very reliable mechanism. There is a delay between loss of body fluids and the sensation of thirst. A 150 pound (about 68 kg) person may lose as much as 1.5 pounds (0.7 kg) of sweat before feeling thirsty. People who take part in endurance activities which make them sweat profusely are generally advised to drink *before* they get thirsty. *See also* **water replacement**.

thought-stopping
A psychological technique often used by sports people to overcome negative attitudes during competition. An athlete is trained to recognize negative thoughts and to replace them with positive, constructive ones. At the start of a slalom, for example, a skier who begins to think

about the disastrous consequences of misjudging a turn, replaces these thoughts with thoughts of how the descent can be completed successfully.

threonine

An essential amino acid, but as it is found in all proteins, a specific deficiency is very unlikely. If taken as a single amino acid supplement, excessive doses of threonine may lead to an increase in urea production and possible toxicity.

thrombosis

The formation of a clot (thrombus) in a blood vessel. A thrombus remains at its site of formation where it restricts or stops blood flow. Regular exercisers are unlikely to suffer from a spontaneous thrombosis (i.e. one not associated with an injury) because their blood tends to have a high concentration of anti-clotting agents. However, thromboses associated with a trauma can sometimes occur. In contact sports, for example, the subclavian or axillary vein can be damaged by a blow to the shoulder or clavicle and a condition known as 'effort thrombosis' may occur. It is characterized by pain, swelling, and sometimes numbness in the affected arm. An effort thrombosis may also result from repetitive overhand movements, for example in racquet sports.

thrower's elbow (pitcher's elbow)

A term given to a number of injuries of the elbow associated with throwing. These are characterized by damage to the triceps muscle, its tendon, and the olecranon process (the end of the ulna which forms the tip of the elbow) which may suffer stress fractures. Loose bodies may form in the joint causing locking and predisposing the injured thrower to osteoarthritis.

Thrower's elbow is often the result of poor throwing technique when forcefully straightening the elbow, resulting in too great a load being imposed. Professional baseball pitchers produce arm speeds of 7000 degrees per second as the arm rotates inwards. The elbow is subjected to violent forces during all phases of the pitching motion, so injuries are no surprise.

Treatment includes correcting faulty technique and removing any loose bodies (this can now be done by keyhole surgery). Although rest, ice, compression, and elevation (see **RICE**) may be sufficient to treat slightly damaged tissue, surgery is often needed for more serious injuries.

thrower's fracture

A fracture of the humerus which occurs when muscle forces generated by a throw are enough to snap the bone. Such dramatic fractures occur rarely, but smaller stress fractures are more common, especially in young throwers and participants in racquet sports. Their immature bones and muscles cannot tolerate the high acceleration forces operating on the humerus during throws. Treatment is based on rest and improvement of technique when throwing is resumed. If the thrower does not rest, a complete fracture is likely. This may require surgery and possibly end a person's ability to throw competitively.

throwing

Throwing forms a central part of many sports, including athletics, baseball, and cricket. The best throwers are usually strong, and have good mobility, balance, and coordination. Mobility is required particularly in the shoulders and hips. Throwers also need a great deal of strength in their throwing arm. They have be able to move the arm very quickly and with great power. To do this effectively, they use the large muscles of the legs and back. Training, therefore, involves strengthening not only the throwing arm, but also the muscles in the abdomen, back, and legs. Throwers subject themselves to tremendous forces and often suffer injuries in the knees, lower back, shoulders, and elbows. To minimize the risk of injury they should:

- warm-up before throwing and cool down afterwards
- do mobility training that develops the flexibility of the back, hips, and shoulders
- strengthen the lower back and abdominal muscles
- adopt a safe and efficient throwing technique.

thrush: *See* candida.

thyroid hormone

A hormone secreted by the thyroid gland, a large gland in the neck. There are two thyroid hormones (thyroxine and tri-iodothyronine), both contain iodine. They regulate the metabolic rate of every cell in the body except those of the brain, spleen, testes, and uterus. They are important regulators of tissue growth and development, particularly of nervous and skeletal tissue. People with an under-active thyroid gland tend to be sluggish and overweight, and to suffer from swollen joints, muscle cramps, puffy faces, and general lassitude. Fortunately, the condition is easily treated with thy-roid hormone replacement tablets or iodine supplements if the problem is due to iodine deficiency. Those with an over-active thyroid gland tend to be thin, hyperactive, and have protruding eyes. Excessive secretion of thyroid hormone can also lead to muscle loss, and cause bones to demineralize and become brittle. The use of thyroid hormones to treat obese people was quite common 30 years ago, but it has grown out of favour because of dangerous and unpleasant side-effects, including muscle loss, heart malfunctions, and mental problems. There is some evidence to show that regu-lar exercise stimulates thyroxine produc-tion. This is just one of the reasons why exercise is beneficial in a weight-loss pro-gramme. *See also* **iodine** and **kelp**.

thyroid stimulating hormone

A hormone secreted by the front part of the pituitary gland. Thyroid stimulating hormone stimulates the production of thyroid hormone from the thyroid gland. It is sometimes taken in drug form to boost metabolism and reduce body weight. *See also* **thyroid hormone**.

thyroxine: *See* thyroid hormone.

tidal volume: *See* lung volume.

time of meals

Many people do not have specific meal times. This is seen by some dietitians as making a major contribution to over-eating: if people eat when they like and food is constantly available, sensible, con-trolled eating is less likely. They are more likely to 'graze' continuously on food and eat too much. Dietitians generally advise people to eat at least three meals at specific times each day. Those on a weight-loss diet are often advised to have as many as six small meals each day. Eating increases metabolic rate (*see* **diet induced thermogenesis**). Consequently, there is less energy available for other body activities (including fat storage) from a number of meals than from one meal containing the same number of calories.

For those who exercise vigorously, the ideal time to consume a meal is 2–3 hours before the activity. Foods high in protein need the maximum time; those high in carbohydrates will require the lower time limit. Although exhaustive exercise may lower the appetite, the best way to replenish energy is by consuming easily absorbable, carbohydrate-rich food or drink immediately after exercise. A delay may result in the body taking up to 48 hours to replenish energy stores. *See also* **breakfast** and **pre-competition meal**.

time-trial

A form of training often used by runners, cyclists, and swimmers, in which they race against the clock to establish how fast they can cover a particular distance. Many coaches believe that racing, even against the clock, should be confined to competition. They argue that time-trials focus on speed at the expense of endurance, and that overexertion during a time-trial may result in injury. However, time-trials below competition distance form an important part of the training programmes of most elite athletes. They provide feedback about the effectiveness of a training programme, and help to develop judgement of pace at racing speed. A major danger with time-trials is that the performer loses confidence because too much importance is placed on the times achieved. Also, there is often an expectation that each time-trial should be faster than the previous one. This is neither possible nor desirable, since a person cannot expect to train hard and perform well simultaneously. It is best to regard time-trials as diagnostic tools and not as measures of ability. Personal-best performances should be saved for competitions.

timing
The ability to perform movements and actions at the most effective moment. It is an important component of skill, and depends on the ability to perceive and respond to a wide variety of factors. For example, correct timing of the swing of a baseball bat depends on visual and auditory cues produced by the pitcher, and on internal stimuli that enable the hitter to make smooth coordinated movements. This ensures the ball is hit on the sweet spot, the area of the bat which exerts the most effective force on the ball.

TMG: *See* **methyl donors.**

tocopherol: *See* **vitamin E.**

tooth decay (dental caries)
A dental disease in which the hard enamel tissue of the tooth is worn away. It is caused mainly by bacterial deposits (known as plaque) on the tooth surface. Bacteria use food, especially fermentable carbohydrates trapped between the teeth, as an energy source, fermenting it to acids which lower the pH of the plaque. If the pH drops below 5.5, the acid reacts with the enamel, dissolving it. Sugars and starches are both fermented by bacteria. Sugar manufacturers say 'Sugar itself does not rot your teeth'; nutritionists reply 'Without it, teeth will not rot!' Studies have shown that foods containing carbohydrates that stick to the teeth are the most likely to cause tooth decay because they remain available to the bacteria for longer. Specifically, sucrose encourages plaque-forming bacteria. Some chewing-gums, marketed as 'tooth-friendly', overcome this problem by replacing sugar with xylitol, a sugar alcohol that does not encourage the growth of the bacteria that cause caries.

torn cartilage: *See* **meniscus.**

torticollis (wryneck)
A painful spasm of muscles in the neck and upper back, causing the neck and head to be drawn to one side. Torticollis can be a congenital condition, but it may also occur in young people who twist their necks violently (for example, when heading a football).

total body stretch
A simple exercise often used as part of a warm-up routine.
■ Lie flat on your back, totally relaxed. Then, with your fingers and toes pointed, slowly and gently extend your arms and legs. Hold the extended position for about 10 seconds, relax, and repeat three or four times.

total hip machine: *See* **fixed-weight machine.**

total thermal load
The sum of all the factors which tend to increase body temperature. The thermal load is determined by exercise intensity, environmental temperature, and environmental evaporative power. Thus, a person has highest thermal loads (and is therefore at greatest risk of heat exhaustion) when exercising intensively in warm, humid environments with little or no wind.

toxicity
The extent to which a substance is poisonous. Toxins in food are usually present in small concentrations. Most toxins in plants are natural and help to protect the plants from pests, disease, and damage. Carcinogenic mycotoxins are produced when moulds and other fungi thrive on food kept in poor storage conditions (*see* **aflatoxins**). Some toxins may also be formed as a result of not cooking food properly. Kidney beans, for example, contain lectins. The beans should be cooked thoroughly to destroy this substance.

Almost any substance in food, air, or water can become toxic if consumed in high enough concentrations. Even some vitamins and minerals, usually beneficial components of the diet, may be toxic in high doses. This applies especially to the fat-soluble vitamins (vitamins A and D) which are stored in the liver, and some water-soluble vitamins (e.g. vitamin B_6 and niacin). If excessive amounts are taken, some of the vitamin spills over into the tissues causing toxic reactions. The amount which induces a reaction depends on an individual's sensitivity, but it is usually a megadose, many times the recommended daily intake.

trace element
An element, usually a metal, required in minute amounts to maintain a healthy body. They are required mainly as components of enzymes and hormones, or are involved in the activation of enzymes. *See also* **fluorine**; **chromium**; **cobalt**; **copper**; **iodine**; **manganese**; and **selenium**.

trainability principle
A basic principle of training which states that the more fully a person is trained with respect to a given fitness component, the less there remains of that component to be trained in the future. Training benefits, therefore, are more easily obtained during the early stages of training than later.

training
An exercise programme designed to help a person acquire skills and improve physical fitness. Training is usually broken down into different phases, typically starting with general whole-body conditioning, then going on to more specific training and psychological preparation (*see also* **periodization**). For every activity, there are many different types of training and a growing body of scientific knowledge to explain their effects. However, this knowledge is far from complete and there are no simple recipes to guarantee success. Individuals rarely respond in exactly the same way to the same type of training. Nevertheless, a number of general training principles have evolved. The following training guidelines are based on basic training principles and the experience of many top-class coaches:

- train regularly all year round, but break the training year down into phases (*see* **periodization**)
- start gently and gradually increase the training intensity (*see* **progression**)
- ensure that you work sufficiently hard in training to improve (*see* **overload principle**)
- train first for endurance, and only later for power or speed

- establish good overall conditioning, and then make training specific (*see* **specific training principle**)
- do not overtrain; listen to your body and rest when you become aware of warning symptoms such as persistent pain (*see* **overuse injury**)
- do not be enslaved by a daily schedule, it may become a recipe for overtraining
- give yourself sufficient rest after a hard training session; alternate a hard training day with an easy day. Include a transition period of reduced training in your yearly schedule
- rest before competition (*see* **peaking** and **tapering down**)
- train with a good coach you trust and respect. The coach will help you to establish appropriate goals (*see* **goal**), provide objective feedback, and maintain motivation
- with your coach, select a training programme you believe in. Persevere even when you do not seem to be improving (*see* **plateau**)
- keep a detailed training log book; it will help you to monitor your fitness and provide a lasting record of your training.

Overtraining may be more harmful than undertraining. Good coaches advise rest between hard training sessions. People who ignore this basic advice are in danger of doing themselves considerable harm (*see* **overtraining** and **overuse injury**). Franz Stampfl (Roger Bannister's coach) said that 'Training is principally an act of faith'. Without belief in a training system, a person will not train over the months or even years needed to acquire maximum training benefits.

training diary
When you start exercising it is a good idea to keep a daily log of your training. The diary does not have to take any special form. A simple notebook is sufficient, with a page or half page dedicated to each day. The following are some of the items that might be included in the daily entries:

- date
- weight
- resting pulse

- training targets
- training location
- actual training achieved
- comments (e.g. how you felt; *see* **perceived exertion**).

The diary will enable you to monitor your progress and set new training goals.

training duration

The optimum duration of each exercise session depends on the intensity of the session and the fitness level of the individual. A minimum period of 15 minutes is required to improve cardiovascular fitness. Most experts recommend that healthy individuals exercising to improve general fitness should start with 20–30 minutes of aerobic exercise. The duration should increase as fitness improves. However, training should not be exhausting. You should feel relaxed and not fatigued within 1 hour of completing your session. Doing too much exercise too soon is one of the main reasons for people giving up. Be patient if you do not seem to be progressing fast enough. It takes at least 12 weeks training to improve aerobic fitness significantly and 8 weeks to improve anaerobic fitness.

training effects

Regular, vigorous exercise affects most parts of the body. Sports scientists and doctors have discovered a long list of benefits gained from regular training. All the benefits listed below have been linked to aerobic exercise, unless otherwise stated.

HEART

- heart muscle enlarged and strengthened, improving the ability to pump blood
- coronary blood supply improved, reducing the risk of heart attack
- resting heart rate lowered
- heart rate needed to perform given workload lowered, reducing stress on the heart

LUNGS

- ventilation of lungs (i.e. ability to breathe) improved
- respiratory muscles strengthened
- blood supply to lungs increased
- ability to extract oxygen from lungs improved

JOINTS

- thickening of articular cartilage with weight-bearing exercises
- increased mobility with flexibility training
- greater stability (less dislocations) with strength training

BONES

- bones thickened, reducing risk of fractures

BLOOD

- blood volume increased
- total volume of red blood cells increased, improving oxygen transport
- high-density (beneficial) lipoproteins increased
- low-density (harmful) lipoproteins lowered
- cholesterol level lowered
- arterial blood pressure lowered
- less tendency for blood to clot spontaneously

MUSCLES

- muscles enlarged and made stronger by strength training
- speed of muscle contraction increased with power training
- myoglobin and muscle glycogen content increased, improving endurance
- mitochondria density increased, improving muscles' ability to use oxygen

BRAIN

- mental alertness improved
- depression and anxiety reduced

WHOLE BODY

- ability to relax and sleep improved
- stress tolerance improved
- lean body mass increased
- metabolic rate increased
- tendency to suffer from obesity and diabetes mellitus decreased

No single form of training produces all of the effects listed, but most of them are gained from regular, vigorous aerobic exercise. It must also be emphasized that individuals vary in their response to exercise. Nevertheless, if performed properly with due regard to individual abilities, regular training has a positive effect on many components of health, and makes weight control easier.

training frequency

The number of times per week training is undertaken. Some athletics coaches advocate training 7 days a week, but recommended frequencies vary considerably. As a rough guideline, it has been suggested that aerobic training should occur three to five times a week (depending on intensity), and anaerobic training (including strength training) no more than three times a week. Optimal exercise frequency to maintain health, rather than to train for competitive sport, was studied by NASA scientists to prepare their astronauts for manned space flights. They concluded that, although some daily exercise is desirable, vigorous aerobic exercises on 3 non-consecutive days per week is sufficient to maintain a good level of personal physical fitness. Exercise frequencies less than this resulted in degeneration of muscles and reduction in cardiovascular fitness.

training heart rate (target heart rate; training zone)

A heart rate reached in training that indicates the level of exercise which produces maximum training effects (figure 64). The

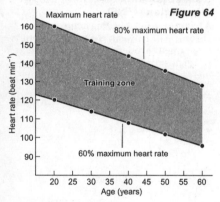

Figure 64

method most commonly used to estimate training heart rate for aerobic exercises on land is to take 60–80 per cent of maximum heart rate (assumed to be 220 minus age). Heart rates in water are naturally lower than on land. This is partly due to the support that the water gives the body. Therefore, for swimming the maximum heart rate is assumed to be 205 minus age, rather than 220. The

training heart rate should be determined in relation to the type of activity and fitness level of the individual. Anaerobic training requires higher heart rates (up to 95 per cent maximum heart rate) sustained for short periods. Unfit people should train at the lower end of the range. For example, a relatively unfit person of 35 years would have a training heart rate (THR) of 60 per cent maximum heart rate, i.e.:

$$THR = (220-35) \times 0.60$$
$$= 111 \text{ beats per minute.}$$

Training heart rates are only estimates. Exercisers should always be aware of symptoms, such as breathlessness, dizziness, and pains in the chest, which indicate that the training level is too high. Those with health problems should seek medical advice concerning their level of activity.

training impulse

A measure of the amount of training performed in one session, calculated from the changes in heart rate experienced during the training, the intensity of the exercises, and the duration of the session.

training intensity

The total amount of effort expended in training. According to the overload principle of training, to improve physical fitness exercise must require more effort than usual. Improvements in flexibility are obtained only if muscles are stretched beyond their normal length; cardiovascular or aerobic fitness is gained only by elevating the heart rate above the normal range; and strength is increased only after training against resistances greater than normal (see **repetition maximum**). Although it is essential to ensure that the training intensity is high enough, it is equally important that the intensity is not so high there is a great risk of overuse injuries and overtraining (see **progression**). A number of methods are used to establish the training intensities which give maximum benefits (see **training heart rate**).

training shoes

Training shoes incorporate features to protect the wearer against the mechanical stresses imposed by the foot striking and moving sideways on the ground (figure 65). Each sport and type of exercise has different requirements. For example, running shoes are designed for forward and backward movements and give little support for the sideways motions experienced in squash. Individuals also have different requirements: heavy people and those with loose tendons and ligaments require a more supportive shoe than light people or those with rigid feet. Modern shoes incorporate the latest technological advances in material science. Some even have gadgets such as rollbars and pumps to inflate bladders which support the upper foot.

In 1995 there were more than 200 types of shoe on the market designed specifically for running. These included high and low mileage shoes; shoes suitable for different terrains; shoes with superior fore and rear foot cushioning for those with high or medium arches; slightly heavier, stability shoes, to limit excessive foot motion; motion control shoes, with supports to correct biomechanical problems (e.g. overpronation); and flexible, lightweight shoes for racing. Unfortunately, choosing the ideal shoe is not easy because two people of similar size and running action can react to the same shoe in completely different ways. The wrong shoe may cause injury by having inadequate shock absorption or inappropriate grip on the sole. Therefore, it is best to seek the advice of a specialist shoe shop when buying training shoes, and to try them on.

training threshold

The minimum amount of exercise needed to improve physical fitness. For exercise to be effective, it must be performed with sufficient frequency, at a high enough intensity, and for a long enough duration. As fitness improves, the threshold level increases. See also **overload principle** and **progression**.

training unit

A single period of training designed to achieve a specific objective. A training session may consist of several units, each with different objectives. In American football, for example, one training session may include sprinting to develop speed, weight training to develop strength, and stretching to develop flexibility.

transcutaneous electrical nerve stimulation (TENS)

A technique for relieving acute and chronic pain. A weak electrical current is discharged through electrodes placed at strategic points on the skin to stop the messages from pain receptors reaching

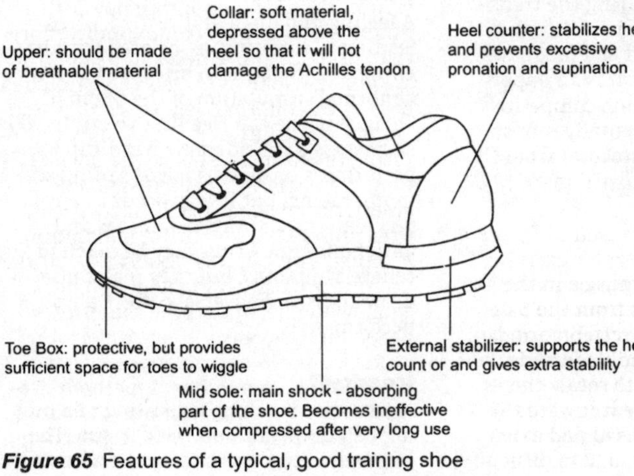

Collar: soft material, depressed above the heel so that it will not damage the Achilles tendon

Upper: should be made of breathable material

Heel counter: stabilizes heel and prevents excessive pronation and supination

Toe Box: protective, but provides sufficient space for toes to wiggle

Mid sole: main shock - absorbing part of the shoe. Becomes ineffective when compressed after very long use

External stabilizer: supports the heel count or and gives extra stability

Figure 65 Features of a typical, good training shoe

the brain. One theory suggests that this current stimulates large nerve fibres in the spinal cord to inhibit or block the transmission along small pain fibres. Another theory proposes that it stimulates the release of chemicals, such as endorphins, that decrease the perception of pain in the same way as opium and morphine. TENS has been used effectively to control the pain caused by some sports injuries, but, because the devices use pulses of short duration, the technique is not well suited to relieving muscle pain.

trans fats: *See* **unsaturated fat**.

transfer
The effect of one form of training on another. The transfer principle emphasizes that the positive effects of different types of training occur only when they share similar components and use the same muscles in the same way. For example, if you learn how to roller-skate, you will probably find it easier to learn ice-skating because the two activities are very alike. Similarly, if you train hard and become physically fit for roller-skating, you are likely to be fit to ice-skate. However, improvements gained from cycling are not so readily passed on to running. *See also* **cross-training** and **specific training principle**.

transition period
An important post-competition phase of a training programme. During the transition period, training intensity is reduced but exercise is continued at a moderate level to maintain fitness. It is an opportunity to participate in non-competitive activities to relax and mentally refresh yourself so that you can recover from the stresses imposed by competition. *See also* **periodization**.

trapezius
A large, flat, triangular muscle in the upper back. It originates from the base of the skull and the upper vertebrae and inserts onto the shoulder blade and collar bone. Its main job is to rotate the shoulder blade and move it inwards. It also helps to rotate the head and extend the neck backwards. If you have difficulty

holding your arms out to the side or over your head, your trapezius may be weak. Back strengtheners (*see* **back extension**) will help to strengthen the trapezius and improve flexibility in the upper back. Overtraining for dance, especially ballet, can tighten the trapezius causing discomfort and restricting movement. Relaxation exercises and physiotherapy may be used to treat the problem, but it is best avoided by not overtraining.

traveller's diarrhoea
A notoriously disabling condition with a number of names depending on the geographical location at which it strikes (e.g. Delhi belly and Montezuma's revenge). It often afflicts tourists in locations where food hygiene is poor. Traveller's diarrhoea is usually caused by certain types of the bacterium *Escherichia coli*. This microbe is a common inhabitant of the gut and is usually harmless. However, in a new locality, the gut may become infected with an unaccustomed strain which upsets the intestinal lining, preventing normal reabsorption of water. Treatment includes drinking plenty of fluids to regain water lost, and sometimes, antibiotics. The condition should be treated more seriously if diarrhoea is accompanied by blood in the stool, or fever. This may indicate a more serious condition, such as dysentery, that requires immediate medical attention.

travel sickness
A feeling of nausea and vertigo, often leading to vomiting, associated with travelling. It is thought to be caused by abnormal stimulation of the organ of balance in the ear. Needless to say, travel sickness is a considerable handicap to performers in sports such as sailing and motor-racing, but it may occur in anyone who travels. Antihistamines and anticholinergic drugs may be taken to relieve symptoms, but they may cause drowsiness and adversely affect physical performance.

treadmill
An exercise machine consisting of a moving belt on which you walk or run. The intensity of the exercise can be adjusted

by altering the speed of the belt or altering its gradient.

Once the preserve of fitness clinics, physiology laboratories, and hospitals, treadmills are becoming more common as an item of home fitness equipment. There has been a phenomenal growth in sales in the USA. Treadmill running now ranks as one of the top activities among Americans. Some treadmills are supplied with computerized equipment to monitor speed, distance travelled, and pulse rate. A video of inspiring scenes and motivational exhortations is often included with the package. You should remember to follow the same precautions when treadmill running as when doing other exercise: warm-up before and cool down after the exercise, and increase your training progressively (*see* **progression**).

Treadmills are used in physiology laboratories to measure fitness. A non-motorized treadmill is commercially available to measure power output during sprint training. The sprinter uses his or her own forces to move the belt. The speed of the belt, and the forces the sprinter exerts to move the belt and to pull against waist-straps (recorded on strain gauges), are used to calculate the power output. Motorized treadmills are more often used to measure aerobic fitness because they demand the use of the arms, torso, and legs, requiring high rates of oxygen consumption. Unfortunately, the test can be so demanding that even healthy individuals have a small risk of sudden cardiac death. Leonard Shapiro in the *Oxford textbook of sports medicine*, estimates the sudden death rate to be once in every 375 000 hours of treadmill activity in healthy individuals, and as high as once in 6000 hours in people with heart disease. So, if you have a healthy bank balance that enables you to buy one of these machines, go to a doctor to ensure that you have an equally healthy heart before you use it.

Motorized treadmills are often used in hospitals to test for cardiovascular disease (*see* **graded exercise test**) although they are losing favour because the results are not very reliable for diagnosis. Many hospital treadmills incorporate electrocardiograms to measure heart activity, and other devices to measure blood pressure and breathing rate. The great advantage of hospital treadmill tests is that there is expert help on hand if anything goes wrong.

triacylglycerol

The chemically correct name for 'triglycerides' but rarely used except by chemists and biochemists. *See* **fat**.

triceps: *See* **triceps brachii**.

triceps brachii

A large fleshy muscle at the back of the arm. It is commonly referred to as the triceps. It opposes the action of the biceps by straightening the arm. This three-headed muscle originates from the humerus and shoulder blade. A single tendon inserts the three heads of the muscle onto the olecranon process, the prominent projection of the ulna in the elbow. This tendon is easily damaged by forceful throwing or when falling on the hand with a fully extended arm. *See also* **thrower's elbow**.

triceps extension

A weight-training exercise that strengthens the elbow extensors (triceps) and the shoulder muscles. It is usually performed at a pull-down station, but it can also be performed with free weights (figure 66). If you are using the pull-down station:

■ Stand upright and grasp the bar with a pronated grip (palms facing forwards). The bar should be about face level, your hands should be close together, and your elbow should be close to your body. Fully extend your elbows, pressing the bar down, then return to the start position.

If you are using free weights, obtain the assistance of a partner so that you can do this exercise safely:

■ In a seated position, with your arms fully extended hold a barbell directly above your head. Hold the bar with an overhand grasp and with your hands close together. Keeping your elbows close to your head, lower the barbell behind your head. Return the barbell to the starting position and repeat.

triceps surae: *See* **soleus**.

Figure 66 Triceps extensions. (a) Using a pull-down station; (b) Using free weights

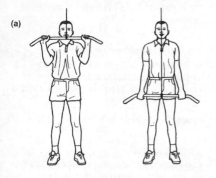

(a)

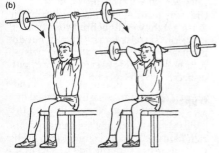

(b)

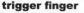

trigger finger
A thickening and hardening of the tendon of the muscle which flexes the trigger finger, resulting from excessive use from pistol- or rifle-shooting. It is still possible to bend the affected finger, but with little strength. Extension of the finger is also impaired but the condition is rarely painful. It can resolve itself spontaneously but it may require surgery.

trigger point
A trigger point usually consists of a small band of muscle which feels knotty. It is sometimes painful when touched, but the pain is often referred to another area of the body. A trigger point in the shoulder, for example, might cause a headache. Trigger points are thought to be due to an accumulation within deep muscle of the waste products of physical activity. This causes localized muscle tension and spasm which may make the points feel like small nodules. Heat treatment with a heat pad or gentle kneading of the trigger point may encourage

removal of the waste products and provide relief from pain.

triglyceride: *See* fat.

trimethylglycine: *See* methyl donors.

triple-jumper's heel
An overuse injury common among triple-jumpers. The triple-jump consists of three phases: the hop, step, and jump. Enormous forces are imposed on the heel during the triple-jump, especially when it is banged into the ground on landing after the hop and step phases. Consequently, the soft tissue in the heels are easily strained. Triple jumper's heel is sometimes accompanied by the development of a bony spur, an abnormal bony outgrowth, on the heel bone.

tri-sets
A weight-training system in which three sets of different exercises are performed before taking a rest. The different exercises may affect different muscles, but body-builders often use tri-sets on a single muscle group to keep blood in the same region of the body and improve muscle appearance. *See also* **flushing methods** and **pumping-up**.

trunk lifts
Two exercises that improve trunk mobility and strengthen the back muscles. Both are performed on a table or bench (figure 67). The lower trunk lift is a specific exercise for the lower back and hips:

■ Lie prone on a firmly fixed bench or table with your legs hanging over the edge. Stabilize your upper body (e.g. by grasping the edges of the table). Slowly raise your legs until they are parallel to the floor, but no further (do not arch your back), then lower your legs slowly.

The upper trunk lift develops the upper back muscles.

■ Lie face down on a table with your upper body hanging over the edge. Place your hands on the top of your head. Get a partner to stabilize your feet and legs while you raise your trunk so that it is parallel to the floor, no further (again, do not arch your back). Return slowly to the start position.

Figure 67 (a) Lower trunk lift; (b) Upper trunk lift

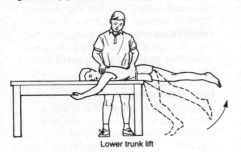

Lower trunk lift

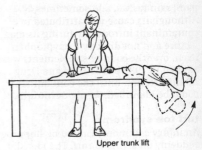

Upper trunk lift

trunk rotation

A simple strengthening exercise for the back and abdominal muscles.

■ With the help of a training partner, hold a weighted barbell behind your head onto your shoulders. Standing upright with a straight back, feet about shoulder width apart and firmly planted on the ground, use your hips to rotate your trunk to the right so that you face sideways. Hold for a few seconds and slowly rotate to the left. Repeat four or five times.

trunk stretcher

A flexibility exercise that stretches the trunk muscles.

■ Stand upright with your feet about shoulder width apart. Stretch your left arm over your head and your right arm in front of your waist. Bend sideways to your right, reaching as far as possible to the right with your left arm, and to the left with your right arm. Do not rotate or twist your trunk. Hold. Return to the starting position and repeat on the other side.

trunk twists

An exercise to tone the abdominal muscles, especially the external obliques; leg and groin muscles are also worked quite hard.

■ Lie on your back with your hands placed lightly on your head, knees bent, and feet firmly secured, (for example, press your toes under a solid object or get a partner to sit on your feet). Use your abdominal and leg muscles to lift your trunk and twist it so that your right elbow is as close as possible to your left knee. Then gently lie back onto the floor and pull upwards again, this time twisting your left elbow towards your right

knee. Repeat the whole routine three or four times, remembering to breathe out on the way up and in on the way down.

Once the technique is mastered, you can grasp a light weight behind your head to make the exercise more difficult, but do not use your hands and arms to force your body upwards because this can put unnecessary pressure on the neck.

tryptophan

An essential component of a balanced diet, this amino acid is found in protein-rich foods, especially legumes (e.g. beans). Once absorbed into the body, some of it is converted into niacin, one of the B complex vitamins needed for efficient respiration and fat metabolism. People whose staple food is maize often suffer from pellagra, a niacin-deficiency disease, mainly because of the low tryptophan content of their food.

Many people take amino acid supplements to stimulate muscle growth artificially or as an aid to health. If the supplement contains high levels of tryptophan, the user may feel drowsy and fatigued because the tryptophan may be converted into serotonin which appears to play a role in sleep inducement. Increased dietary intake of tryptophan increases brain levels of serotonin, reducing the time taken to go to sleep by as much as 50 per cent. High levels of tryptophan may also cause faeces to be smelly as the tryptophan is broken down by intestinal bacteria into two odoriferous chemicals, indole and skatole. More worrying, in the USA a few years ago several hundred people who took tryptophan supplements developed a rare blood disease (eosinophil myalgia syndrome, EMS) which caused excruciating muscular pain, skin rashes, and sometimes death. Although its cause was attributed to a contaminant introduced during its manufacture and not directly to tryptophan itself, over-the-counter supplements were banned in 1989 by the Food and Drug Administration until the contaminant could be identified. *See also* **serotonin**.

turf toe syndrome
An injury commonly caused by stopping suddenly on artificial turf. The foot slides forward in the shoe, bending the big toe upward and stretching ligaments. This usually results in swelling and pain at the base of the big toe, but if the movement is particularly violent, the toe-nail may be damaged (*see* **black nail**) and bones may be fractured.

twister
A simple exercise for stretching upper body muscles. It is often used as part of a warm-up routine.

■ Stand with your feet astride and firmly fixed on the ground. Interlock your hands and raise both elbows to shoulder height. Slowly and smoothly rotate your trunk first one way then the other. Use your elbows to exert some extra tension.

type A behaviour
A form of behaviour exhibited by people who tend to be aggressive, competitive, tense, time-conscious, and generally hostile. Although not all people who exhibit type A behaviour have an increased risk of heart attacks, those who are chronically hostile or cynical are twice as likely to suffer coronary heart disease as people who have a more relaxed and tolerant attitude. The reasons for the relationship between hostile behaviour and heart disease are not clear.

It has been suggested that the hormones produced during hostility may do some physical damage, or that people who exhibit such negative behaviour do not maintain good health habits, such as exercising and eating a balanced diet. *Compare* **type B behaviour**.

type B behaviour
A type of behaviour exhibited by an easy-going, non-aggressive, and non-competitive person. Such people may be less prone to heart disease. *Compare* **type A behaviour**.

Type I diabetes: *See* **diabetes**.

Type II diabetes: *See* **diabetes**.

Type I fibre: *See* **muscle fibre types**.

Type II fibre: *See* **muscle fibre types**.

tyramine
A toxic chemical derived from the amino acid tyrosine. It is present in some fermented cheeses, fermented sausages (such as pepperoni), chocolate, pickled or fermented fish (particularly herring), sauerkraut, yeast extracts, red wine, and some strong beers. These foods may provoke an allergic reaction in people who are highly sensitive to tyramine. The chemical acts as a stimulant, raising blood pressure in a manner similar to adrenaline. Tyramine has been linked to headaches and migraines. The effect is amplified by some drugs (e.g. monoamine oxidase inhibitors used in the treatment of depression), sometimes resulting in fatally high blood pressures.

tyrosine
A non-essential amino acid. It can be made in the body from phenylalanine, which is an essential amino acid.

ulcer: *See* peptic ulcer.

ulnar compression syndrome: *See* compression neuropathy.

ultrasound

Very high frequencies of sound, above 20 kHz. Ultrasound is used in both diagnosis and treatment. Ultrasonography uses echoes of the sound waves to produce images of structures within the body. Continuous ultrasound is a common treatment for deep, soft-tissue injuries. The high-frequency sound waves are believed to vibrate and loosen scar tissue, accelerating the healing process. The vibrations also heat deep tissues and relieve pain. If a swelling occurs, pulsed ultrasound is used because, unlike continuous ultrasound, it does not heat up the tissues. Ultrasound may also be used in a process called phonophoresis to drive anti-inflammatory drugs through the skin into underlying tissue.

ultraviolet light

People who exercise out of doors may be exposed to ultraviolet (UV) light for long periods and are at particular risk from its damaging effects. UV light can penetrate the skin and burn underlying tissues. Certain wavelengths disrupt normal cell activity and are linked with the development of skin cancers (e.g. melanoma). There are a number of sensible precautions that participants in outdoor activities should take:

- wear a hat or cap to shade the head and back of the neck, particularly for long-duration activities such as 18 holes of golf or a marathon
- keep your arms, torso, and, if possible, legs covered with pale-coloured clothing to reflect the light
- apply a suitable barrier on exposed parts of the body (*see* **sun-protection factor**)
- wear sunglasses which protect the eyes from damaging UV rays; this is especially important at high altitudes where UV light is especially intense
- exercise outdoors when the UV light is less intense, before 10 a.m. and after 4 p.m.
- seek medical advice if any persistent sores develop or if moles change appearance.

undereating

Eating less food than the body demands to maintain weight. Mild undereating is a necessary part of a planned weight-loss regime, but it should not be severe. It is important that undereating results in a lower calorie intake but not a reduction in essential nutrients (especially vitamins and minerals). This usually means reducing the fat content of meals. Once the ideal weight is achieved, the dieter should revert to a well-balanced maintenance diet. Prolonged or severe undereating results not only in weight loss but also potentially dangerous muscle wasting. It may also lead to metabolic and psychological disturbances. *See also* **starvation**.

underload principle

A basic principle of training which states that if exercise intensity is regularly below the threshold to stimulate improvements, muscles will gradually become weaker and other training effects will be lost. It is summed up in the phrase 'If you don't use it, you will lose it'.

underweight

A person is significantly underweight if he or she is more than 10 per cent below their optimal body weight. It must be stressed that this optimal weight varies from individual to individual (see **ideal weight**).

Some people are constitutionally thin and their optimum weight will be lower than those who are more comfortable, fit, and healthy at a higher weight. Some athletes, such as long-distance runners, are thin by nature and suffer no ill-effects from being thin. However, such is the pressure for success in sport, that many athletes are unnaturally thin by design rather than by nature. Many exercisers, particularly young female runners and gymnasts, take great pains to keep their weight low. There is no doubt that their high power to weight ratio gives them a competitive advantage, but this may be at a cost to health if taken to extremes.

An obsessive desire for thinness can lead to eating disorders. A survey of more than 4000 recreational runners found that 8 per cent of the men and 24 per cent of the women had attitudes to food similar to those of people suffering anorexia or bulimia nervosa. Many of the women had irregular periods (see **amenorrhoea**) and, although weight-bearing exercise offers partial protection, some may be in danger of suffering brittle bone disease in later life (see **osteoporosis**). In addition, low food intake may result in malnourishment and all its attendant problems, including greater risk of sports injuries. Extreme underweight is often associated with an insufficient intake of the vitamins and minerals required to maintain health.

If you are underweight, your first priority should be to ensure that you are obtaining adequate nutrients. If you wish to increase your weight to its ideal level, you should do this gradually. Aim to gain about 1 pound (0.5 kg) per week by increasing your intake of lean meat, complex carbohydrates, and low-fat dairy products. These foods, combined with a

well-devised exercise programme, will help you gain muscle, not fat.

unfitness

Condition of a person unable to meet the demands of his or her way of life. It can be caused by illness, physical injury, or by social, emotional, and psychological maladjustment. However, it is most commonly due to a combination of lack of exercise and a poor diet.

unhappy triad

A classic knee injury, first described in American footballers. The medial collateral ligament, the anterior cruciate ligament, and the medial cartilage in the knee are ripped apart. This is a devastating injury, usually caused by falling awkwardly after a tackle, and can put an end to a sporting career.

unilateral muscular hypertrophy

The unequal development of muscle so that one side of the body is more bulky. It is common in participants of 'one arm' activities, such as tennis, shotputting, and throwing. See also **tennis shoulder**.

United States Recommended Daily Allowance (US RDA)

A dietary standard used on food labels in the USA until 1995, when the 1991 Nutrition, Labelling, and Education Act came into force. The US RDA is an estimate of the amount of nutrient needed by the population group with the highest demand for that particular nutrient. US RDAs have been replaced by Daily Values. See also **Recommended Dietary Allowance**.

unsaturated fat

A fat which is not fully saturated with hydrogen. Each molecule contains at least one double bond between two carbon atoms because these carbon atoms have not combined with all the hydrogen atoms they could carry. They are more reactive than saturated fats and combine relatively easily with oxygen to become rancid.

There are two main types of unsaturated fats: cis fats and trans fats. Cis fats have molecules with irregular shapes that do not allow them to pack closely together, consequently they are liquid at room temperature. Most natural vegetable oils contain cis fats. Trans fats form straight-chained molecules that can pack tightly together. Trans fats have properties similar to those of saturated fats, making them more harmful to health than cis fats. Butter, milk fat, and some vegetable oils that have been hydrogenated contain significant amounts of trans fats. *See also* **monounsaturated fat** and **polyunsaturated fat**.

upright rowing

An excellent exercise for strengthening muscles in the shoulders and the biceps in the arms. It can be performed using a pulley or free weights (figure 68).

■ Stand close to the pulley with your feet about shoulder width apart. Grasp the bar and pull upwards making sure that you keep your elbows flared. Lower the bar slowly.

If you are using free weights:

Figure 68

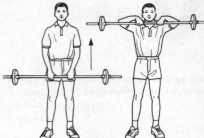

■ Stand upright with your feet about shoulder width apart. With your arms extended, hold a barbell at waist level with an overhand grip. Your hands should be close together near the centre of the bar. Keeping your elbows above the bar and the bar close to your body, lift the barbell up to shoulder level. Lower to the starting position.

US RDA: *See* **United States Recommended Daily Allowance**.

V

....

valgus

Abnormal shape of a part of the body so that it curves outwards from its proximal end (point nearest to the trunk) to its distal end (point furthest from the centre of the trunk). For example, femoral valgus results in a bow-legged appearance. Extra stress is placed on the inside of the hips and on the outside of the knee which can give rise to injuries. A valgus of the forearm involving a pathological bony change in the elbow is an overuse injury of throwers. It can be avoided by using a proper throwing technique.

valine

An essential amino acid found in all proteins. It is one of three branched-chain amino acids. It is seldom deficient in the diet.

Valsalva's manoeuvre

A manœuvre first described by an Italian, A.M. Valsalva (1666–1723). It occurs when the breath is held while muscles in the abdomen and chest are contracted. The chest contents become compressed, increasing gas pressure in the cavity of the thorax and blood pressure in the blood vessels. When breathing is restarted, a reflex reaction causes the heart to slow down, sometimes resulting in dizziness and fainting. Weight-lifters may unintentionally perform a Valsalva's manoeuvre if they hold their breath during a lift. It can cause dizziness, blackouts, and inguinal hernias. This is why weight-lifters are instructed to breathe normally when performing their exercises and never to hold their breath. It is not unknown for children to perform the Valsalva manoeuvre intentionally in

order to induce a fainting attack. They, and anyone else performing the manœuvre, should be strongly discouraged because the increase in intrathoracic pressure can provoke a heart attack in people with a weak heart.

vanadium

An essential trace element which has several metabolic functions. Deficiency causes sterility in certain animals. However, there is as yet no record of deficiency symptoms in humans so no recommended intakes have been established. Dietary sources of vanadium include wholegrain breads, cereals, nuts, shellfish, and liver.

variable resistance exercise

An exercise, usually performed on a special machine, in which the resistance varies throughout the range of movement of the muscles involved. The ability of the muscles of a particular joint system to exert a force changes as the angles of the joint change. Thus the amount of resistance that can be moved is limited by the weakest point in the range of movement. Variable resistance exercise machines adjust the resistance to the muscle's ability to exert a force. It is claimed that these machines bring about a faster and greater increase of strength through the whole range of movement than exercises using a constant resistance.

varices: *See* varicose veins.

varicose veins (varices)

Veins, commonly in the legs, which have become distended and twisted as a result of weakening of their walls and valves.

Because they protrude, they are ruptured relatively easily. Ruptured veins bleed heavily, but the application of firm pressure usually brings the bleeding under control quickly. Obese individuals, pregnant women, those who regularly stand for prolonged periods, and the physically inactive are particularly susceptible. As long as varicose veins are not associated with other symptoms that may indicate a more sinister condition, a controlled programme of physical exercise may improve circulation and benefit sufferers.

varus
Abnormal curving of a part of the body inwards, from the proximal end (nearest the trunk) to the distal end (farthest from the centre of the trunk). Knock-knees is caused by a varus of the thigh bone (femoral varus). It results in stress being placed on the outside of the hips and the inside of the knees, increasing the likelihood of injury. Varus is relieved by strengthening the hip muscles and the quads at the front of the thigh.

vastus intermedius: *See* quadriceps.

vastus lateralis: *See* quadriceps.

vastus medialis: *See* quadriceps.

vegan
A person who eats only food of plant origin. Strict vegans eat no dairy products, eggs, or even honey. Their diet of cereals, vegetables, fruit, and nuts must provide all the essential nutrients. With careful planning this is possible, but there is a risk of vitamin B_{12} deficiency because no plants contain this vitamin. Vegans are usually advised to take B_{12} supplements made by bacterial fermentation.

Spirulina, a blue-green alga used as a staple food by the Aztecs of Mexico and by inhabitants around Lake Chad, Africa, is sold in some health food shops as a high-protein food supplement, rich in minerals and vitamins (including B_{12}). It is true that *Spirulina* contains B_{12}-related compounds that act as growth factors for *Lactobacillus* (the legal definition of vitamin B_{12}), but these compounds do not appear to have B_{12} activity in humans; they may even act as antivitamins.

Vitamin B_{12} activity obtained from some *Spirulina* extracts or concentrates may be due to contamination with faecal bacteria, some of which do form active vitamin B_{12}. Vegans who use *Spirulina* as their source of B_{12} should be cautious.

Some vegans may also need zinc supplements if their diet has a high content of phytates, chemicals that can reduce the availability of zinc. Vegans who exercise a lot may be especially susceptible to a zinc deficiency because of large losses in sweat and urine. However, excessive zinc consumption can produce several harmful effects (including inhibition of copper absorption that can lead to anaemia), so zinc supplementation should not exceed 15 milligrams per day.

Most research indicates that vegans tend to be healthier than people who eat animal products. They also have a lower risk of heart disease, certain cancers, and metabolic and digestive disorders. *See also* **vegetarian**.

vegetarian
A person who does not eat meat. There are different degrees of vegetarianism, from strict vegans who omit all animal products from their diet to semi-vegetarians who eat some animal products. Pescovegetarians eat fish; lacto-vegetarians consume milk but not eggs; lacto-ovovegetarians consume both eggs and milk; and ovo-vegetarians eat eggs. So-called new vegetarians restrict their meat intake to the occasional fish or white meat (e.g. chicken) dish, but avoid red meat and processed foods.

There are many reasons for adopting a vegetarian diet. Some people are vegetarian for religious and cultural reasons; others avoid eating meat for ethical, environmental, or health reasons. Some people do not eat meat for the simple reason that they dislike the taste. The recent upsurge in interest in vegetarian diets has been fuelled by reports in the press about animal cruelty and the potential dangers of eating meat. Media reports associating red meat consumption with heart disease, or about mad cow disease (*see* **bovine spongiform encephalopathy**), increase the number of converts to vegetarianism.

There is much debate about the

nutritional adequacy of vegetarian diets, but it is not possible to say that they are all 'good' or 'bad' because they vary so much in nutrient composition. Nevertheless, well-planned vegetarian diets can provide adequate amounts of all the required nutrients and may be more beneficial to health than an omnivorous diet (studies in the United States indicate that vegetarians have heart attacks on average 10 years later in life than meat eaters). However, the diets of vegans have a greater risk of deficiencies and vegans have to be particularly careful to consume a variety of foods. Vegans may also need to supplement their diets with vitamin B_{12} and possibly calcium to ensure adequate intakes. Poor nutritional health in vegetarians does occur, but is usually a result of poor dietary planning.

It has been estimated recently that there are about 5 million vegetarians in the UK with a growing number of adherents under 16 years of age. The food industry is responding to the increased demand by providing a greater variety of highly nutritious, competitively priced, convenience foods for vegetarians. This is likely to encourage a further expansion in vegetarianism in the future.

ventilation rate: *See* lung volume.

versa-ball

A weighted ball used for throwing exercises. Versa-ball exercises can be used to strengthen the rotator cuff muscles in the shoulders of baseball pitchers and other throwers susceptible to shoulder injuries. The thrower lies on the back, bends the elbow at 90 degrees and throws the ball to a partner. The throw is made by rotating the shoulder and the elbow remains bent at 90 degrees.

vertical jump test: *See* Sargent jump test.

very low calorie diet

A very low calorie diet (VLCD) provides less than 800 Calories per day. Some contain as little as 400 Calories. VLCDs were first introduced in the 1920s to replace fasting as a means of treating overweight people. Some take the form of a drink made from powder and water. So-called

'liquid protein diets' were freely available in the 1970s and gained considerable notoriety after they were linked to a number of deaths. It was discovered that the protein they contained was mainly collagen derived from cowhides. The diets were nutritionally inadequate. Deficiencies of certain essential amino acids and potassium were thought to have caused a loss of lean muscle mass, weakening of heart muscle, and heart irregularities which probably contributed to the death of at least 60 people in the United States. Such liquid protein diets are no longer generally available. Most modern VLCDs are designed to be nutritionally sound and provide the recommended daily intake of proteins, vitamins, and minerals to sustain health.

VLCDs can be dangerous if not used properly, or if taken by certain groups of people. Pregnant women and people with an eating disorder, psychiatric illness, a history of high blood pressure, diabetes, or heart, liver, kidney, or gall bladder disease, should not use a VLCD. Children, breast-feeding women, and the elderly should only take one if medically advised to do so. The general consensus is that VLCDs are safe if used under medical supervision and that they should be used only by those who are medically classified as obese (i.e. have a body mass index of at least 31). Many doctors believe they should be used only by the morbidly obese (BMI greater than 40). In Canada, laws ensure that VLCDs can be used only with a medical prescription; similar laws are being considered in the United States. Potential side-effects, even when VLCDs are used under medical supervision, include gastro-intestinal problems, fatigue, and muscle cramping. The risk of suffering side-effects is reduced by drinking plenty of fluids (at least eight glasses a day).

VLCDs have high rates of short-term success, with the majority of dieters losing 9 kg (about 20 lb). However, people usually stick to the diets only for a short time. They lose weight rapidly, but fail to maintain the loss. One British survey of VLCD users found that less than 20 per cent stayed with the diet for more than two weeks. The better VLCDs include regimes of exercise, nutrition education, and support groups to increase their long-term effectiveness.

VLCDs include the Cambridge Diet or Cambridge Health Plan, which has been used by more than 15 million people worldwide (*see* **Cambridge diet**).

very low-density lipoprotein: *See* lipoprotein.

viropause

A term coined by the popular media for the mid-life changes experienced by some men between the ages of 35 and 45 years. These middle-aged men report that they feel depressed and lack vitality. They complain that their body fat increases and their physical capacity decreases. A few doctors have linked these changes to a critical period when testosterone levels decrease. They argue that the changes are physiological and equivalent to the female menopause (the viropause is sometimes called the 'male menopause'). However, most experts believe that viropause is a myth. They believe that the reported changes are more psychological than physiological. Testosterone levels decline gradually with age and there is no critical drop.

visceral fat deposition

Storage of excess fat around the internal organs, especially the liver and gut. This type of fat deposition is predominant in males and has been linked to a higher risk of heart disease and diabetes. *See also* **android fat distribution**.

visualization (imaging)

A method of training and preparation for performing a physical activity. You create a vivid, controlled image of a situation and imagine yourself coping successfully with it. Before David Hemery won the gold medal for the 400 metres hurdles in the 1968 Mexico Olympics, he visualized himself running in every lane, and imagined how he would cope with the race under different circumstances, but in every instance he pictured himself winning the race. Psychologists believe that visualization establishes neural pathways in the brain which act as a blue-print to be followed in the actual performance. There are different types of visualization:

in external imaging, you imagine that you are an external observer watching yourself perform; in internal imaging, you imagine how you would feel if you performed a particular skill successfully. One computer program available in the USA is designed to help people to visualize how they would like to perform a particular activity. Users can create and modify their own images on the computer screen. The images can then be fixed in the mind prior to visualization. European bobsleigh teams already use virtual reality-type techniques for practice runs.

You can test your powers of visualization by imagining an experience (e.g. making a successful putt at golf) and then rate the vividness of your images using the following scale:

VIVIDNESS OF IMAGES	RATING
clear and vivid as the actual experience	5
moderately clear and vivid	4
not clear but recognizable	3
dim and hardly recognizable	2
thinking of experience but no image	1

If your rating was poor, you can improve your powers of visualization by relaxing and clearing your mind. Sit in a comfortable chair and listen to the sounds around you before visualizing so that the sounds do not distract you during visualization.

vital capacity

The maximal volume of air forcefully expelled from the lungs after a maximal inspiration. It is a measure of the maximum amount of air the lungs can breathe in or out. At rest, values vary from about 3.5–6.0 litres, according to age, sex, and height. Measurements of vital capacity are used as part of a fitness assessment. A person whose vital capacity is less than 75 per cent of the expected value, is generally advised to consult a doctor for further testing before exercising vigorously. *See also* **lung volume**.

vitamin

One of a group of potent, non-protein, organic compounds required in small amounts for the maintenance of normal health and metabolic integrity.

Deficiency leads to specific clinical signs that respond only to restoration of the vitamin. They are essential in the diet because they cannot be made in the body (with the exception of vitamin D and niacin). So far, 13 compounds have been classed as true vitamins. Several other substances, such as laetrile and pangamic acid, have been described as vitamins but these compounds do not meet the strict definition of a vitamin. Although vitamins form a diverse and chemically unrelated group, they are classified as fat-soluble vitamins or water-soluble vitamins.

FAT-SOLUBLE VITAMINS
- vitamin A (retinol; carotene is an important precursor of vitamin A)
- vitamin D (ergocalciferol and cholecalciferol)
- vitamin E (tocopherol)
- vitamin K (phylloquinone from plants; menaquinone from gut bacteria)

WATER-SOLUBLE VITAMINS
- vitamin B_1 (thiamin)
- vitamin B_2 (riboflavin)
- vitamin B_6 (pyridoxine)
- vitamin B_{12} (cobalamin)
- niacin (nicotinic acid and nicotinamide)
- pantothenic acid
- biotin
- folic acid
- vitamin C (ascorbic acid)

Each vitamin has a specific function; one vitamin cannot substitute for another. Lack of any one vitamin in the diet leads to ill health and eventually a deficiency disease. In addition, many body functions require the interaction of several vitamins, and the lack of one may undermine the function of others.

The relationship between vitamin requirements and exercise is complex, and the subject of much debate. There is some dispute about whether active people require more of every type of vitamin. However, it is generally agreed that requirements of the B-complex vitamins, which play many diverse roles in energy metabolism, are directly related to calorie expenditures of up to 5000 Calories per day. On this basis, some coaches believe that very active people may need at least twice the recommended daily amounts of these vitamins. Many sports nutritionists maintain that this increased demand for vitamins can be satisfied by eating a well-balanced diet. They argue that, as energy expenditure increases, food intake and therefore vitamin intake will also increase. On the other hand, some coaches advocate the use of vitamin supplements, arguing that increased dietary intake alone cannot guarantee a sufficient vitamin intake. *See also* **vitamin supplementation**.

vitamin A (retinol; carotene)
A fat-soluble vitamin which helps with normal functioning of the mucus membranes of the eye and respiratory tract, and the formation of visual pigments in the eye. It is also essential for normal tissue growth and differentiation. Vitamin A can be manufactured in the body from beta-carotene, found in a variety of foods, particularly green vegetables and carrots. Vitamin A deficiency increases the risk of all infections, especially those of the respiratory, digestive, and urinogenital tracts, and causes a number eye disorders, including night blindness. It is the most prevalent vitamin deficiency, affecting more than 200 million people worldwide. It is the commonest preventable cause of blindness in the world. However, in economically developed countries, most people can acquire adequate amounts from a well-balanced diet. There is little evidence to support the use of vitamin A supplements, even for athletes whose demands would be expected to be considerably higher than normal. Excessive intakes of vitamin A can lead to nausea, vomiting, anorexia, headaches, hairlessness, bone and joint pain, and bone fragility. (This toxicity applies only to preformed retinol; carotene is not toxic in excess.) Women who are, or might become, pregnant are advised not to take vitamin A supplements, unless advised to do so by their doctor. The safe upper limit in pregnancy (3300 micrograms per day) is considerably lower than for non-pregnant women (7500 micrograms per day) because there may be a risk to the developing baby.

The US Recommended Daily Allowance is 5000 IU or 750 microgram retinol equivalents (the UK adult Reference Nutrient Intake is 700 micrograms for males and 600 micrograms for females). A footballer, acting on the premise that more is better, attempted to improve his performance by consuming 100 000 IU of vitamin A a day in cod liver oil, liver, milk, and vitamin supplements. The huge amounts of vitamin A taken over a period of more than two months resulted in the footballer's legs swelling and becoming stiff, and his bones changing structure. Fortunately, the changes were reversed within a month of the diet being discontinued.

vitamin B complex
A group of vitamins including thiamin (vitamin B_1), riboflavin (vitamin B_2), niacin, pyrodoxine (vitamin B_6), pantothenic acid, folic acid, cobalamin (vitamin B_{12}), and biotin. These vitamins play an essential role in the release of energy from food, making them of great interest to exercisers. Prolonged aerobic exercise depends on a sustained production of energy, so deficiencies impair endurance performance. However, there is no evidence for beneficial effects of supplements over and above the amounts required to prevent deficiency.

vitamin B_1 (aneurine, thiamin)
A water-soluble vitamin first extracted and isolated from rice polishings. It is also found in lean meat, liver, eggs, wholegrains, and milk. It plays a very important role in releasing energy from foods rich in carbohydrates. Gross deficiency causes the potentially fatal disease known as beriberi. Mild deficiencies cause fatigue, loss of appetite, muscle weakness, and digestive disturbances. Deficiency is also associated with chronic alcohol abuse which may lead to derangement of the central nervous system, enlargement of the heart, and death by heart failure. Vitamin B_1 is rapidly destroyed by heat and is stored in the body in very small amounts. In the UK, the Reference Nutrient Intake for adults is 1.0 mg each day for males and 0.8 mg for females. Physically active people may need more thiamin than inactive people. Increased intakes may also be required by those on high carbohydrate diets, during pregnancy, and in other stressful situations.

vitamin B_2 (riboflavin)
A water-soluble vitamin present in the body as coenzymes which play a central role in releasing energy from food. It is obtained from a wide variety of foods including wholegrains, yeast, liver, eggs, and milk. Riboflavin is quickly decomposed by heat and when exposed to light it is converted to lumiflavin which destroys vitamin C. Thus milk left outside for long periods in bright sunlight will lose much of its riboflavin activity. The Reference Nutrient Intake (UK) ranges from 0.4 mg in babies to 1.6 mg in breast-feeding women. Deficiency causes ariboflavinosis, characterized by cracked skin and eye problems including blurred vision. Riboflavin is used as a food colouring agent; an example of a food additive that has a considerable beneficial effect.

vitamin B_3: *See* niacin.

vitamin B_5: *See* pantothenic acid.

vitamin B_6 (pyridoxine)
A water-soluble vitamin obtained from meat, poultry, and eggs. It acts as a coenzyme to over 60 enzymes and plays a vital role in protein metabolism. Those on high protein diets may require more vitamin B_6. The vitamin is essential for efficient nerve and muscle function. It is also involved in the initial breakdown of glycogen, and in the formation of antibodies and haemoglobin. Deficiency, although relatively rare, causes nervous irritability, anaemia, convulsions in infants, and sores around the eyes and mouth in adults. Excessive intake results in depressed tendon reflexes and loss of sensation in the fingers and toes. Intakes greater than 500 mg per day are associated with permanent sensory nerve damage. In the UK, the adult Reference Nutrient Intake is 1.4 mg per day for males, and 1.2 mg per day for females.

vitamin B_{12} (cobalamin; cyanocobalamin)
A complex water-soluble vitamin containing cobalt. Vitamin B_{12} can be obtained from liver, fish, and some dairy products.

It is the only member of the B complex
that cannot be obtained from yeast.
Vitamin B_{12} acts as a coenzyme. It is
involved in DNA synthesis and the formation of red blood cells. Vitamin B_{12} and
folic acid interact: deficiency of B_{12} leads
to functional deficiency of folic acid. In
addition, a glycoprotein (known as intrinsic factor) produced by the stomach is
needed for absorption of Vitamin B_{12}
across the membrane of the intestine
into the bloodstream. Lack of B_{12}, or
intrinsic factor, or folic acid, may cause
pernicious anaemia and weight loss.
Vitamin B_{12} is regarded as an ergogenic
aid by many coaches who believe it
improves energy metabolism in muscle
cells. Supplementation, often by injection into the buttocks, is common even
though most research has shown no
significant benefits where a B_{12} deficiency
does not exist. Toxic effects of vitamin B_{12}
are virtually unknown, but allergic reactions occasionally occur from injections.
In the UK, the Reference Nutrient Intake
for adults is 1.5 micrograms per day.

vitamin B_{15}: *See* pangamic acid.

vitamin B_{17}: *See* laetrile.

vitamin C (ascorbic acid)
A water-soluble vitamin essential for the
formation of collagen (a major component of skin, muscles, and bone) and the
healthy functioning of tissues containing
collagen. It is required for the repair of
joint tissues which are often damaged
during high levels of physical activity.
Vitamin C acts as a stimulant for body
defence mechanisms, and protects vitamin A, vitamin E, and dietary fats from
oxidation (*see* **antioxidants**). Vitamin C
also plays an important role in the
absorption of iron from plant foods. Mild
deficiencies can cause fleeting joint
pains, poor tooth and bone growth, poor
wound healing, and an increased susceptibility to infection. The Nobel Prize winner, Linus Pauling, and others claimed
that doses 10 to 100 times greater than
normal are effective in preventing the
common cold. This claim is still very controversial, but there is some evidence to
support it. In the test-tube, vitamin C has
been shown to detoxify histamine—a

product of stress (including the common
cold). It is not clear whether the vitamin
has the same ability in a living person.
An extreme deficiency of vitamin C
causes scurvy. In the UK, the Reference
Nutrient Intake (RNI) is 40 mg per day for
adults, but this should be increased for
those under any stress and those who are
physically active. The RNI for pregnant
women is 50 mg per day, and for lactating mothers is 70 mg per day. The USA
recommendations are higher.
Vitamin C toxicity is unlikely, therefore
many coaches feel free to advocate sub-
stantial supplementation for athletes.
The whole topic is controversial; there is
little unequivocal research to support
large supplementation, and there may be
some problems not yet fully reported.
Most nutritionists recommend taking
vitamin C naturally in the diet rather
than as artificial supplements. Vegetables
(especially green peppers) and citrus
fruits are good sources. The richest
source is acerola cherry juice (3390 mg of
vitamin C per 100 g of juice).

vitamin D (anti-rachitic factor)
A fat-soluble vitamin that enhances the
absorption of calcium and phosphorus
from the intestine and, with parathyroid
hormone, mobilizes their deposition in
bones. Vitamin D is relatively stable when
exposed to heat and light. It is stored in
the liver and, to a lesser extent, in the
fatty tissue in the skin. Vitamin D occurs
in two forms: vitamin D_2 and vitamin D_3.
Vitamin D_2 (ergocalciferol or calciferol) is
obtained in the diet from foods such as
oily fish, eggs, and margarine. Vitamin D_3
(cholecalciferol) is the main form of the
vitamin and is produced in the skin by
the action of ultraviolet light on another
compound, 7-dehydrocholesterol.
Vitamin D deficiency causes a loss of muscle tone, restlessness, and irritability. It
also causes rickets in children, and demineralization and softening of the
bones (osteomalacia) in adults.
In the UK, no Dietary Reference Values
are given for adults with normal sunlight
exposure because the main source of vitamin D is from the action of sunlight on
skin. However, for those confined indoors
during the winter months, the Reference
Nutrient Intake is 10 micrograms for

adults (18–65 years) and 7 micrograms for children. In the USA, a daily intake of 10 micrograms throughout life is recommended. As with vitamin A, vitamin D can be toxic if large amounts are consumed over a long period of time. Calcium may be deposited in the organs and soft tissues of the body damaging, for example, the kidneys. Vitamin D supplements have been used to treat rheumatoid arthritis and they may reduce the risk of osteoporosis, but the evidence is conflicting: most studies show no benefit, and some even show an adverse effect. Nevertheless, vitamin D supplements in the elderly will prevent osteomalacia which may occur together with, or independently of, osteoporosis.

vitamin deficiency disease

A disease due to a lack of a vitamin in the body. It may be caused by a dietary deficiency or as a secondary disease associated with anorexia, vomiting, or diarrhoea. Vitamin deficiency disease may also result from the increased metabolic demands for vitamins imposed by fever or stress, including the stress of vigorous, prolonged physical exertion. A substance which interferes with the activity of a vitamin may also cause a deficiency disease.

It is now generally recognized that certain groups within the population have a greater risk of deficiency diseases because of their increased vitamin requirements. They include pregnant women, nursing mothers, those following a weight-reducing diet, convalescents, the elderly, athletes in hard training, and those in physically demanding jobs. These groups may benefit from carefully managed vitamin supplementation.

vitamin E (anti-sterility factor; fertility vitamin)

A group of related compounds called tocopherols which maintain the integrity of cell membranes. Vitamin E is an antioxidant and mutually protects vitamins A and C. Some coaches claim that it increases muscular development and function; this claim is hotly disputed, but there is considerable support for the suggestion that vitamin E reduces the oxygen requirements of muscles and so enhances performance. It has been suggested that physical endurance at high altitudes may be increased, and oxygen debt reduced, by taking 1200 IU of vitamin E per day. Such high doses can be toxic and should be taken only under medical supervision. Vitamin E is widely available in the diet. The richest sources include wheatgerm oil, sunflower oil, and roasted peanuts. Natural sources of Vitamin E are almost twice as potent as synthetic vitamin E. Natural and synthetic forms can be identified by subtle differences in the names of their main components: natural forms are known as 'd-alpha tocopherol' and the synthetic ones as 'dl-alpha tocopherol'. Vitamin E deficiencies are rare, but when they do occur they may lead to destruction of red blood cells and anaemia. Deficiencies impair the reproductive ability of rats and causes muscle wasting in pigs, but vitamin E has no effect on human fertility or libido. There is a growing body of good evidence that vitamin E supplements may offer some protection against atherosclerosis and heart disease. It has also been suggested that supplements may reduce the risk of miscarriages, but this suggestion is disputed.

vitamin F: *See* linoleic acid.

vitamin K (anti-haemorrhagic vitamin)

A fat-soluble vitamin which occurs in two main forms: one of plant origin (phytomenadione or phylloquinone), and the other of animal origin (menaquinone). Dietary sources include green leafy vegetables, some vegetable oils, and liver. Some vitamin K is derived from bacterial activity in the gut, but it is not clear how active this form of vitamin K is compared with phylloquinone. Bacterial synthesis is not adequate to maintain normal blood clotting if no phylloquinone is obtained from the diet. Vitamin K is needed to manufacture prothrombin, a substance essential for the normal clotting of blood. Deficiency is rare but may result from taking antibiotics which interfere with the activity of gut bacteria. Symptoms include easy bruising and prolonged clotting time, leading to excessive bleeding and haemorrhage.

vitamin supplementation

Additional vitamins taken to make up a deficit, to avoid a vitamin deficiency disease, or to enhance athletic performance. There is much controversy concerning the value of vitamin supplements as ergogenic aids. There is little evidence to support the notion that extra vitamins improve the physical performance of athletes already eating a balanced diet and not suffering from a vitamin deficiency. However, high doses of vitamins may improve athletic performance by acting as drugs in, as yet, undefined ways.

There is general agreement that physical activity increases vitamin requirement, but many sports nutritionists believe that the increased requirement can be satisfied by a balanced diet. As exercise increases, food intake will increase and so should vitamin intake if the right foods are eaten. Nevertheless, because the difference between success and failure in sport may be very finely balanced, many coaches like to ensure that their athletes are taking sufficient vitamins, particularly the energy-related B vitamins, and advocate moderate multivitamin supplementation. Those taking supplements should be aware of the risk of toxicity from overdoses. This especially applies to the vitamins A, B_6, D, and niacin. Vitamin B complex tablets, particularly those containing nicotinic acid, should not be taken immediately before a prolonged bout of exercise because nicotinic acid can impair endurance by preventing mobilization of free fatty acids used as an energy source.

volleyball

Volleyball is a dynamic game requiring high levels of aerobic endurance, power, flexibility, speed, and agility. The most important of these is endurance, because without this a player is unable to maintain skill and effort throughout a game. A well-balanced training programme includes aerobic fitness (e.g. running), weight training, agility drills, and jump training (*see* **plyometrics**) to provide the explosive power the game requires. Much of the formal training of a volleyball team focuses on court skills, technique, and strategy, leaving each player to take responsibility for developing individual fitness. However, it is essential for players to train for general fitness so that they can perform to their maximum ability and reduce the risk of injury. The shoulder is the part of the body most commonly injured in volleyball, followed by the back and ankle. The most common chronic ailment of volleyball players is probably inflammation of the tendon that crosses the kneecap. These injuries can be reduced by an adequate warm-up and a programme of good flexibility exercises.

waist-hip ratio

The circumference of the body at the level of the navel divided by the circumference at the widest point around the buttocks. The waist-hip ratio is used as a convenient method of assessing the distribution of body fat. Men tend to have high ratios indicating that most fat is distributed around the waist; women have low ratios indicating fat distribution around the hips. These sex differences in fat distribution are thought to be due to hormonal effects during puberty. High oestrogen levels in women encourage the deposition of fat around the buttocks and hips, while high testosterone levels in men encourages deposition around the waist. Accumulation of fat around the waist increases the risk of certain diseases. Men with waist–hip ratios greater than 1.0, and women with ratios greater than 0.8, have an increased risk of cardiovascular illness.

According to a theory supported by Professor Devendra Singh of the University of Texas, USA, the waist–hip ratio holds the key to sex appeal in women. Tests showed that women become more attractive to men as the waist becomes smaller in relation to the hip, with the ideal ratio in healthy premenopausal women being between 0.67 and 0.80. This belief was supported by studies of Ms America contestants and *Playboy* playmates between 1957 and 1987, all of whom had waist–hip ratios between 0.68 and 0.71. In addition to being a sexual attractant, the high stores of fat in the buttocks are used during the last stages of pregnancy and during breast-feeding to support the baby.

Women with low waist–hip ratios also have a lower risk of heart disease and diabetes. *See also* **android fat distribution** and **gynoid fat distribution**.

walking

Walking is one of the most popular exercises. It has many benefits. It is a low-impact exercise with very little risk of injury; it requires the minimum of special equipment (good shoes and loose-fitting clothing are usually sufficient); the whole family can take part; and it has the added advantage of being socially acceptable for women and older people.

Many people believe that only strenuous exercise has health benefits. This is not true. Exercise no more exhausting than a brisk walk can lower blood cholesterol levels and reduce the risk of coronary heart disease. Walking about 10 miles (16 kilometres) per week at about 60 per cent maximum aerobic capacity, is enough for the heart to benefit, and, cardiologists estimate, may reduce the risk of heart attack by half.

Walking can improve aerobic fitness, as long as it is done fast enough. As you walk faster, you can expect to improve your aerobic fitness at a higher rate. Strolling at 20 minutes per mile pace is likely to improve your maximum aerobic capacity (VO_2 max) by no more than 5 per cent; walking at 15 minutes per mile pace may almost double that improvement; and if you walk very fast (at 12 minutes per mile pace), your VO_2 max may improve as much as 15 per cent. Benefits gained from fast walking can be as good as those derived from running, cycling, or swimming. Very fast walking is sometimes called power walking. Some people use hand weights to increase the resistance and to develop upper body muscles. These weights are generally not effective unless they are used in an exaggerated way that disturbs the stride pattern and increases the risk of injury.

If you wish to walk to improve health:

• walk at least three times a week
• start with a 1 mile (1.6 km) and walk at a slow pace (20 minutes per mile)
• add a quarter of a mile (400 m) a week until you can walk three miles easily.

This will be enough to improve your health, but if you wish to improve your aerobic fitness you will need to increase your pace gradually. Aim to do one of the three miles in 15 minutes, then two, and finally all three. When you have achieved this, aim to do one mile in 12 minutes, and so on. Be patient. It will take about six months before you feel the real benefits of your training.

warm down: *See* cool down.

warm-up
A routine used before strenuous activity to attain optimal body temperature, and to prepare physically and mentally for the activity. Body temperature can be raised by aerobic activities called pulse raisers. These are usually followed by mobility exercises or callisthenics (gentle movements to loosen joints) and static stretching of all the major muscle groups. Warm-ups improve the body's ability to transport oxygen and fuel to active muscles, increase the speed of muscle contraction, and reduce the risk of muscle and joint injuries.

water
Water is the most abundant chemical in the body, making up roughly 60 per cent of body weight. It is an essential nutrient although it provides no energy. It has excellent solvent properties enabling it to act as a transport medium for many chemicals. It is involved in many chemical reactions including digestion of food.

Evaporation of water as sweat is essential for cooling the body. However, failure to replace water losses results in dehydration. This can adversely affect physical

performance even if relatively slight. Each 1 per cent loss of water results in a 2 per cent reduction in aerobic capacity. Water loss causes the heart rate to spiral upwards. A loss of 6 per cent of total body water is serious; and loss of more than 10 per cent can be fatal. The amount of water an individual drinks depends on water losses (*see* **water replacement**).

Hardness of water varies with geographical location. There is statistical evidence that heart disease is more common in areas with soft drinking water than in those with hard water. However, the link between type of water and heart disease is not proven.

The quality of drinking water varies. In most areas of the USA and the UK, tap water is safe, but in some areas it can become contaminated with bacteria, nitrates, or other pollutants. Some people drink bottled water because they are worried about pollutants, but others drink it because they prefer the taste, or believe that bottled water has health-giving properties. Ironically, bottled water is not always healthy. Some contain high levels of sodium and the same pollutants as tap water.

water balance (fluid balance)
The relationship between the water taken into the body by all routes (e.g. food and drink) and the water lost by all routes (e.g. sweat, vomit, urine, and faeces). An inadequate water balance has immediate and serious debilitating effects on physical activity. *See also* **dehydration** and **water intoxication**.

water intoxication (dilutional hyponatremia; hypotonic hydration)
A condition of water imbalance which may result from a kidney disorder or from drinking large amounts of water in a short time. The water dilutes the fluid surrounding cells and causes them to swell. This may result in metabolic disorders, nausea, vomiting, muscular cramps, and, in extreme cases, death. In February 1995, a twenty-year-old man from Derby in the United Kingdom drank himself to death after taking a single tablet of the drug ecstasy. It was estimated that he drank 26 pints of water which, according to a pathologist, caused brain damage

and death. Such extreme cases are very rare, but mild water intoxication can occur when people try to replenish fluid losses by drinking too much water, too quickly. *See also* **hyponatremia**.

water replacement
To reduce the risk of dehydration, water should be replaced during vigorous physical exercises lasting more than about 50 minutes. Replacement is particularly important for children and adolescents because their body temperature rises faster than that of adults. The best form of replacement is a cold drink (8–13°C); low in sugars (sugar retards gastric emptying and inhibits the absorption of water); and with a salt concentration less than that of the body fluids. The main purpose of the salts is to speed up the transfer of water through the small intestine into the body. Water lost due to sweating during exercise results in weight loss, and a loss of muscle strength and endurance. As a rough guide, a person should drink two cups of fluid for every pound of weight lost. The rate of replacement should not exceed the maximum absorption rate (about 800 ml per hour). *See also* **thirst**.

water retention: *See* **fluid retention**.

water tablets
Tablets used to increase the elimination of water from the body (*see* **diuretics**).

weight belt
Certain weight-lifting exercises put a lot of pressure on the spine, actually compressing it. A tightly-fastened weight belt helps to alleviate this; the belt supports the spine and also, by keeping the stomach in, prevents the spine from bending inwards.

weight cycling
A cycle of weight changes associated with alternating periods of dieting (restricted food intake) and periods of normal eating with weight gain. The basal metabolic rate (BMR, a measure of the body's energy consumption at complete rest) of people on a weight-loss diet is usually reduced. The body adapts to the lower intake of food by using the limited supply of energy more efficiently. It appears that this reduction in BMR is more pronounced in those who exhibit weight cycling, making it increasingly difficult to lose weight and much easier to regain it. There is also evidence that weight cycling over several years increases the risk of coronary heart disease. *See also* **Yo-Yo diet**.

weight-gain diet
Theoretically, to put on weight, a person should eat about 500 Calories more each day than are required to maintain a constant weight. In practice, some people put on weight easily while others seem unable to gain weight even after eating extravagantly over a long period. A healthy weight-gain diet is usually low in fats and not especially high in proteins. Most of the extra calories should be in the form of carbohydrates which will provide the energy required for muscle growth. Excess protein is not stored as muscle. Muscles grow only in response to increased demands of exercise. Specific exercises, such as weight training, should be performed to ensure that the diet promotes muscle growth rather than fat deposition. *See also* **body building**.

weight-lifter's headache: *See* **headache**.

weight-loss maintenance
Maintenance of a relatively constant body weight after a successful weight-loss programme. It is relatively easy to lose weight, but much more difficult to maintain the weight at a lower level. Most dieters return to their original weight within one year. Weight-loss maintenance is easier if dieters adopt exercise as part of their lifestyle. It is also more likely if dieters have lost weight slowly and steadily. Dieters should aim to lose about 1–2 lb (0.5–1.0 kg) per week. Successful weight-loss maintenance usually requires considerable effort in planning balanced, nutritious, and interesting meals. The following tips may help you maintain your ideal weight:

- weigh yourself regularly (once a week), but do not worry about fluctuations of a few pounds, this may be due to variations in water retention
- plan your meals and try to eat only at meal times

- have at least three meals each day
- choose foods with a high nutrient density
- keep an eating diary recording when and what foods are eaten
- have a good breakfast and avoid eating heavy meals in the evening
- if you need to have a snack, eat fruit or other nutrient-rich foods rather than sweets which contain empty calories
- avoid foods with a high fat content
- eat plenty of complex carbohydrates, such as wholewheat pasta, wholemeal bread, and jacket potatoes
- cut down sugar intake
- include small portions of favourite foods on a regular basis
- drink plenty of watery fluids (about eight glasses of water each day)
- exercise regularly (for example, by walking briskly for 20 minutes each day).

Once an ideal weight is achieved, it is just as important not to allow it to go down as it is to prevent it from going up.

weight training

A form of strength training involving the use of either free weights or a weight-training machine. There are many weight-training systems including the blitz system, burns, pyramid system, multi-set system, superset system, and multi-poundage system. In addition, there is a long list of weight-training exercises which train specific muscles or muscle groups.

Pumping iron is no longer the preserve of the young. It has been shown that pensioners can benefit from regular weight-training sessions designed to improve leg strength. Weight training for 45 minutes every other day for 10 weeks, can double muscle strength, even in frail octogenarians. Weight training has helped older people walk more quickly and to climb stairs, and to discard the Zimmer frames on which they previously relied.

If you wish to start weight training, you should obtain proper instruction from a qualified trainer. You should also be confident that you can cope with strenuous physical exertion. If you have been inactive or ill, see your doctor to obtain approval. The following are some other guidelines to help you train safely:

- plan ahead what you want to do; set achievable goals
- warm-up for at least 5 minutes before you start a session and cool down afterwards
- incorporate slow, static stretches in your routines
- start your session slowly with light weights
- position yourself properly; e.g. when standing and lifting free weights
  - spread your feet shoulder width apart
  - position yourself close to the weights
  - bend your knees a little
  - avoid twisting your body
  - do not bend at the waist
- focus on performing skillful movements rather than lifting heavy weights
- train with relatively high repetitions (8–12) and moderate loads
- do not try to lift weights that are too heavy
- do not use bouncing movements
- breathe normally during lifts; do not hold your breath
- train muscles on all sides of a joint
- vary exercises and routines
- use spotters (partners who assist with the weights).

weight-training machine

A specialized device that provides support for a person trying to overcome a resistance. Weight-training machines can be designed to produce resistances at a particular angle of pull for a specific muscle, or to provide variable resistances for isokinetic exercises which are performed at a constant speed. There have been claims that these machines bring about faster and greater increases in strength than other types of weight training. Although this may be true in some cases, most exercise physiologists agree that each type of training method has advantages and disadvantages, and as long as basic training principles (particularly the overload principle) are adhered to, it is possible to make strength gains using machines or free weights.

whiplash injury

Damage to the nerves and ligaments in the neck caused by a sudden, uncontrolled, and usually unexpected movement of the head. Players of rugby and American football may sustain a whiplash injury when tackled by two players simultaneously, one at the back and the other at the front. Rear-end vehicle collisions are notorious for causing neck strains as the vulnerable neck vertebrae are first extended and then fully flexed. Treatment usually includes wearing a restricting neck collar. Neck injuries should always be treated with great respect and, with the exception of obviously minor injuries, medical advice should be sought to ensure there is no serious injury. The risk of serious injury from a whiplash can be reduced by adherence to the rules (for example, no high tackles in rugby), wearing appropriate protective equipment, and special strength training for the neck.

whirlpool treatment

Immersion in warm water agitated by high-pressure jets of water that provide an underwater massage. Whirlpool treatment may relax muscles and relieve aches and pains temporarily, but they can be harmful if the temperature is excessively high (above 37°C), causing birth defects in pregnant women and temporary infertility in men. It is also important to ensure that the water is not contaminated with bacteria because warm water is an ideal environment for them.

white adipose tissue

Normal fat stored under the skin and between organs. It is relatively inactive and difficult to break down, making it an efficient energy store. Its biological efficiency is a great disadvantage to overweight people trying to get rid of excess weight. *Compare* **brown fat**.

white fibre: *See* **muscle fibre types**.

wind: *See* **flatulence**.

winding

A common injury in contact sports resulting from a blow to the abdomen that overstimulates the solar plexus,

causing nervous shock. Typically, a winded person doubles up and has difficulty breathing because the diaphragm is momentarily paralysed and the abdominal muscles go into a spasm. Drawing the knees up to the abdomen is a popular treatment that may help to relax the abdominal muscles and relieve the pain. Even without special treatment a winded person usually recovers quickly without any residual symptoms. If symptoms persist, there may be a serious internal injury requiring expert medical attention.

windmills

A stretching exercise often used as part of a warm-up routine.

■ Stand upright with arms extended. Circle your arms backwards alternately, making sure that you bring your upper arm close to your ear. Repeat the exercise, but this time circling both arms together. Start with about 20 circles in each direction and build up to about 40.

As with all stretching, windmills should be performed slowly. Windmills are often used as rehabilitation exercises for tennis players who have had a shoulder injury. The windmills are performed very slowly, first without a tennis racket and then with a tennis racket. When using a tennis racket, it is a good idea to hold a racket in each hand to ensure balanced muscle development.

Work Related Upper Limb Disorder: *See* **repetitive strain injury**.

wrestler's bridge

An exercise that develops the neck muscles and strengthens the back and spine (figure 69).

Figure 69

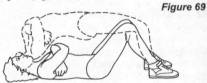

■ Lie on your back with your head resting on a cushion and your feet drawn up close to your buttocks. Fold your arms, then slowly arch your body up until you are supported by the top of your head and feet only.

Figure 70 Wrist curl

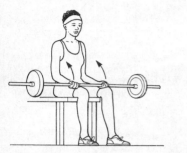 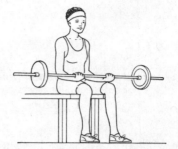

This is a difficult exercise and should be performed only after expert instruction. If performed incorrectly, or by someone who is not sufficiently fit, there is a danger of damaging the neck.

wrist curl

A weight-training exercise for strengthening the muscles of the wrist (figure 70).

■ Sit on a bench or chair with your elbows resting on your thighs just behind your knees. With palms facing upwards and your arms parallel to the floor, grip a barbell in your hands. Slowly raise and lower the barbell using only the muscles in your wrists; do not move your arms.

wryneck: *See* **torticollis**.

X

"If we had not tasted honey, we would think figs far sweeter."
Xenophanes of Colophon, c. 570–475 BC, Greek poet and philosopher.

xanthines
A group of compounds that include caffeine found in tea and coffee. Xanthines act as diuretics, causing you to eliminate more water than usual in your urine, temporarily reducing your weight. *See also* **caffeine** and **diuretics**.

xerophthalmia
A disease caused by deficiency of vitamin A. It is characterized by drying of the tear ducts resulting in degeneration of the transparent part of the eye, leading to ulceration of the cornea and blindness. It is the commonest preventable cause of blindness worldwide.

X-ray
Radiation that can penetrate body structures to varying degrees. X-rays are used in radiography to produce photographic images of internal structures. They are used in the diagnosis of sports injuries where there is a suspected fracture.

xylitol
A sugar alcohol extracted from birch wood, corn cobs, and peanuts. It is used to make sugar-free sweets, such as chewing gums and mints. Xylitol does not cause dental caries, in fact it actually inhibits the growth of bacteria which cause tooth decay. Although rich in calories, xylitol may have a small advantage over sugars in calorie controlled diets because it has a lower calorie yield and is more slowly absorbed. Its slow absorption also makes it more suitable for diabetics because it produces little or no stress on the pancreas.

xylose
A sugar involved in carbohydrate metabolism. It occurs in some high fibre foods.

Y

"I thought no more was needed
Youth to prolong
Than dumb-bell and foil
To keep the body young.
O who would have foretold
That the heart grows old?"

W. B. Yeats, 1865–1939. A song, quoted in (1979) *The Oxford dictionary of quotations.*
Oxford University Press, Oxford.

yang: *See* macrobiotic diet.

Yerkes-Dodson curve
A curve depicting the relationship between arousal and performance. *See also* **catastrophe theory** and **inverted U hypothesis**.

ying: *See* macrobiotic diet.

yoga
A philosophical system attributed to the Hindu, Patanjali, who lived in India in about 150 BC In Sanskrit, the word 'yoga' means 'union'. The yoga philosophy is based on developing a mystical union between yourself and a personal deity through a combination of self-hypnosis, meditation, the adoption of special postures (asanas), and ascetic practices. In the West, the meditation and special postures have been adapted as a system of physical exercise and relaxation techniques. The exercises consist of slow stretching movements performed in harmony with breathing. Yoga tones all the muscles, flexes the joints and strengthens the body. Some of the exercises have been incorporated in a new form of aerobic activity called 'yogacise'.

yogacise: *See* yoga.

Yo-Yo diet
An eating pattern that results in wild swings in body weight (figure 71). Rapid

Figure 71

Diet

Diet

Regain

Regain

Weight

Time

weight loss is followed by equally rapid weight gain. The final body weight is often higher than the original body weight. Yo-Yo diets include many short-term, very low calorie diets which encourage rapid fasting. Weight is lost, but when the period of dieting ends, the dieter often binges in an effort to satisfy the body's craving for food. Yo-Yo diets are now known to be associated with an increased risk of coronary heart disease.

young runner's heel
An injury of the growing points of the heel bone resulting in pain as the heel strikes the ground. It is common in young runners who overtrain.

Z

Zatopek phenomenon: *See* tapering down.

Zen macrobiotic diet

An extreme form of vegetarianism that progresses through 10 stages of dietary restriction with the gradual elimination of animal products, fruits, and vegetables. The initial stages may meet minimum nutritional requirements. However, the highest stages allow only cereals (mainly brown rice) in the diet and are nutritionally inadequate. The diet of the last three stages is poor in proteins, calcium, and vitamins B_{12} and C. Deficiencies of these nutrients may cause growth retardation in children and can be fatal in adults. *See also* **macrobiotic diet**.

zero fat diet

A diet containing no fat. If you eat natural foods, it is almost impossible to have a zero fat intake. Consequently, zero fat diets are composed of artificial foods, usually in the form of powders and drinks. They are bought in the mistaken belief that all fat is bad for you. On the contrary, certain fats are an essential part of a balanced diet. A truly zero fat diet is harmful and would result in potentially fatal metabolic disorders. *See also* **essential fatty acid**.

zinc

An essential trace element that works in close association with vitamins and over 100 enzymes. It is, therefore, involved in almost every physiological function in the body. It forms part of a protein (gustin) in saliva and plays a role in taste and smell. It also helps to heal wounds.

Although there is only a little evidence that taking extra zinc can improve athletic performance, some weight-lifters take zinc supplements in the belief that it increases stamina by prolonging muscle contractions.

Zinc deficiency may cause loss of taste and smell, and a reduction of appetite. A deficiency can slow down the healing of wounds (zinc oxide ointment is applied to abrasions to accelerate healing), retard growth in children, and reduce the sperm count of adult males (the concentration of zinc in semen is 100 times greater than in the blood plasma).

The US recommended dietary allowance (RDA) for adults is 15 mg for males and 12 mg for females. The UK Reference Nutrient Intake for adults is 9.5 mg for males and 7.0 mg for females (lactating mothers require higher amounts). Zinc can be obtained from seafood (especially oysters and other shellfish), cereal crops, legumes, wheat germ, and yeast products. Zinc may bind to some constituents of dietary fibre, interfering with its absorption from the gut. Consequently, vegetarians may require a higher than normal intake of this element. As zinc is lost in urine and sweat, exercisers (especially those who train intensively) may also need zinc supplementation. However, zinc supplementation should not exceed the RDA because excessive amounts can have harmful effects including inhibition of copper absorption, which may lead to anaemia.

zinc oxide ointment

An ointment used as a skin protector, preventing the penetration of ultraviolet light. It is also applied to abrasions to accelerate healing.

zone of optimal functioning

A range of arousal levels that produces the best performances in physical activities. The zone of optimal arousal differs for different activities. Weight-lifters, for example, benefit from high levels of arousal so they can generate maximum power during the lift. Marksmen, on the other hand, benefit from low levels so that they can perform controlled, delicate movements. *See also* **catastrophe theory**.

Appendix 1: Recommended Dietary Allowances and Intakes

Estimated safe and adequate daily dietary intakes of selected vitamins and minerals[a]

| Category | Age (years) | Vitamins | | Trace elements[b] | | | | |
		Biotin (µg)	Pantothenic acid (mg)	Copper (mg)	Manganese (mg)	Fluoride (mg)	Chromium (µg)	Molybdenum (µg)
Infants	0.0–0.5	10	2	0.4–0.6	0.3–0.6	0.1–0.5	10–40	15–30
	0.5–1.0	15	3	0.6–0.7	0.6–1.0	0.2–1.0	20–60	20–40
Children and adolescents	1–3	20	3	0.7–1.0	1.0–1.5	0.5–1.5	20–80	25–50
	4–6	25	3–4	1.0–1.5	1.5–2.0	1.0–2.5	30–120	30–75
	7–10	30	4–5	1.0–2.0	2.0–3.0	1.5–2.5	50–200	50–150
	11+	30–100	4–7	1.5–2.5	2.0–5.0	1.5–2.5	50–200	75–250
Adults		30–100	4–7	1.5–3.0	2.0–5.0	1.5–4.0	50–200	75–250

[a]Because there is less information on which to base allowances, these figures are not given in the main table of RDA and are provided here in the form of ranges of recommended intakes.

[b]Because the toxic levels for many trace elements may be only several times usual intakes, the upper levels for the trace elements given in this table should not be habitually exceeded.

Reprinted with permission from *Recommended Dietary Allowances, 10th Edition*. © 1989 by the National Academy of Sciences. Published by National Academy Press, USA.

Food and Nutrition Board, National Academy of Sciences – National Research Council Recommended Dietary Allowances,[a] Revised 1989 (Designed for the maintenance of good nutrition of practically all healthy people in the United States)

Age (years) or condition	Weight[b] (kg)	Weight[b] (lb)	Height[b] (cm)	Height[b] (in.)	Protein (g)	Fat-soluble vitamins				Water-soluble vitamins							Minerals						
						Vitamin A (µg R.E.)[c]	Vitamin D (µg)[d]	Vitamin E (mg α-T.E.)[e]	Vitamin K (µg)	Vitamin C (mg)	Thiamin (mg)	Riboflavin (mg)	Niacin (mg N.E.)[f]	Vitamin B6 (mg)	Folate (µg)	Vitamin B12 (µg)	Calcium (mg)	Phosphorus (mg)	Magnesium (mg)	Iron (mg)	Zinc (mg)	Iodine (µg)	Selenium (µg)
Infants																							
0.0–0.5	6	13	60	24	13	375	7.5	3	5	30	0.3	0.4	5	0.3	25	0.3	400	300	40	6	5	40	10
0.5–1.0	9	20	71	28	14	375	10	4	10	35	0.4	0.5	6	0.6	35	0.5	600	500	60	10	5	50	15
Children																							
1–3	13	29	90	35	16	400	10	6	15	40	0.7	0.8	9	1.0	50	0.7	800	800	80	10	10	70	20
4–6	20	44	112	44	24	500	10	7	20	45	0.9	1.1	12	1.1	75	1.0	800	800	120	10	10	90	20
7–10	28	62	132	52	28	700	10	7	30	45	1.0	1.2	13	1.4	100	1.4	800	800	170	10	10	120	30
Males																							
11–14	45	99	157	62	45	1000	10	10	45	50	1.3	1.5	17	1.7	150	2.0	1200	1200	270	12	15	150	40
15–18	66	145	176	69	59	1000	10	10	65	60	1.5	1.8	20	2.0	200	2.0	1200	1200	400	12	15	150	50
19–24	72	160	177	70	58	1000	10	10	70	60	1.5	1.7	19	2.0	200	2.0	1200	1200	350	10	15	150	70
25–50	79	174	176	70	63	1000	5	10	80	60	1.5	1.7	19	2.0	200	2.0	800	800	350	10	15	150	70
51+	77	170	173	68	63	1000	5	10	80	60	1.2	1.4	15	2.0	200	2.0	800	800	350	10	15	150	70

National Research Council Recommended Dietary Allowances—continued

Age (years) or condition	Weight[b] (kg)	Weight[b] (lb)	Height[b] (cm)	Height[b] (in.)	Protein (g)	Fat-soluble vitamins				Water-soluble vitamins								Minerals						
						Vitamin A (µg R.E.)[c]	Vitamin D (µg)[d]	Vitamin E (mg α-T.E.)[e]	Vitamin K (µg)	Vitamin C (mg)	Thiamin (mg)	Riboflavin (mg)	Niacin (mg N.E.)[f]	Vitamin B6 (mg)	Folate (µg)	Vitamin B12 (µg)	Calcium (mg)	Phosphorus (mg)	Magnesium (mg)	Iron (mg)	Zinc (mg)	Iodine (µg)	Selenium (µg)
Females																							
11–14	46	101	157	62	46	800	10	8	45	50	1.1	1.3	15	1.4	150	2.0	1200	1200	280	15	12	150	45
15–18	55	120	163	64	44	800	10	8	55	60	1.1	1.3	15	1.5	180	2.0	1200	1200	300	15	12	150	50
19–24	58	128	164	65	46	800	10	8	60	60	1.1	1.3	15	1.6	180	2.0	1200	1200	280	15	12	150	55
25–50	63	138	163	64	50	800	5	8	65	60	1.1	1.3	15	1.6	180	2.0	800	800	280	15	12	150	55
51+	65	143	160	63	50	800	5	8	65	60	1.0	1.2	13	1.6	180	2.0	800	800	280	10	12	150	55
Pregnant					60	800	10	10	65	70	1.5	1.6	17	2.2	400	2.2	1200	1200	320	30	15	175	65
Lactating 1st 6 months					65	1300	10	12	65	95	1.6	1.8	20	2.1	280	2.6	1200	1200	355	15	19	200	75
2nd 6 months					62	1200	10	11	65	90	1.6	1.7	20	2.1	260	2.6	1200	1200	340	15	16	200	75

[a]The allowances, expressed as average daily intakes over time, are intended to provide for individual variations among most normal persons as they live in the United States under usual environmental stresses. Diets should be based on a variety of common foods in order to provide other nutrients for which human requirements have been less well defined. See text for detailed discussion of allowances and of nutrients not tabulated.

[b]Weights and heights of reference adults are actual medians for the U.S. population of the designated age, as reported by NHANES II. The median weights and heights of those under 19 years of age were taken from Hamill et al. (1979). The use of these figures does not imply that the height to weight ratios are ideal.

[c]Retinol equivalents. 1 retinol equivalent = 1 µg retinol or 6 µg β-carotene. See text for calculation of vitamin A activity of diets as retinol equivalents.

[d]As cholecalciferol, 10 µg cholecalciferol = 400 I.U. of vitamin D.

[e]α-Tocopherol equivalents. 1 mg d-α tocopherol = 1 α-T.E.

[f]1 N.E. (niacin equivalent) is equal to 1 mg of niacin or 60 mg of dietary tryptophan.

*Reprinted with permission from Recommended Dietary Allowances, 10th Edition. © 1989 by the National Academy of Sciences. Published by National Academy Press, USA.

Estimated sodium, chloride, and potassium minimum requirements of healthy persons[a]

Age	Weight (kg)[a]	Sodium (mg)[ab]	Chloride (mg)[ab]	Potassium (mg)[c]
Months				
0–5	4.5	120	180	500
6–11	8.9	200	300	700
Years				
1	11.0	225	350	1000
2–5	16.0	300	500	1400
6–9	25.0	400	600	1600
10–18	50.0	500	750	2000
>18[d]	70.0	500	750	2000

[a]No allowance has been included for large, prolonged losses from the skin through sweat.

[b]There is no evidence that higher intakes confer any health benefit.

[c]Desirable intakes of potassium may considerably exceed these values (3500 mg for adults).

[d]No allowance included for growth. Values for those below 18 years assume a growth rate at the 50th percentile reported by the National Center for Health Statistics (Hamill et al., 1979) and averaged for males and females.

Reprinted with permission from Recommended Dietary Allowances, 10th Edition. © 1989 by the National Academy of Sciences. Published by National Academy Press, USA.

Appendix 2: Reference Nutrient Intakes (RNIs) per day for selected nutrients

	Protein (g)	Vit. B_1 (mg)	Vit. B_2 (mg)	Niacin (mg)	Vit. B_6 (mg)	Vit. B_{12} (mg)	Folate (mg)	Vit. C (mg)	Vit. A (mcg)	Calcium (mg)	Iron (mg)	Zinc (mg)
Males												
1–3 years	14.5	0.5	0.6	8	0.7	0.5	70	30	400	350	6.9	5.0
4–6 years	19.7	0.7	0.8	11	0.9	0.8	100	30	500	450	6.1	6.5
7–10 years	28.3	0.7	1.0	12	1.0	1.0	150	30	500	550	8.7	7.0
11–14 years	42.1	0.9	1.2	15	1.2	1.2	200	35	600	1000	11.3	9.0
15–18 years	55.2	1.1	1.3	18	1.5	1.5	200	40	700	1000	11.3	9.5
19–50 years	55.5	1.0	1.3	17	1.4	1.5	200	40	700	700	8.7	9.5
50+ years	53.3	0.9	1.3	16	1.4	1.5	200	40	700	700	8.7	9.5
Females												
1–3 years	14.5	0.5	0.6	8	0.7	0.5	70	30	400	350	6.9	5.0
4–6 years	19.7	0.7	0.8	11	0.9	0.8	100	30	500	450	6.1	6.5
7–10 years	28.3	0.7	1.0	12	1.0	1.0	150	30	500	550	8.7	7.0
11–14 years	41.2	0.7	1.1	12	1.0	1.2	200	35	600	800	14.8**	9.0
15–18 years	45.0	0.8	1.1	14	1.2	1.5	200	40	600	800	14.8**	7.0
19–50 years	45.0	0.8	1.1	13	1.2	1.5	200	40	600	700	14.8**	7.0
50+ years	46.5	0.8	1.1	12	1.2	1.5	200	40	600	700	8.7	7.0
Pregnancy	+6	+0.1*	+0.3	–	–	–	+100	+10	+100	–	–	–
Lactation												
0–4 months	+11	+0.2	+0.5	+2	–	+0.5	+60	+30	+350	+550	–	+6.0
4+ months	+8	+0.2	+0.5	+2	–	+0.5	+60	+30	+350	+550	–	+2.5

– no increase

* last trimester only

** insufficient for women with high menstrual losses

From: (1990) *Dietary reference values for food energy and nutrients for the United Kingdom.* HMSO, London. Reproduced with the permission of the Controller, HMSO.

Appendix 3: Composition of selected foods

Each value is the amount per 100 g of the edible part of the food described.

Food	Inedible waste (%)	Water (g)	Energy (kJ)	Energy (kcal)	Protein (g)	Total fat (g)	Saturated (g)	Carbohydrate (g)	Total sugar (g)	Fibre NSP (\g)	Calcium (mg)	Iron (mg)	Sodium (mg)	Vitamin A (µg)	Thiamin (mg)	Vitamin C (mg)
Almonds, flesh only	63	4.2	2534	612	21.1	55.8	4.7	6.9	4.2	7.4	240	3	14	0	0.21	0
Apples, eating, raw	11	84.5	199	47	0.4	0.1	11.8	11.8	11.8	1.8	4	0.1	3	3	0.03	6
Avocado	29	72.5	784	190	1.9	19.5	4.1	1.9	0.5	3.4	11	0.4	6	3	0.1	6
Bananas	34	75.1	403	95	1.2	0.3	0.1	23.2	20.9	1.1	6	0.3	1	3	0.04	11
Beans, baked	0	71.5	355	84	5.2	0.6	0.1	2.2	2	2	10	1.4	2	12	0.02	4
Beef, minced, stewed	0	59.1	955	229	23.1	15.2	6.5	0	0	0	18	3.1	320	0	0.05	0
Beefburgers, frozen, fried	0	53	1099	264	20.4	17.3	8	7	1.4	ND	33	3.1	880	0	0.02	0
Beer, bitter, keg	0	93.5	129	31	0.3	0	0	2.3	2.3	0	8	0.01	8	0	0	0
Bolognese sauce	0	74.7	602	145	8	11.1	3.1	3.7	3.3	1	23	1.4	430	213	0.07	4
Brie	0	48.6	1323	319	19.3	26.9	16.8	0	0	0	540	0.8	700	320	0.04	0
Butter	0	15.6	3031	737	0.5	81.7	54	0	0	0	15	0.2	750	887	0	0
Cabbage, raw	23	90.1	109	26	1.7	0.4	0.1	4.1	4	2.4	52	0.7	5	64	0.15	49
Celery, raw	9	95.1	32	7	0.5	0.2	0	0.9	0.9	1.1	41	0.4	60	8	0.06	8
Cheddar	0	36	1708	412	25.5	34.4	21.7	0.1	0.1	0	720	0.3	670	363	0.03	0
Chocolate biscuits	0	2.2	2197	524	5.7	27.6	16.7	67.4	43.4	2.1	110	1.7	160	0	0.03	0

Food	Inedible waste (%)	Water (g)	Energy (kJ)	Energy (kcal)	Protein (g)	Total fat (g)	Saturated (g)	Carbohydrate (g)	Total sugar (g)	Fibre NSP (\g)	Calcium (mg)	Iron (mg)	Sodium (mg)	Vitamin A (µg)	Thiamin (mg)	Vitamin C (mg)
Chocolate, milk	0	2.2	2214	529	8.4	30.3	17.8	59.4	56.5	0	220	1.6	120	7	0.1	0
Coca-cola	0	89.8	168	39	0	0	0	10.5	10.5	0	4	0	8	0		0
Coconut, dessicated	0	2.3	2492	604	5.6	62	53.4	6.4	6.4	13.7	23	3.6	28	0	0.03	0
Coffee, infusion	0	ND	8	2	0.2	0	0	0.3	0.3	0	2	0	0	ND	0	0
Coffee, instant	0	3.4	424	200	14.6	0	0	11	6.5	0	160	4.4	41	ND	0	0
Corn flakes	0	3	1535	360	7.9	0.7	0.1	85.9	8.2	0.9	15	6.7	1110	0	1	0
Cream crackers	0	4.3	1857	440	9.5	16.3	ND	68.8	0	2.2	110	1.7	610	0	0.23	0
Cream, fresh, single	0	73.7	817	198	2.6	19.1	11.9	4.1	4.1	0	91	0.1	490	336	0.04	1
Cucumber	3	96.4	40	10	0.7	0.1	0	1.5	1.4	0.6	18	0.3	3	10	0.03	2
Currant buns	0	27.7	1250	296	7.6	7.5	ND	52.7	15.1	ND	110	1.9	230	ND	0.37	0
Digestive biscuits	0	2.5	1978	471	6.3	20.9	8.6	68.6	13.6	2.2	92	3.2	600	0	0.14	0
Eggs, chicken, boiled	0	75.1	612	147	12.5	10.8	3.1	0	0	0	57	1.9	140	190	0.07	0
Fish fingers, grilled	0	56.2	899	214	15.1	9	2.8	19.3	0	0.7	52	0.8	380	0	0.1	0
Flour, plain, white	0	14	1450	341	9.4	1.3	0.2	77.7	1.5	3.1	140	2	3	0	0.31	0
Fromage frais, fruit	0	71.9	551	131	6.8	5.8	3.6	13.8	13.8	0	86	0.1	35	ND	0.02	0
Fruit cake, rich	0	17.6	1438	341	3.8	11	3.4	59.6	48.4	1.7	82	1.9	200	125	0.08	0
Fruit crumble	0	54.8	835	198	2	6.9	2.1	34	21.3	1.7	49	0.6	68	88	0.05	3
Grapefruit, raw	32	89	126	30	0.8	0.1	0	6.8	6.8	1.3	23	0.1	3	3	0.05	36
Grapes, seedless	5	81.8	257	60	0.4	0.1	0	15.4	15.4	0.7	13	0.3	2	3	0.05	3
Haddock, steamed	24	75.1	417	98	22.8	0.8	0.2	0	0	0	55	0.7	120	0	0.8	0
Honey	0	23	1229	288	0.4	0	0	76.4	76.4	0	5	0.4	11	0	0	0
Kiwi fruit, no skin	14	84	207	49	1.1	0.5	ND	10.6	10.3	1.9	25	0.4	4	6	0.01	59
Lager, bottled	0	94.9	120	29	0.2	0	0	1.5	1.5	0	4	0	4		0	0
Low-fat spread	0	49.9	1605	390	5.8	40.5	11.2	0.5	0.5	0	39	0	650	501	0	0
Mackeral fried	0	65.5	828	199	20.4	13	3.7	0	0	0	33	1.2	170	34	0	0

Margarine, polyunsaturated	0	16	3039	739	0.2	81.6	16.2	1	1	0	4	0.3	800	946	0	0
Marmite	0	25.4	730	172	39.7	0.7	ND	1.8	0	0	95	3.7	4500	0	3.1	0
Muesli, Swiss style	0	7.2	1540	363	9.8	5.9	0.8	72.2	26.2	6.4	110	5.8	380	0	0.5	0
Mushrooms, raw	3	92.6	55	13	1.8	0.5	0.1	0.4	0.2	1.1	6	0.6	5	0	0.09	1
Mycoprotein, Quorn	0	75	360	86	11.8	3.5	0.6	2	1.1	4.8	ND	ND	240	0	36.6	0
Onions, raw	9	89	150	36	1.2	0.2	0	7.9	5.6	1.4	25	0.3	3	2	0.13	5
Orange juice	0	89.2	153	36	0.5	0.1	0	8.8	8.8	0.1	10	0.2	10	3	0.08	39
Oranges, no seeds	30	86.1	158	37	1.1	0.1	0	8.5	8.5	1.7	47	0.1	5	5	0.11	54
Pate, liver	0	50.6	1308	316	13.1	28.9	8.4	1	0.3	0	15	7.1	790	7352	0.13	ND
Peppers, green, raw	16	93.3	65	15	0.8	0.3	0.1	2.6	2.4	1.6	8	0.4	4	44	0.01	120
Potato crisps	0	1.9	2275	546	5.6	37.6	9.2	49.3	0.7	4.9	37	1.8	1070	0	0.11	27
Potatoes, old, baked inc. skin	0	62.6	581	136	3.9	0.2	0	31.7	1.2	2.7	11	0.7	12	0	0.37	14
Potatoes, old, boiled, no salt	0	80.3	306	72	1.8	0.1	0	17	0.7	1.2	5	0.4	7	0	0.18	6
Potatoes, old, roast	0	64.7	630	149	2.9	4.5	0.4	25.9	0.6	1.8	8	0.7	9	0	0.23	8
Prawns, boiled	0	70	451	107	22.6	1.8	0.4	0	0	0	150	1.1	1590	0	0.02	0
Prunes, ready to eat	0	31.1	601	141	2.5	0.4	ND	34	34	5.7	34	2.6	11	23	0.09	0
Rice, brown, boiled	0	66	597	141	2.6	1.1	0.3	32.1	0.5	0.8	4	1	1	0	0.14	0
Salami	0	28	2031	491	19.3	45.2	ND	1.9	0	0.1	10	1	1850	0	0.21	ND
Semi-skimmed milk	0	89.8	195	46	3.3	1.6	1	5	5	0	120	0.05	55	23	0.04	1
Soy sauce	0	67.6	266	64	8.7	0	0	8.3	ND	0	19	2.7	5720	0	0.05	0
Spirits, 40% volume	0	63.3	919	222	0	0	0	0	0	0	0	0	0	0	0	0
Strawberries, raw	5	89.5	113	27	0.8	0.1	0	6	6	1.1	16	0.4	6	1	0.03	77
Sugar, white	0	0	1680	394	0	0	0	105	105	0	2	0	0	0	0	0
Sunflower seed oil	0	0	3696	899	0	99.9	11.9	0	0	0	0	0	0	0	0	0
Tea, Indian, infusion	0	ND	2	0	0.1	0	0	0	0	0	0	0	0	0	0	0

Food	Inedible waste (%)	Water (g)	Energy (kJ)	Energy (kcal)	Protein (g)	Total fat (g)	Saturated (g)	Carbohydrate (g)	Total sugar (g)	Fibre NSP (\g)	Calcium (mg)	Iron (mg)	Sodium (mg)	Vitamin A (µg)	Thiamin (mg)	Vitamin C (mg)
Tofu, steamed	0	85	304	73	8.1	4.2	0.5	0.7	0.3	ND	510	1.2	4	0	0.06	0
Tomatoes, raw	0	93.1	73	17	0.7	0.3	0.1	3.1	3.1	1	7	0.5	9	105	0.09	17
Tomato ketchup	0	64.8	420	98	2.1	0	0	24	22.9	0.9	25	1.2	1120	38	1	2
Trifle	0	67.2	674	160	3.6	6.3	3.1	22.3	16.8	0.5	79	0.5	53	75	0.06	4
Turkey roast inc. skin	0	65	717	171	28	6.5	2.1	0	0	0	9	0.9	52	ND	ND	0
Watercress	38	92.5	94	22	3	1	0.3	0.4	0.4	1.5	170	2.2	49	420	0.16	62
Weetabix	0	5.6	1498	352	11	2.7	0.4	75.7	5.2	9.7	35	7.4	270	0	0.9	0
White bread	0	37.3	1002	235	8.4	1.9	0.4	49.3	2.6	1.5	110	1.6	520	0	0.21	0
Wholemeal bread	0	38.3	914	215	9.2	2.5	0.5	41.6	1.8	5.8	54	2.7	550	0	0.34	0
Whole milk	0	87.8	275	66	3.2	3.9	2.4	4.8	4.8	0	115	0.06	55	55	0.03	1
Wine, red	0	88	284	68	0.2	0	0	0.3	0.3	0	7	0.9	10	0	0	0
Wine, white, medium	0	86.3	311	75	0.1	0	0	3.4	3.4	0	4	0.9	10	0	0	0
Yogurt, low fat, fruit	0	77	382	90	4.1	0.7	0.4	17.9	17.9	ND	150	0.1	64	11	0.05	1

Each value is the amount per 100 g of the edible part of the food described. Information based on the 5th edition of McCance. From (1995) *Manual of nutrition*. HMSO, London.

ND–not deformined

Appendix 4:
Ratings for activities and sports

Activity/sport	Stamina	Suppleness	Strength	Weight-control	Injury risk
aerobic dance	good	excellent	fair	good	low
aerobics	good	good	fair	good	low
American football	fair	poor	good	fair	very high
aquarobics	good	good	good	poor	very low
archery	poor	fair	good	poor	very low
badminton	good	good	fair	good	moderate
baseball and softball	fair	fair	fair	fair	moderate
basketball	excellent	poor	fair	good	high
body building	poor	good	excellent	good	moderate
bowling	poor	poor	poor	poor	very low
boxercise	good	fair	good	good	low
boxing	fair	fair	good	good	very high
bungee jumping	poor	poor	poor	poor	high
calisthenics	good	good	good	good	low
canoeing and kayaking	good	fair	good	fair	moderate
circuit training	good	good	good	good	moderate
climbing	good	good	good	fair	high
cricket	poor	fair	poor	poor	moderate
cross-country skiing	excellent	poor	fair	excellent	low
cycling (hard)	excellent	poor	fair	good	low
dance	fair	fair	poor	fair	very low
fencing	fair	fair	fair	fair	moderate
golf	fair	fair	poor	fair	moderate
gymnastics	fair	excellent	excellent	good	high
hockey	good	fair	fair	fair	moderate
horse-riding	poor	fair	fair	poor	moderate
ice hockey	good	fair	fair	good	very high
jogging	excellent	poor	fair	good	high on roads
martial arts	poor	good	good	fair	high
medau	good	good	poor	good	low
netball	good	fair	poor	fair	low
orienteering	excellent	fair	fair	good	low
rope jumping	good	good	poor	good	low
rowing	excellent	fair	good	good	low
rugby	good	fair	good	fair	very high

Activity/sport	Stamina	Suppleness	Strength	Weight-control	Injury risk
SCUBA diving	fair	fair	fair	poor	high
skiing, downhill	poor	poor	fair	poor	high
slide training	good	fair	low	good	moderate
soccer	good	fair	fair	good	moderate
squash	good	good	fair	fair	high
step aerobics	good	good	poor	good	moderate
swimming	excellent	excellent	excellent	fair	low
tai chi	poor	excellent	fair	poor	very low
tennis	good	fair	fair	fair	moderate
volleyball	fair	fair	fair	fair	moderate
walking (brisk)	excellent	fair	poor	excellent	low
weight training	poor	fair	excellent	fair	moderate
yoga	fair	excellent	fair	fair	very low

The benefits acquired from each activity will depend on the skill and intensity of performance.

Appendix 5:
Average energy expenditure of various activities and sports

Activity/sport	Energy expenditure in kilocalories per hour according to body mass.				
	50 kg	60 kg	70 kg	80 kg	90 kg
aerobic dance	270	310	350	380	420
aerobics	260	300	340	370	410
American football	240	270	305	340	370
aquarobics	235	290	310	360	400
archery	190	220	250	270	300
badminton	270	310	350	385	420
baseball and softball	220	250	285	315	350
basketball (half court)	240	270	305	340	370
basketball (competition)	480	545	610	670	740
body building	375	427	480	530	585
bowling	215	230	275	305	335
boxercise	260	310	340	370	410
boxing (sparring)	190	220	250	270	300
calisthenics	190	220	250	270	300
canoeing and kayaking (4 mph)	240	270	350	385	420
circuit training	263	300	335	375	410
climbing (mountain)	480	545	610	680	745
cricket (fielding)	240	270	350	385	420
cross-country skiing	560	635	715	790	870
cycling (moderate speed)	165	190	214	240	260
dance (social)	223	255	285	315	350
fencing	240	270	305	340	370
golf (walking with bag)	200	230	255	280	310
gymnastics	255	280	315	350	380
hockey	430	490	550	610	670
horse-riding	190	220	250	270	300
ice hockey	280	270	355	395	435
jogging (9km/h)	520	590	660	735	806
martial arts	250	280	315	350	385
netball	250	290	325	360	395
orienteering	520	590	660	735	806
rope jumping (continuous)	560	635	715	790	870
rowing (recreational)	190	220	250	270	300
rugby	430	490	550	610	670
running (16 km/h)	719	820	920	1016	1116

Activity/sport	Energy expenditure in kilocalories per hour according to body mass.				
	50 kg	60 kg	70 kg	80 kg	90 kg
skiing (downhill)	480	545	610	680	745
soccer	430	490	550	610	670
squash	480	545	610	680	745
swimming (laps)	255	290	326	361	395
tennis	335	380	430	475	520
volleyball	280	270	355	395	435
walking (brisk)	240	280	315	350	385
weight training	375	427	480	530	585

Energy expenditure will depend on the skill of the performer, the intensity of the activity, the weather, and so on.

Appendix 6: Benefits of exercises

For details, see text.

Exercise	Flexibility	Strength	Upper body	Lower body	Apparatus needed
abdominal contraction		■	■		none
abdominal hold		■	■		none
abductor raise		■		■	none
Achilles stretch	■			■	none
adductor stretch	■	■		■	none
ankle stretchers	■			■	none
arm curl		■	■		weights
arm lifts	■	■	■		none
arm sprints		■	■		bench
arm stretch	■		■		none
back and leg stretch	■			■	none
back extension	■	■			bench/table
back scratcher stretch	■		■		none
bench blasts		■		■	bench
bench press		■	■		weights
bent arm pullover		■	■		weights
bent over row		■	■	■	weights
biceps curl		■	■		weights
Billig's exercise	■			■	doorway
calf raise	■	■		■	wood block
cat stretch	■		■	■	none
chest stretch	■		■		none
chin-up		■	■		bar
chinnies		■		■	none
chinning		■	■		bar
curl-up		■	■		none
dead-lift		■	■	■	weights
dips		■	■		chairs/bars
dumbbell curls		■	■		weights
dumbbell punch		■	■		weights
Eastern prayer	■		■	■	none
foetal stretch	■		■	■	none
gluteal lift	■	■	■	■	none
half-squats		■		■	none
hamstring stretcher	■			■	none

Exercise	Flexibility	Strength	Upper body	Lower body	Apparatus needed
heel raise	■	■		■	wood block
hip stretch	■			■	none
hug	■		■		none
hurdle stretch	■			■	none
iliopsoas stretcher	■			■	none
jumping jack	■	■	■	■	none
knee raises	■			■	none
kneeling kickback	■	■		■	none
lateral arm raise		■	■		weights
lateral pull-down		■	■		weights
leg curl		■		■	weights
leg extension		■		■	weights
leg lift		■	■		none
leg presses	■	■		■	none
leg raises	■	■	■	■	bar
low back stretcher	■		■		none
lower leg lift		■		■	none
lunges	■	■		■	none
military press		■	■		weights
neck extension exercise	■	■	■		none
neck flexion	■	■	■		none
neck flexion & extension		■	■		weights
neck rotation	■	■	■		none
neck shrugging	■		■		none
neck stretches	■		■		none
Nieder press		■	■		weights
pectoral stretch	■	■	■		doorway
pelvic floor lift	■	■		■	none
pelvic tilt	■	■	■		none
power clean		■	■	■	weights
preacher curls		■	■		weights
press		■	■		weights
press-up		■	■		none
pull-up		■	■		bar
push-up		■	■		none
quad stretch	■			■	none
recumbent leg press		■		■	weights
shin stretcher	■			■	none
shoulder lifts	■	■	■		none
shoulder shrugs		■	■		weights

Exercise	Flexibility	Strength	Upper body	Lower body	Apparatus needed
side bends	■		■		none
side leg raises		■		■	none
side twist	■		■		none
sitting tucks		■	■	■	none
sit-up	■	■	■		none
ski jump	■	■	■	■	none
squat		■		■	none
squat thrust	■	■		■	none
star jumps	■	■	■	■	none
stationary leg change	■	■		■	none
stomach curl		■	■		none
stretch-and-curl	■		■	■	none
stride jumps	■	■		■	none
stride stretch	■			■	none
total body stretch	■		■	■	none
triceps extension		■	■		weights
trunk lifts	■	■	■		table
trunk rotation		■	■		none
trunk stretcher	■		■		none
trunk twists	■		■		none
twister	■		■		none
upright rowing		■	■		weights
windmills	■		■		none
wrestler's bridge	■	■	■		none
wrist curl		■	■		weights

Thematic Index

Themes

Diet

- Diets and dietary regimes
- Drinks and food ingredients
- Diet-related disorders

Exercise

- Sports and activities
- Exercises: stretches and strengtheners
- Training methods and equipment
- Fitness and exercise physiology
- Exercise-related injuries
- Sports injury treatments

Diet and Exercise

- Body structures and movements
- Disorders and diseases
- Drugs and chemicals
- Other topics

Entries

Diet

Diets and dietary regimes
absorption
adiposis *See* liposis.
adipostat
Air Force diet *See* ketogenic diet.
appestat
appetite suppressant
appetite
aromatherapy
Atkins diet
Atwater factor
balanced diet
BBC diet
beta-oxidation
Beverly Hills diet
body wraps
breakfast
breast-feeding
calorie counting
Cambridge diet
carbohydrate addict's diet
carbohydrate loading
carboloading *See* carbohydrate loading.
colonic fermentation
Columbus Nutrition Plan
combining diets *See* food combining diets.
comfort eating
crash diet
detox diets *See* detoxication.
detoxication
detoxification
 See detoxication.
diet
diet induced thermogenesis
digestion
digestive juices
Doctor's Quick Weight Loss Diet: *See* high protein diet.
duodenum
eating diary
elastic belt
elimination diet
emulsification

enteric bacteria *See* gut bacteria.
enzyme
Eskimo diet
fad diet
faeces
fasting
fat blockers
fat loading
fat mobilization
Feingold diet
fermentation
food combining diets
food diary *See* eating diary.
food transit time
foodie
F-plan diet
fruitarian
grapefruit pills
grazing
gut bacteria
high protein diet
hip and thigh diet *See* spot theory of fat reduction.
inflatable belt *See* elastic belt.
Italian football diet
ketogenic diet
ketone bodies *See* ketogenic diet.
ketosis *See* ketogenic diet.
lacto-ovo vegetarian diet
laxative
lipolysis
liposis
liposuction
liposurgery
liquid protein diet
low carbohydrate diet
low-density lipoprotein *See* lipoproteins.
low fat diet
macrobiotic diet
magic formula
making weight
mammaplasty
meal replacement diet
Mediterranean diet
mud treatment *See* body wraps.
muscle glycogen loading *See* carbohydrate loading.
Nutron diet
one food diets
plastic surgery
pre-activity meal *See* pre-competition meal.
pre-competition meal
Pritikin diet
protein-sparing modified fast
PSMF *See* protein sparing modified fast.

purging
reconstructive surgery *See* plastic surgery.
Revolutionary Three in One Diet *See* aromatherapy.
rotation diet
rubber suit
sauna suit *See* rubber suit.
Scarsdale diet
self-starvation syndrome *See* anorexia nervosa.
semi-vegetarian
set point theory
skin patches *See* slimming patch.
slimming patch
slimming pills
spot-reducing *See* spot theory of fat reduction.
spot theory of fat reduction
starvation
stomach stapling
supercompensation *See* carbohydrate loading.
thermic effect of food *See* diet induced thermogenesis.
time of meals
vegan
vegetarian
very low calorie diet
weight-gain diet
weight-loss maintenance
yang *See* macrobiotic diet.
ying *See* macrobiotic diet.
Yo-Yo diet
Zen macrobiotic diet
zero fat diet

Drinks and food ingredients
acesulfame-K
additive *See* food additive
aflatoxins
alanine
alcohol
amino acids
amino acid supplements
amygdalin *See* laetrile.
animal starch *See* glycogen.
antihaemorrhagic vitamin *See* vitamin K.
antinutrients
antioxidant
anti-rachitic factor *See* vitamin D.
anti-sterility factor *See* vitamin E.
arginine
arsenic
artificial colours
artificial fats

artificial flavours
artificial sweeteners
ascorbic acid
aspartame
aspartates
aspartic acid *See* aspartates.
avidin *See* biotin.
azo dyes
B complex
BCAA *See* branched-chain amino acids
bee pollen
beta-carotene
BHA
BHT *See* butylated hydroxyanisole.
biotin
boron
branched-chain amino acids
bromelain
bulk *See* fibre.
bulking agents
calciferol *See* vitamin D.
calcium
carbohydrates
carnitine
carotenes
cellulose
cholecalciferol *See* vitamin D.
cholesterol
chromium
cis *See* unsaturated fat
cobalamin *See* vitamin B$_{12}$.
cobalt
coenzyme Q
coffee *See* caffeine.
complete protein
complex carbohydrate
copper
creatine
cyanocobalamin *See* vitamin B$_{12}$.
cyclamate
Daily Values
designer foods
dextrin
dextrose
diastase
dietary exchange lists
dietary fibre
Dietary Reference Values
dimethylglycine *See* methyl donors.
dimethylnitrosamine *See* nitrosamines.
disaccharide
DMG *See* methyl donors.
double sugar *See* disaccharide.
eicosapentaenoic acid
electrolyte drink

empty calories
emulsifiers
encephalins *See* endorphins.
endotoxin
energy drink
energy nutrient
enriched foods
E-numbers *See* food additives.
EPA *See* eicosapentaenoic acid.
ergocalciferol *See* vitamin D.
essential amino acid
essential fat
essential fatty acid
Estimated Average Requirement *See* Dietary Reference Values.
exotoxin
fast foods
fat
fat-soluble vitamins
fatty acids
fermented foods
fertility vitamin *See* vitamin E.
fibre
fibre supplements
fish-oil supplements
flavour enhancers
fluoride *See* fluorine.
fluorine
folacin *See* folic acid.
folic acid
food additives
food exchange system *See* dietary exchange lists.
food group
food guide pyramid
food labelling
formula diet
fortified foods
free fatty acid *See* fatty acid.
free radicals
fructose
galactose
gamma-aminobutyric acid
gammalinolenic acid
garlic
gelatin *See* collagen.
ginseng
GLA *See* gamma-linolenic acid.
gliadins *See* gluten.
glucose
glucose polymers
glutamate *See* glutamic acid.
glutamic acid
glutathione
glutathione peroxidase *See* glutathione.
gluten
glutenin *See* gluten.
glycaemic index

glycerol
glycine
guar gum
haem iron
hexose
hidden fat
histidine
hydrogenation
hypertonic drink *See* electrolyte drink.
hypotonic drink *See* electrolyte drink.
incomplete proteins
inosine monophosphate
inositol
insoluble fibre *See* fibre.
insulin
intrinsic factor
iodine
iodized salt *See* table salt.
iron
isoleucine
isotonic drink *See* electrolyte drink.
junk food
kelp
lactose
laetrile
lecithin
lectins
lentils
linoleic acid
lipid
lysine
macromineral
macronutrient
magnesium
maltose
manganese
medium chain triglycerides *See* fatigue.
megadoses
megavitamin
methionine
methyl donors
micromineral *See* mineral.
milk sugar *See* lactose.
minerals
mixers *See* emulsifiers.
molybdenum
monosaccharide
monosodium glutamate.
monounsaturated fat
MSG *See* monosodium glutamate
mumie
muscle triglyceride
mycoprotein
negative calories
neutral fat *See* fat.
niacin

nicotinamide *See* niacin.
nicotine
nicotinic acid *See* niacin.
nitrates
nitrites *See* nitrates.
nitrosamine
non-haem iron
non-starch polysaccharide
nutrient
nutrient density
octacosanol
omega-3 fatty acids
organic food
orotic acid
oxalic acid
PABA
pangamic acid
pantothenic acid
para-aminobenzoic acid *See* PABA.
pectin
pH control agents
phenylalanine
phenylbutazone
phosphatidylcholine *See* lecithin.
phosphorus
phytic acid
polyunsaturated fat
polyunsaturates *See* polyunsaturated fat.
potassium
PPA *See* phenylpropanolamine.
preservatives
protective protein theory
protein supplement
protein efficiency ratio
protein
P/S
pteroyl-L-glutamic acid *See* folic acid.
pyridoxine *See* vitamin B_6.
Quorn *See* mycoprotein.
RDA *See* Recommended Dietary Allowance.
Recommended Daily Amounts *See* Recommended Dietary Allowance.
Recommended Daily Intake *See* Recommended Dietary Allowance.
Recommended Dietary Allowance
recommended dietary goal
Reference Nutrient Intake *See* Dietary Reference Values.
replacement drink
resistant starch
retinol *See* vitamin A.
riboflavin *See* vitamin B_2.

saccharin
Safe Intake *See* Dietary
    Reference Values.
salicylates
salicylic acid *See* salicylates.
salt
salt replacement
salt substitute
salt tablet
saponins
saturated fat
selenium
simple carbohydrate
snack
sodium
sodium bicarbonate
solanine
soluble fibre *See* fibre.
spreads
starch blockers
starch gum *See* dextrin.
starch sugar *See* dextrin.
starch
sucrose
sugar
sugar fix
sugar-free food
sulphites
sulphur
sulphur dioxide *See* sulphites.
supplements
table salt
tannins
texturizers
thiamin *See* vitamin B_1.
threonine
TMG *See* methyl donors.
tocopherol *See* vitamin E.
trace element
trans fat *See* unsaturated fat.
trimethylglycine *See* methyl
    donors.
tryptophan
tyramine
tyrosine
United States Recommended
    Daily Allowance
unsaturated fat
US RDA *See* United States
    Recommended Daily
    Allowance.
valine
vanadium
vitamin
vitamin A
vitamin B complex
vitamin B_1
vitamin B_2
vitamin B_5 *See* pantothenic
    acid.
vitamin B_3 *See* niacin.

vitamin B_{12}
vitamin B_{15} *See* pangamic acid.
vitamin B_{17} *See* laetrile.
vitamin C
vitamin D
vitamin E
vitamin F *See* linoleic acid.
vitamin K
vitamin supplementation
water replacement
water
water retention *See* fluid
    retention.
water balance
xanthines
xylitol
xylose
zinc

Diet-related disorders

activity-induced anorexia
    See anorexia.
anal fissure
anal itching
anaphylactic shock
anaphylaxis
anorexia *See* anorexia nervosa.
anorexia nervosa
appendicitis *See* appendix.
banded gastroplasty
beriberi
binge eating
binge–purge syndrome
    See bulimia nervosa.
blue baby syndrome
    See nitrates.
botulism
bovine spongiform
    encephalopathy
breast reduction
    See mammaplasty.
BSE *See* bovine spongiform
    encephalopathy.
bulimia nervosa
caffeinism
campylobacteriosis
candida
candidiasis *See* candida.
cellulite
Chinese restaurant syndrome
chocoholic
coeliac disease
compulsive overeating
constipation
cosmetic surgery
Creutzfeldt-Jakob disease
Crohn's disease
cytotoxic testing
dental caries *See* tooth decay.
diarrhoea
digestive disorders

diverticulitis
diverticulosis
dysentery
dyspepsia *See* indigestion.
eating disorder
eating disorder not otherwise
    specified
fat malabsorption
flatulence
fluid retention
food allergy *See* allergy.
food aversion
food intolerance
food poisoning
gall bladder
gallstones
gastric balloons
gastritis
gastroenteritis
glucose tolerance test
gluten intolerance *See* coeliac
    disease.
glycosuria
gout
gut *See* alimentary canal.
hunger
hydrolipodystrophy
    See cellulite.
hyperglycaemia
hypervitaminosis
hypoglycaemia
indigestion
insulin rebound
irritable bowel syndrome
jaw wiring
kwashiorkor
lactase *See* lactose.
lactose intolerance
    See lactose.
listeria
listeriosis *See* listeria.
malabsorption
malnutrition
marasmus
meal tolerance test
mesotherapy *See* cellulite.
NOS *See* eating disorder not
    otherwise specified.
obesity
obesity gene
overweight
pancreas
pancreatitis *See* pancreas.
parahaemolyticus food
    poisoning
pellagra
peptic ulcer
pica
proteinuria
pseudo-allergy *See* food
    intolerance.

rebound hypoglycaemia
See insulin rebound.
rickets
salicylism See salicylates.
salmonellosis
salt depletion
scurvy
shigellosis
sprue See coeliac disease.
staphylococcal food poisoning
stomach ulcer See peptic ulcer.
sugar malabsorption
tooth decay
toxicity
traveller's diarrhoea
ulcer See peptic ulcer.
undereating
underweight
vitamin deficiency disease
water intoxication
wind See flatulence.
xerophthalmia

Exercise

Sports and activities

adapted physical exercise
aerobic dance See dance.
aerobic exercise
aerobic points
aerobics
aerobox See boxercise.
American football
anaerobic exercise
aquarobics
aqua running See aquarobics.
archery
athletics
badminton
balanced exercise programme
baseball and softball
basketball
body building
bowling
bowls See bowling.
boxercise
boxing
bungee jumpingcalisthenics
canoeing and kayaking
circuit training
climbing
contact sport
continuous exercise
Cooper points See aerobic
points.
cricket
cross-country skiing See
skiing.

cross-training
cycling.
dance
distance running See jogging.
dropout
fencing
football See American Football
and soccer.
gamesmanship
golf
gymnastics
hockey
horse-riding
ice hockey
International Olympic
Committee
jiu-jitsu See martial arts.
jogging
judo See martial arts.
jumping
karate See martial arts.
kayaking See canoeing and
kayaking.
kung-fu See martial arts.
long-slow distance training
low impact activity
martial arts
medau
netball
orienteering
pattering
physical recreation
play
power sport
rock-climbing See climbing.
Rockport Fitness Walking Test
rope jumping
rowing
Royal Canadian 5BX and XBX
Programs
rugby
SCUBA diving
skiing
slide training
soccer
soft workouts
sport
sporting behaviour
sprint
squash
stage training See circuit
training.
steady state exercise
See aerobic exercise.
step aerobics
swimming
t'ai chi
tae kwon do See martial arts.
tenpin bowling See bowling.
tennis
thinness-demand sport

throwing
volleyball
walking
warm-up
weight training
yoga
yogacise See yoga.

Exercises: stretches and strengtheners

abdominal contraction
abdominal hold
abductor raise
abnormal quadriceps pull
See Q-angle.
Achilles stretch See Achilles
tendon.
adductor stretch See adductor
muscle.
ankle stretchers
arm curl
arm lift
arm sprints
arm stretch
back and leg stretch
back extension
back scratcher stretch
ballistic stretching
bare foot exercise
bench blasts
bench press
bent arm pullover
bent over row
biceps curl See arm curl.
Billig's exercise
blitz system See body building.
calf raise
cat stretch
chest stretch
chinnies
chinning See chin-up.
chin-up
contraindicated
crunch programme
curl-up
dead-lift
descending sets
dips
dumbbell curls
dumbbell punch
Eastern prayer
ergometer
exercise
foetal stretch
gluteal lift
half-squats
hamstring stretcher
heel raise
hip stretch
hug
hurdle stretch

iliopsoas stretcher
isometrics
jumping jack
knee raises
kneeling kickback
lateral arm raise
lateral pull-down
leg curl
leg extension
leg lift
leg press
leg raise
lifting
   See stretching.
low back stretcher
lower leg lift
lunges
military press
multigym
muscle pumping
   See pumping.
neck extension exercise
neck flexion
neck flexion and extension
neck rotation exercise
neck shrugging
neck stretches
Nieder press
passive exercise
pectoral stretch
pelvic floor exercises
pelvic floor lift
pelvic tilt
Pilates
plyometrics
PMR *See* progressive muscle
   relaxation.
PNF *See* proprioceptive
   neuromuscular facilitation.
power clean
power lifting
pre-exhaustion system
pre-fatigue method
preacher curls
press *See* military press.
press-up
progressive muscle relaxation
progressive resistance exercise
proprioceptive
   neuromuscular facilitation
pull-up *See* chin-up.
pulse raiser
pumping-up
push-up *See* press up.
quad stretch
recumbent leg press *See* fixed-
   weight machine.
resistance exercise
set system
shin stretcher
shoulder lifts
shoulder shrugs

side bends
side leg raises
side twist
sitting tucks
sit-up
ski jump
split routine
squat
squat thrust
standing toe-touch test
star jumps *See* stride jumps.
static stretching
   See stretching.
stationary leg change
step test
stepping-stone test
stick test *See* reaction time.
stomach curl
stretch-and-curl
stretching
stride jumps
stride stretch
super-set system
total body stretch
total hip machine *See* fixed-
   weight machine.
treadmill
triceps extension
trunk lifts
trunk rotation
trunk stretcher
trunk twists
twister
upright rowing
variable resistance exercise
vertical jump test *See* Sargent
   jump test.
windmills
wrestler's bridge
wrist curl

**Training methods and
equipment**
acceleration sprint
active rest
adaptogen
air resistance
altitude
altitude training
anxiety
arousal
arrested progress *See* plateau.
barbell
base training
bench
blood doping
butterfly machine *See* fixed-
   weight machine.
cheating
clo unit
clothing

coach
conditioning
cool down
cycle training
deinhibition training
DIRT
double progressive system
dumbbell
duration of exercise
   See training duration.
dynamometer
ergogenic aid
ergogens *See* ergogenic aid.
exercise band *See* resistance
   exercise.
exercise diary *See* training
   diary.
exercise duration *See* training
   duration.
exercise frequency
   See training frequency.
exercise intensity *See* training
   intensity.
exercise machine
exercise modification
exercise prescription
fartlek training
fixed-weight machine
flushing methods
forced repetitions *See* forced
   reps.
forced reps
free weight
frequency of exercise
   See training frequency.
gloves *See* clothing.
graded exercise test
gripping aids
gumshield
hill training
hollow sprints
hydrafitness *See* omnikinetic
   resistance machine.
imagery relaxation
imaging *See* visualization.
incline bench
incremental run
individual differences
   principle
instructor *See* coach.
intensity of exercise
interval sprinting
interval training
isolation stress
locomotives
macrocycle *See* cycle training.
medicine ball
mental practice
mesocycle *See* cycle training.
microcycle *See* cycle training.
mode of exercise

motivational strategies
See motivation.
multi-poundage system
multi-set system
multi-weight sets
See descending sets.
negative-resistance training
'no pain, no gain'
omnikinetic resistance
machine
overdistance training
overload principle
peaking
pec deck
pep talk
performance plateau
See plateau.
periodization
pressure training
principle of progression
See progression.
programme-setting
progression
pyramid system
Ratzeburg method
recovery
recovery period
repetition maximum
repetitions
repetition training
resistance
rest
rest-pause training
reversibility principle
SAID principle
segmenting
SERP See Sports Emotional-
Reaction Profile.
set
shock exercises
shuttle test
sit-and-reach test
Specific Adaptations to
Imposed Demands
principle See SAID principle.
specific-training principle
speed play See fartlek training.
speed chute
sport psychologist
sports clothes See clothing.
sports medicine
spotter
stepper
strength training
stress inoculation training
tapering down
tempolauf
time-trial
trainability principle
training
training diary

training duration
training effects
training frequency
training heart rate
training impulse
training intensity
training shoe
training threshold
training unit
transfer
transition period
underload principle
versa-ball
visualization
warm down See cool down.
weight belt
weight cycling
weight-training machine
Zatopek phenomenon
See tapering down.
zone of optimal functioning

**Fitness and exercise
physiology**
absolute strength
See strength.
acclimation
See acclimatization.
acclimatization
accommodation principle
adaptation energy
adaptation
adenosine triphosphate
aerobic capacity
aerobic energy system
See aerobic respiration.
aerobic fitness
aerobic power
aerobic respiration
aerobic threshold
aerobic training zone
aerobic work capacity
See aerobic power.
agility
alkalosis See alkali.
altitude acclimatization
anabolism
anaerobic threshold
athlete's heart
athletic pseudonephritis
See proteinuria.
ATP See adenosine
triphosphate.
ATP-PCr system
See phosphagen.
back extension test
balance
benign hypermobility
See hypermobility.
bent arm hang
blind stork test

blood
blood glucose
blood lactate
blood platelets See blood.
blood pressure
body awareness
body fuels
body temperature See core
temperature.
bomb calorimeter
bonking
Borg scale See perceived
exertion.
born athlete See athlete.
bradycardia
breathing
butterflies
caloric balance See energy
balance.
caloric equivalence See heat
equivalence.
calorimetry
Canadian home fitness test
Canadian trunk strength test
cardiac output
cardiorespiratory endurance
See aerobic fitness.
cardiovascular fitness
See aerobic fitness.
carotid pulse See carotid
artery.
carotid sinus See carotid
artery.
citric acid cycle See Krebs
cycle.
comfort index
comfort zone
concentric contraction
See muscle contraction.
conversational index
Cooper twelve-minute test
coordination
core temperature
creatine phosphate
See phosphagen system
detraining effects
diastolic blood pressure
See blood pressure.
dynamic strength
See strength.
dynamogeny
eccentric contraction
See muscle contraction.
ECG See electrocardiogram.
EEG See
electroencephalogram.
elastic strength See strength.
electrocardiogram
electroencephalogram
electrogoniometer
See goniometer.

endurance
energy continuum
energy expenditure
excess postexercise oxygen
consumption *See* oxygen
debt.
exercise adherence
exhaustion *See* general
adaptation syndrome.
expedition-type endurance
fibre splitting *See* muscle
growth.
fitness
flexibility
flow
forced expiratory volume
form
gaseous exchange
glycogen
glycogen overshoot
See carbohydrate loading.
glycolysis
goniometer
GXT
haemoglobin
Harvard step test *See* step test.
health-related fitness
heart rate
heart test
heat acclimatization
heat balance
heat equivalence
hexagon test
homeostasis
hypermobility
hypertension
hyperventilation
iceberg profile *See* Profile of
Mood States.
Illinois agility run *See* agility.
inversion
isokinetic contraction
See muscle contraction.
isometric contraction
See muscle contraction.
isotonic contraction
See muscle contraction.
jump height
kinaesthesis
kinesiology
Krebs cycle
lactate *See* lactic acid.
lactate threshold *See* lactic
acid.
lactic acid
lung volume
maximal heart rate
maximal oxygen
consumption
maximum passive range
See range of movement.

McCutchen's weeping
lubrication theory
MET *See* metabolic equivalent.
metabolic equivalent
metabolism
mobility
muscle contraction
muscle growth
muscle fibre types
muscle strength *See* strength.
myoglobin
negative sit-up test
OBLA *See* lactic acid.
onset of blood lactate
accomolation *See* lactic
acid.
oxygen cost
oxygen debt
oxymyoglobin *See* myoglobin.
PAR-Q
peak experience
perceived exertion
perspiration *See* sweating.
phosphagen
phosphagen system
phosphocreatine
See phosphagen system.
Physical Activity Level
Physical Activity Ratio
physical fitness
physical work capacity
physiological limit
plateau
pooling
posture
psychoneuromuscular
theory
pulse
radial pulse *See* pulse.
rate–pressure product
rating of perceived exertion
See perceived exertion.
reaction time
relative strength *See* strength.
respiration
respiratory quotient
ruler drop test *See* reaction
time.
runner's high
Sargent jump test
skill
spasm
speed
speed-accuracy trade off
Sport Emotional Reaction
Profile
stamina *See* endurance.
steadiness
strength
strength endurance
stretch reflex

stretch stress
stroke volume
suppleness
sweating
tetany
thermogenesis
thirst
tidal volume *See* lung
volume.
timing
total thermal load
ventilation rate *See* lung
volume.
vital capacity

Exercise-related injuries

Achilles tendinitis *See* Achilles
tendon.
acute injury
acute muscle soreness
See muscle soreness.
ankle sprain
anterior compartment
syndrome
atrophy
backache
baseball finger
black nail
blister
bone injury
bone scan *See* bone injury.
boredom
bouncing breast syndrome
boxer's arm
boxer's fracture
boxer's knuckle
bowler's hip
bowler's thumb
breaststroker's knee
bruise
bunion
burnout
burns
bursitis *See* bursa.
cardiac rehabilitation
carpal tunnel syndrome
chafing
choking
chondromalacia patellae
compartment syndrome
compression neuropathy
concussion
conjunctivitis
contusion *See* bruise.
corn
cramp
cut *See* laceration.
dart thrower's elbow
dehydration
delayed onset muscle soreness
See muscle soreness.

dementia pugilistica
  See punch-drunk syndrome.
detached retina
dilutional hyponatremia
  See water intoxication.
dislocation
distraction strain See muscle
  strain.
distraction rupture See muscle
  strain.
double jointed See
  hypermobile joint disease.
ectopic heartbeat
encephalopathy See punch-
  drunk syndrome.
epiphyseal avulsion
exercise addiction
exercise-induced asthma
exercise-induced headache
  See headache.
exercise risks
eye injury
fallen arches
fatigue
fatigue index
fibrositis
flat feet See fallen arches.
footballer's ankle
footballer's migraine
  See headache.
fracture
friction burn
frostbite
frostnip See frostbite.
frozen shoulder
gamekeeper's thumb
  See skier's thumb.
glass jaw
golfer's elbow
golfer's toe
groin pain See groin.
groin strain See groin.
gymnast's fracture
haematoma
haematuria
hammer toe
hand injuries
handlebar palsy See hand
  injuries.
head injuries
heat collapse
heat cramps
heat exhaustion
heat neurasthenia See heat
  exhaustion.
heat stroke
heat syncope
housemaid's knee
hypermobile joint disease
  See hypermobility.
hyperthermia

hypothermia
impingement exostosis
  See footballer's ankle.
indisposition See run down.
inguinal hernia See hernia.
inguinocrural pain See groin.
injury See sports injury.
intertrigo See chafing.
javelin thrower's elbow
  See golfer's elbow.
jock itch
jogger's nipple
jogger's trots See food transit
  time.
joint injury
joint mice See joint injury.
joint stiffness
judo elbow
jumper's knee
jumper's heel
knee disorders See knee.
knockout See concussion.
laceration
loafer's heart theory
locking
luxation
mallet finger
march fracture
march haemoglobinuria
  See haematuria.
mat burns See friction burn.
medial epicondylitis
  See golfer's elbow.
microtrauma
muscle hernia See fascial
  hernia.
muscle strain
muscle poops See fascial
  hernia.
muscle pull See muscle strain.
muscle soreness
muscle tear See muscle strain.
orthostatic hypotension
  See postural hypotension.
orthostatic proteinuria
  See postural proteinuria.
Osgood-Schlatter's disease
osteitis pubis See groin pain.
osteophytes See footballer's
  ankle.
overpronation See pronation.
overreaching
overtraining
overuse injury
pain
pain cycle
patellar tendinitis
  See jumper's knee.
patellofemoral disorders
  See knee disorders.
patellofemoral malalignment

periostitis See periosteum.
peritendinitis
peritonitis
pitcher's elbow See thrower's
  elbow.
plantar fasciitis
postural hypotension
postural proteinuria
prepatellar bursitis
  See housemaid's knee.
priapism
prolapsed intervertebral disc
protective muscle spasm
punch-drunk syndrome
repetitive strain injury
rider's strain
run down
runner's knee
runner's haemolysis
  See haematuria.
runner's haematuria
  See haematuria.
runner's toe See black nail.
sciatica
second wind
shallow-water black-out
  See oxygen poisoning.
shin fracture
shin splints
skier's thumb
slipped disc
snow-blindness
soccer toe See black nail.
soft tissue injury
spinner's finger
spondylolithesis
  See spondylolysis.
spondylolysis
sports injury
sprain
stiffness
stitch
strain See muscle strain.
stress fracture
subluxation See dislocation.
sudden immersion injury
sudden death
sunburn
sunstroke
surfer's ear See swimmer's ear.
swimmer's ear
swimmer's shoulder
tachycardia
tendinitis
tendinosis
tendon injuries
tennis elbow
tennis leg
tennis toe See black nail.
tetanus
thrower's elbow

thrower's fracture
torn cartilage See meniscus.
torticollis
travel sickness
trigger finger
triple-jumper's heel
turf toe syndrome
ulnar compression syndrome
   See compression
   neuropathy.
unhappy triad
unilateral muscular
   hypertrophy
valgus
Valsalva's manoeuvre
varus
weight-lifter's headache
   See headache.
whiplash injury
winding
Work Related Upper Limb
   Disorder See repetitive
   strain injury.
wryneck See torticollis.
young runner's heel

Sports injury treatments
acupuncture
Alexander technique
arthroscopy
balneotherapy
baths
CAT scan See computerized
   tomography.
chiropractic
cold therapy
computerized tomography
connective tissue massage
   See massage.
contrast baths
cross-frictional massage
   See massage.
cryotherapy
deep friction massage
   See massage.
deep stroking See massage.
diathermy
effleurage See massage.
effluage See massage.
electric muscle stimulator
electrotherapy
elevation
exercise therapy
fanning See massage.
flotation therapy
heat treatment
hydrocollator
hydrotherapy
hyperbaric oxygen therapy
ibuprofen
jostling See massage.

kneading See massage.
liniment
local cross-fibre stroke
   See massage.
manipulation
massage
massager
orthotics
phonophoresis See ultrasound.
physiotherapy
rehabilitation
RICE
sauna baths
scintigraphy
short wave diathermy
   See diathermy.
SPF See sun-protection factor.
steam treatment
sun-protection factor
SWD See diathermy.
taping
TENS See transcutaneous
   electrical stimulation.
transcutaneous electrical
   nerve stimulation
ultrasound
whirlpool treatment
X-ray
zinc oxide ointment

Diet and
exercise

**Body structures and
movements**
abdominal muscles
abduction See body
   movements.
abductor
Achilles tendon
adduction See body
   movements.
adductor muscles
adipocyte
adipose tissue
alimentary canal
appendix
antagonist
anterior cruciate ligaments
anthropometry
antigravity muscle
apocrine glands See sweat
   glands.
android fat distribution
apple-shaped obesity
   See android fat distribution.
arches

athlete's foot
biceps
biceps brachii
biceps femoris See hamstrings.
bioelectrical impedance
biomechanics
BMI See body mass index.
body composition
body mass
body mass index
body size
body movements
body fat
bone
bone marrow See bone.
bony spur
boxer's muscle
bowel
brown fat
brown adipose tissue
   See brown fat.
bursa
cardiac muscle
cardiovascular system
carotid artery
circumduction See body
   movements.
clavicle See collar bone.
collagen
collar bone
collateral circulation
compartment See
   compartment syndrome.
connective tissue
constitutional theory
   See somatotype.
cruciate ligaments
deltoid muscle
delts See deltoid muscle.
disc
eccrine glands See sweating
ectomorph See somatotype.
elbow joint
emergency muscle
end point See range of
   movement.
extension See body
   movements.
extensor
fascia
fat cells See adipocytes.
fatfold test See skinfold
   measurements.
fat-free body mass See lean
   body mass.
fat-free body weight
fat pad
flexion See body movements.
flexor See body movements.
functional short leg See short
   leg.

gluteal muscle
gluteus medius *See* gluteal
  muscle.
gluteus minimus *See* gluteal
  muscle.
gluteus maximus *See* gluteal
  muscle.
groin
gynoid fat distribution
hamstrings
heart
hydrostatic weighing
hyperplasia *See* growth.
hypertrophy *See* growth.
ideal weight
infraspinatus *See* rotator cuff.
involuntary muscle
joint stability
kneecap
knee
lean body mass
loose bodies *See* joint injuries.
meniscus
mesomorph
mitochondrion
muscle
muscle balance
muscle-bound
muscle bulk
muscle group
normal active range *See* range
  of movement.
os trigonum
paratenon *See* peritendinitis.
parathyroid glands
  See parathormone.
parathyroid hormone
patella *See* kneecap.
pear-shaped obesity *See* gynoid
  fat distribution.
pecs *See* pectoral muscles.
pectoral muscles
pelvic floor muscles
periosteum
phantom
pituitary
ponderal index *See* body size.
pot belly
prime mover
pronation
pronator
Q-angle
quadriceps
Quetelet index *See* body mass
  index.
range of motion *See* range of
  movement.
range of movement
rectus femoris *See* quadriceps.
reference man and woman
relative weight

rotator cuff
sciatic nerve *See* sciatica.
serratus anterior *See* boxer's
  muscle.
Sheldon's constitutional
  theory *See* somatotype.
short leg
skeletal muscle
skeleton
skin
skinfold measurements
slow-twitch fibre *See* muscle
  fibre type.
small intestine *See* alimentary
  canal.
smooth muscle *See* muscle.
somatotype
spare tyre
spleen
stability *See* joint stability.
stomach muscles
  See abdominal muscles.
storage fat
supination
supinator
suprascapularis *See* rotator
  cuff.
supraspinatus *See* rotator cuff.
Syndrome X
tendon
trapezius
triceps *See* triceps brachii.
triceps brachii
triceps surae *See* soleus.
trigger point
Type I fibre *See* muscle fibre
  types.
Type II fibre *See* muscle fibre
  types.
vastus lateralis *See* quadriceps.
vastus medialis
  See quadriceps.
vastus intermedius
  See quadriceps.
visceral fat deposition
waist–hip ratio
white fibre *See* muscle fibre
  type.
white adipose tissue

Disorders and diseases

adult onset diabetes
  See diabetes.
adult onset obesity
  See obesity.
allergy
altitude sickness
Alzheimer's disease
amenorrhoea
anaemia
angina

anhydrosis
arteriosclerosis
arthritis
asthma
atherosclerosis
autoimmunity *See* immunity.
brittle bone disease
  See osteoporosis.
bronchitis
cardiac hypertrophy
cardiac arrest
cardiac arrhythmia
cardiovascular disease
chest pain
childhood onset obesity
  See obesity.
cholera
cold
coronary heart disease risk
  factor
coronary heart disease
coronary-prone personality
coryza *See* cold.
counter-conditioning
desensitization
diabetes
diabetes insipidus
diabetes mellitus *See* diabetes.
diuresis
duodenal ulcer
dysmenorrhoea
dyspepsia *See* indigestion.
dyspnoea
eczema
emphysema
endometriosis
epilepsy
fainting
fascial hernia
fever
fulminant exertional
  rhabdomyolosis *See* sickle
  cell disease.
fungal infections
haemorrhoids
headache
health risk
health-risk appraisal
heart attack
heartburn
heart overload
hernia
herniated disc *See* prolapsed
  intervertebral disc.
hidrosis
high altitude pulmonary
  oedema
hypernatremia
hypokinetic disease
hyponatremia
hypotension

hypotonic hydration *See* water
   intoxification.
hypoxia
indigestion
insulin-dependent diabetes
   See diabetes.
insulin-independent diabetes
   See diabetes.
juvenile-onset diabetes
   See diabetes.
kidney stones
lordosis
mad cow disease *See* bovine
   spongiform
   encephalopathy.
metabolic acidosis
   See acidosis.
migraine *See* headache.
myocardial infarction
   See heart attack.
myocarditis
nephrolithiasis *See* kidney
   stones.
non-insulin-dependent
   diabetes *See* diabetes.
oesophagitis
osteoarthritis
osteoporosis
oxygen poisoning
palpitation
paunch *See* pot belly.
pernicious anaemia
phenylketonuria
piles *See* haemorrhoids.
pyrexia *See* fever.
pyrosis *See* heartburn.
renal stones *See* kidney stones.
respiratory acidosis
   See acidosis.
rheumatoid arthritis
rupture *See* hernia.
shock
sickle cell disease
stress incontinence
stroke
syncope *See* fainting.
thrombosis
thrush *See* candida.
Type I diabetes *See* diabetes.
Type II diabetes *See* diabetes.
varices *See* varicose veins.
varicose veins

Drugs and chemicals

acetylsalicylic acid
   See aspirin.
adrenaline
alkali
alkalinizer *See* alkali.
aluminium
amphetamines

anabolic steroids
anaesthetic
androgen
anorexiant drug
antacid
antibiotic
antihistamine
antihypertensive
anti-inflammatory
antiperspirant
aspirin
atropine *See* belladonna.
banned substance
barbiturates
belladonna
betablockers
bicarbonate *See* alkali.
bile
buffer
bute *See* phenylbutazone.
caffeine
cholesterol-lowering drugs
cholesterol-testing kits
   See cholesterol.
chymotrypsin
clenbuterol
cocaine
corticosteroids
cortisone
cyproheptadine
   hydrochloride
diet pill *See* slimming pills.
dimethyl sulphoxide
diuretic
DLPA *See* DL-phenylalanine
DL-phenylalanine
DMSO *See* diemthyl
   sulphoxide
doping
dose regime
drugs
endorphins
entramine *See* serotonin.
ephedrine
EPO *See* erythropoietin. ,
erythropoietin
fenfluramine
ferritin
fibrin
fluoxetine *See* prozac.
gamma-oryzanol
glucagon
GO *See* gamma-oryzanol.
growth hormone
histamine
human chorionic
   gonadotrophin
hyaluronic acid
   See hyaluronidase.
hyaluronidase
hydrocortisone

hydroxyproline *See* muscle
   soreness.
lipoprotein
marijuana
methaemoglobin *See* nitrates.
narcotic
neohesperidine
non-steroidal anti-
   inflammatory drug
noradrenaline
norepinephrine
   See noradrenaline.
oestrogen
opiate
opium *See* opiate.
oxygen
ozone
paracetamol
parathormone *See* parathyroid
   hormone.
pep pills *See* amphetamines.
peptide hormones
phenylpropanolamine
phytochemical
probenecid
prostaglandin
prozac
PTH *See* parathormone.
relaxin
renin
rennin
secretin
serotonin
SOD *See* superoxide
   dismutase.
steroid
stevioside
stimulants
stress hormone
strychnine
superoxide dismutase
testosterone
thyroid stimulating hormone
thyroid hormone
thyroxine *See* thyroid
   hormone.
triacylglycerol
triglyceride *See* fat.
very low-density lipoprotein
   See lipoprotein.
water tablets

Other topics

acidosis
acquired ageing *See* ageing.
acquired immune deficiency
   syndrome
addiction
adolescence
advertisements
ageing

AIDS *See* acquired immune
deficiency syndrome.
air pollutants
Apgar scores
athlete
autoconditioning
See biofeedback training.
autogenic training
aversion therapy
Bandura's self-efficacy theory
basal metabolic rate
behaviour therapy
biofeedback training
blood
biorhythm
body image
body schema *See* body image.
calorie
cancer
catastrophe theory
cerebrotonic trait
See somatotype.
childhood
circadian rhythm
concentration
confidence
contraception
contraceptive pill
See contraception.
control group
cult of slenderness
depression
development *See* growth.
drive
emotions
energy balance
extrinsic motivation
See motivation.
fashion
FDA
feedback
Food and Drug
Administration *See* FDA.
framing *See* segmenting.
gastroporn

gender
gender role stereotyping
See gender.
gene *See* genetic endowment.
general adaptation syndrome
genetic endowment
goal
goal displacement *See* goal.
goal setting *See* goal.
growth
hair
handicapped
Hawthorne effect
health screening
health
healthy lifestyle
high-density lipoproteins
See lipoproteins.
hormone
hormone replacement
therapy *See* menopause.
hypnotherapy
immune system
incentive
incontinence
infancy
insomnia
intelligence
intrinsic motivation
See motivation.
inverted U hypothesis
IQ *See* intelligence.
joule
libido
lipid deposit theory
longevity
male menopause
See viropause.
maturation *See* growth.
medical screening *See* health
screening.
menarche
menopause
menstruation
mental health

mood swings
motivation
negative-change goal
personality
phospholipids
placebo
plumpness
praise
pregnancy
premenstrual tension
Profile Of Mood States
psyche
psyched-out *See* psyche.
psyching-up *See* psyche.
puberty
relaxation
resistance stage *See* general
adaptation.
syndrome.
SAD *See* seasonal affective
disorder.
seasonal affective disorder
self-concept
self-confidence
self-efficacy *See* self-
confidence.
self-esteem
self-image *See* self-concept.
self-talk *See* self-confidence.
sex and exercise
sex differences
shaping
sleep
smoking
sports science
state anxiety *See* anxiety.
stress
synergist
synergythought-stopping
type A behaviour
type B behaviour
ultraviolet light
unfitness
viropause
Yerkes-Dodson curve

Index

A

abdominal contraction
abdominal hold
abdominal muscles
abduction *See* body
   movements.
abductor
abductor raise
abnormal quadriceps pull
   See Q-angle.
absolute strength
   See strength.
absorption
acceleration sprint
acclimation
   See acclimatization.
acclimatization
accommodation principle
acesulfame-K
acetylsalicylic acid *See* aspirin
Achilles stretch *See* Achilles
   tendon.
Achilles tendinitis *See* Achilles
   tendon.
Achilles tendon
acidosis
acquired ageing *See* ageing.
acquired immune deficiency
   syndrome
active rest
activity-induced anorexia
   See anorexia.
acupuncture
acute injury
acute muscle soreness
   See muscle soreness.
adaptation
adaptation energy
adapted physical exercise
adaptogen
addiction
additive *See* food additive.
adduction *See* body
   movements.
adductor muscles
adductor stretch *See* adductor
   muscles.
adenosine triphosphate
adipocyte
adipose tissue
adiposis *See* liposis.
adipostat
adolescence
adrenaline
adult onset diabetes
   See diabetes.

adult onset obesity *See* obesity.
advertisements
aerobic capacity
aerobic dance *See* dance.
aerobic energy system
   See aerobic respiration.
aerobic exercise
aerobic fitness
aerobic points
aerobic power
aerobic respiration
aerobics
aerobic **training** threshold
aerobic training zone
aerobic work capacity
   See aerobic power.
aerobox *See* boxercise.
aflatoxins
ageing
agility
AIDS
aikido *See* martialarts.
Air Force diet *See* ketogenic
   diet.
air pollutants
air resistance
alanine
alcohol
Alexander technique
alimentary canal
alkali
alkalinizer *See* alkali.
alkalosis *See* alkali.
allergy
altitude
altitude acclimatization
   See altitude.
altitude sickness *See* altitude.
altitude training *See* altitude.
aluminium
Alzheimer's disease
amenorrhoea
American football
amino acids
amino acid supplements
amphetamines
amygdalin *See* laetrile.
anabolic steroids
anabolism
anaemia
anaerobic exercise
anaerobic threshold
anaesthetic
anal fissure
anal itching
anaphylactic shock

anaphylaxis
androgen
android fat distribution
angina
anhydrosis
animal starch *See* glycogen.
ankle sprain
ankle stretchers
anorexia *See* anorexia nervosa.
anorexia nervosa
anorexiant drug
antacid
antagonist
anterior compartment
   syndrome
anterior cruciate ligaments
anthropometry
antibiotic
antigravity muscle
antihaemorrhagic vitamin
   See vitamin K.
antihistamine
antihypertensive
anti-inflammatory
antinutrients
antioxidant
antiperspirant
anti-rachitic factor *See* vitamin
   D.
anti-sterility factor *See* vitamin
   E.
anxiety
Apgar scores
apocrine glands *See* sweat
   glands.
appendicitis *See* appendix.
appendix
appestat
appetite
appetite suppressant
apple-shaped obesity
   See android fat distribution.
aquarobics
aqua running *See* aquarobics.
archery
arches
arginine
arm curl
arm lift
arm sprints
arm stretch
aromatherapy
arousal
arrested progress *See* plateau.
arsenic
arteriosclerosis

arthritis
arthroscopy
artificial colours
artificial fats
artificial flavours
artificial sweeteners
ascorbic acid *See* vitamin C.
aspartame
aspartates
aspartic acid *See* aspartates.
aspirin
asthma
atherosclerosis
athlete
athlete's foot
athlete's heart
athletic pseudonephritis
See proteinuria.
athletics
Atkins diet
ATP *See* adenosine
   triphosphate.
ATP–PCr system
   See phosphagen system.
atrophy
atropine *See* belladonna.
Atwater factor
autoconditioning *See*
   biofeedback training.
autogenic training
autoimmunity *See* immunity.
aversion therapy
avidin *See* biotin.
azo dyes

B

backache
back and leg stretch
back extension
back extension test
back scratcher stretch
badminton
balance
balanced diet
balanced exercise programme
ballistic stretching
balneotherapy
banded gastroplasty
Bandura's self-efficacy theory
   See self-confidence.
banned substance
barbell
barbiturates
bare foot exercise
basal metabolic rate
baseball and softball
baseball finger
base training
basketball
baths
BBC diet

BCAA *See* branched-chain
   amino acids
B complex vitamins
bee pollen
behaviour therapy
belladonna
bench
bench blasts
bench press
benign hypermobility
   See hypermobility
bent arm hang
bent arm pullover
bent over row
beriberi
beta-blockers
beta-carotene
beta-oxidation
Beverly Hills diet
BHA
BHT *See* butylated
   hydroxyanisole.
bicarbonate *See* alkali.
bicarbonate loading
   See sodium bicarbonate.
biceps
biceps brachii
biceps curl *See* arm curl.
biceps femoris *See* hamstrings.
bile
Billig's exercise
binge eating
binge–purge syndrome
   See bulimia nervosa.
bioelectrical impedance
biofeedback training
biomechanics
biorhythm
biotin
black nail
blind stork test
blister
blitz system *See* body building.
blood
blood doping
blood glucose
blood lactate
blood platelets *See* blood.
blood pressure
blue baby syndrome
   See nitrates.
BMI *See* body mass index.
BMR *See* basal metabolic rate.
body awareness
body building
body composition
body fat
body fuels
body image
body mass
body mass index

body movements
body schema *See* body image.
body size
body temperature *See* core
   temperature.
body wraps
bomb calorimeter
bone
bone injury
bone marrow *See* bone.
bone scan *See* bone injury.
bonking
bony spur
boredom
Borg scale *See* perceived
   exertion.
born athlete *See* athlete.
boron
botulism
bouncing breast syndrome
bovine spongiform
   encephalopathy
bowel
bowler's hip
bowler's thumb
bowling
bowls *See* bowling.
boxercise
boxer's arm
boxer's fracture
boxer's knuckle
boxer's muscle
boxing
bradycardia
branched-chain amino acids
breakfast
breast-feeding
breast reduction
   See mammaplasty.
breast-stroker's knee
breathing
brittle bone disease
   See osteoporosis.
bromelain
bronchitis
brown adipose tissue
   See brown fat.
brown fat
bruise
BSE *See* bovine spongiform
   encephalopathy.
buffer
bulimia nervosa
bulk *See* fibre
bulking agents
bungee jumping
bunion
burn out
burns
bursa
bursitis *See* bursa.

bute *See* phenylbutazone.
butterflies
butterfly machine *See* fixed-weight machine.
butylated hydroxyanisole
  See BHA.

C

caffeine
caffeinism
calciferol *See* vitamin D.
calcium
calf raise
calisthenics
caloric balance *See* energy balance.
caloric equivalence *See* heat equivalence.
calorie
calorie counting
calorimetry
Cambridge diet
campylobacteriosis
Canadian home fitness test
Canadian trunk strength test
cancer
candida
candidiasis *See* candida.
canoeing and kayaking
carbohydrate addict's diet
carbohydrate loading
carbohydrates
carboloading *See* carbohydrate loading.
cardiac arrest
cardiac arrhythmia
cardiac hypertrophy
cardiac muscle
cardiac output
cardiac rehabilitation
cardiorespiratory endurance *See* aerobic fitness.
cardiovascular disease
cardiovascular fitness *See* aerobic fitness.
cardiovascular system
carnitine
carotenes
carotid artery
carotid pulse *See* carotid artery.
carotid sinus *See* carotid artery.
carpal tunnel syndrome
catastrophe theory
CAT scan *See* computerized tomography.
cat stretch
cellulite
cellulose

cerebrotonic trait *See* somatotype.
chafing
cheating
chest pain
chest stretch
childhood
childhood onset obesity *See* obesity.
Chinese restaurant syndrome
chinnies
chinning *See* chin-up.
chin-up
chiropractic
chocoholic
choking
cholecalciferol *See* vitamin D.
cholera
cholesterol
cholesterol-lowering drugs
cholesterol-testing kits *See* cholesterol.
chondromalacia patellae
chromium
chymotrypsin
circadian rhythm
circuit training
circumduction *See* body movements.
cis *See* unsaturated fat.
citric acid cycle *See* Krebs cycle.
clavicle *See* collar bone.
clenbuterol
climbing
clothing
clo unit
coach
cobalamin *See* vitamin B_{12}.
cobalt
cocaine
coeliac disease
coenzyme Q
coffee *See* caffeine.
cold
cold therapy
collagen
collar bone
collateral circulation
colonic fermentation
Columbus Nutrition Plan
combining diets *See* food combining diets.
comfort eating
comfort index
comfort zone
compartment *See* compartment syndrome.
compartment syndrome
complete protein

complex carbohydrate
compression neuropathy
compulsive overeating
computerized tomography
concentration
concentric contraction *See* muscle contraction.
concussion
conditioning
confidence
conjunctivitis
connective tissue
connective tissue massage *See* massage.
constipation
constitutional theory *See* somatotype.
contact sport
continuous exercise
contraception
contraceptive pill *See* contraception.
contraindicated
contrast baths
control group
contusion *See* bruise.
conversational index
cool down
Cooper points *See* aerobic points.
Cooper twelve-minute test
coordination
copper
core temperature
corn
coronary heart disease
coronary heart disease risk factor
coronary-prone personality
corticosteroids
cortisone
coryza *See* cold.
cosmetic surgery
counter-conditioning
cramp
crash diet
creatine
creatine phosphate *See* phosphagen system.
Creutzfeldt-Jakob disease
cricket
Crohn's disease
cross-country skiing *See* skiing.
cross-frictional massage *See* massage.
cross-training
cruciate ligaments
crunch programme
cryotherapy
cult of slenderness

curl-up
cut *See* laceration.
cyanocobalamin *See* vitamin B₁₂.
cyclamate
cycle training
cycling
cyproheptadine hydrochloride
cytotoxic testing

D

Daily Values
dance
dart thrower's elbow
dead-lift
deep friction massage *See* massage.
deep stroking *See* massage.
dehydration
deinhibition training
delayed onset muscle soreness *See* muscle soreness.
deltoid muscle
delts *See* deltoid muscle
dementia pugilistica *See* punch-drunk syndrome.
dental caries *See* tooth decay.
depression
descending sets
desensitization
designer foods
detached retina
detox diets *See* detoxication.
detoxication
detoxification *See* detoxication.
detraining effects
development *See* growth.
dextrin
dextrose
diabetes
diabetes insipidus
diabetes mellitus *See* diabetes.
diarrhoea
diastase
diastolic blood pressure *See* blood pressure.
diathermy
diet
dietary exchange lists
dietary fibre
Dietary Reference Values
diet induced thermogenesis
diet pill *See* slimming pills.
digestion
digestive disorders
digestive juices
dilutional hyponatremia *See* water intoxication.

dimethylglycine *See* methyl donors.
dimethylnitrosamine *See* nitrosamine.
dimethyl sulphoxide
dips
DIRT
disaccharide
disc
dislocation
distance running *See* jogging.
distraction strain *See* muscle strain.
distraction rupture *See* muscle strain.
diuresis
diuretic
diverticulitis
diverticulosis
DLPA *See* DL-phenylalanine
DL-phenylalanine
DMG *See* methyl donors.
DMSO *See* diemthyl sulphoxide.
Doctor's Quick Weight Loss Diet *See* high protein diet.
doping
dose regime
double-jointed *See* hypermobility.
double progressive system
double sugar *See* disaccharide.
drive
dropout
drugs
dumbbell
dumbbell curls
dumbbell punch
duodenal ulcer
duodenum
duration of exercise *See* training duration.
dynamic strength *See* strength.
dynamogeny
dynamometer
dysentery
dysmenorrhoea
dyspepsia *See* indigestion.
dyspnoea

E

Eastern prayer
eating diary
eating disorder
eating disorder not otherwise specified
eccentric contraction *See* muscle contraction.

eccrine glands *See* sweating.
ECG *See* electrocardiogram.
ectomorph *See* somatotype.
ectopic heartbeat
eczema
EEG *See* electroencephalogram.
effleurage *See* massage.
effluage *See* massage.
eicosapentaenoic acid
elastic belt
elastic strength *See* strength.
elbow joint
electric muscle stimulator
electrocardiogram
electroencephalogram
electrogoniometer *See* goniometer.
electrolyte drink
electrotherapy
elevation
elimination diet
emergency muscle
emotions
emphysema
empty calories *See* sugar.
emulsification
emulsifiers
encephalins *See* endorphins.
encephalopathy *See* punch-drunk syndrome.
endometriosis
endorphins
endotoxin
end point *See* range of movement.
endurance
energy balance
energy continuum
energy drink
energy expenditure
energy nutrient
enriched foods
enteric bacteria *See* gut bacteria.
entramine *See* serotonin.
E-numbers *See* food additives.
enzyme
EPA *See* eicosapentaenoic acid.
ephedrine
epilepsy
epiphyseal avulsion
EPO *See* erythropoietin.
ergocalciferol *See* vitamin D.
ergogenic aid
ergogens *See* ergogenic aid.
ergometer
erythropoietin
Eskimo diet
essential amino acid
essential fat

essential fatty acid
Estimated Average
    Requirement *See* Dietary
    Reference Values.
excess postexercise oxygen
    consumption *See* oxygen
    debt.
exercise
exercise addiction
exercise adherence
exercise band *See* resistance
    exercise.
exercise diary *See* training
    diary.
exercise duration *See* training
    duration.
exercise frequency
    See training frequency.
exercise-induced asthma
exercise-induced headache
    See headache.
exercise intensity *See* training
    intensity.
exercise machine
exercise modification
exercise prescription
exercise risks
exercise therapy
exhaustion *See* general
    adaptation syndrome.
exotoxin
expedition-type endurance
extension *See* body
    movements.
extensor
extrinsic motivation
    See motivation.
eye injury

F

fad diet
faeces
fainting
fallen arches
fanning *See* massage.
fartlek training
fascia
fascial hernia
fashion
fast foods
fasting
fat
fat blockers
fat cells *See* adipocytes.
fatfold test *See* skinfold
    measurements.
fat-free body mass *See* lean
    body mass.
fat-free body weight
fatigue
fatigue index

fat loading
fat malabsorption
fat mobilization
fat pad
fat-soluble vitamins
fatty acids
FDA
feedback
Feingold diet
fencing
fenfluramine
fermentation
fermented foods
ferritin
fertility vitamin *See* vitamin E.
fever
fibre
fibre splitting *See* muscle
    growth.
fibre supplements
fibrin
fibrositis
fish-oil supplements
fitness
fixed-weight machine
flat feet *See* fallen arches.
flatulence
flavour enhancers
flexibility
flexion *See* body
    movements.
flexor
flotation therapy
flow
fluid retention
fluoride *See* fluorine.
fluorine
fluoxetine *See* prozac.
flushing methods
foetal stretch
folacin *See* folic acid.
folic acid
food additives
food allergy *See* allergy.
Food and Drug
    Administration *See* FDA.
food aversion
food combining diets
food diary *See* eating diary.
food exchange system
    See dietary exchange lists.
food group
food guide pyramid
foodie
food intolerance
food labelling
food poisoning
food transit time
football *See* American football
    and soccer.
footballer's ankle

footballer's migraine
    See headache.
forced expiratory volume
forced repetitions *See* forced
    reps.
forced reps
form
formula diet
fortified foods
F-plan diet
fracture
framing *See* segmenting.
free fatty acid *See* fatty
    acids.
free radicals
free weight
frequency of exercise
    See training frequency.
friction burn
frostbite
frostnip *See* frostbite.
frozen shoulder
fructose
fruitarian
fulminant exertional
    rhabdomyolosis *See* sickle
    cell disease.
functional short leg *See* short
    leg.
fungal infections

G

GABA *See* gamma-
    aminobutyric acid
galactose
gall-bladder
gallstones
gamekeeper's thumb *See*
    skier's thumb.
gamesmanship
gamma-aminobutyric acid
gamma-linolenic acid
gamma-oryzanol
garlic
gaseous exchange
gastric balloons
gastritis
gastroenteritis
gastroplasty *See* banded
    gastroplasty.
gastroporn
gelatin *See* collagen.
gender
gender role stereotyping
    See gender.
gene *See* genetic endowment.
general adaptation syndrome
genetic endowment
ginseng
GLA *See* gamma-linolenic acid.
glass jaw

gliadins *See* gluten.
gloves *See* clothing.
glucagon
glucose
glucose polymers
glucose tolerance test
glutamate *See* glutamic acid.
glutamic acid
glutathione
glutathione peroxidase
  See glutathione.
gluteal lift
gluteal muscle
gluten
gluten intolerance *See* coeliac
  disease.
glutenin *See* gluten.
gluteus maximus *See* gluteal
  muscle.
gluteus medius *See* gluteal
  muscle.
gluteus minimus *See* gluteal
  muscle.
glycaemic index
glycerol
glycine
glycogen
glycogen overshoot *See*
  carbohydrate loading.
glycolysis
glycosuria
GO *See* gamma-oryzanol.
goal
goal displacement *See* goal.
goal setting *See* goal.
golf
golfer's elbow
golfer's toe
goniometer
gout
graded exercise test
grapefruit pills
grazing
gripping aids
groin
groin pain *See* groin.
groin strain *See* groin.
growth
growth hormone
guar gum
gumshield
gut *See* alimentary canal.
gut bacteria
GXT
gymnastics
gymnast's fracture
gynoid fat distribution

H

haematoma
haematuria

haem iron
haemoglobin
haemorrhoids
hair
half-squats
hammer toe
hamstrings
hamstring stretcher
handicapped
hand injuries
handlebar palsy *See* hand
  injuries.
Harvard step test *See* step test.
Hawthorne effect
HCG *See* human chorionic
  gonadotrophin.
headache
head injuries
health
health-related fitness
health risk
health risk appraisal
health screening
healthy lifestyle
heart
heart attack
heartburn
heart overload
heart rate
heart test
heat acclimatization
heat balance
heat collapse
heat cramps
heat equivalence
heat exhaustion
heat neurasthenia *See* heat
  exhaustion.
heat stroke
heat syncope
heat treatment
heel raise *See* calf raise.
hernia
herniated disc *See* prolapsed
  intervertebral disc.
hexagon test
hexose
hidden fat
hidrosis
high altitude pulmonary
  oedema
high-density lipoproteins
  See lipoproteins.
high protein diet
hill training
hip and thigh diet *See* spot
  theory of fat reduction.
hip stretch
histamine
histidine
hockey

hollow sprints
homeostasis
hormone
hormone replacement
  therapy *See* menopause.
horse-riding
housemaid's knee
HRmax *See* maximal heart
  rate.
hug
human chorionic
  gonadotrophin
hunger
hurdle stretch
hyaluronic acid
  See hyaluronidase.
hyaluronidase
hydrafitness *See* omnikinetic
  resistance machine.
hydrocollator
hydrocortisone
hydrogenation
hydrolipodystrophy
  See cellulite.
hydrostatic weighing
hydrotherapy
hydroxyproline *See* muscle.
  soreness.
hyperbaric oxygen therapy
hyperglycaemia
hypermobile joint disease
  See hypermobility.
hypermobility
hypernatremia
hyperplasia *See* growth.
hypertension
hyperthermia
hypertonic drink
  See electrolyte drink.
hypertrophy *See* growth
hyperventilation
hypervitaminosis
hypnotherapy
hypoglycaemia
hypokinetic disease
hyponatremia
hypotension
hypothermia
hypotonic drink
  See electrolyte drink.
hypotonic hydration *See* water
  intoxication.
hypoxia

I

ibuprofen
iceberg profile *See* Profile of
  Mood States.
ice hockey
ideal weight
iliopsoas stretcher

Illinois agility run *See* agility.
imagery relaxation
imaging *See* visualization.
immune system
impingement exostosis
  See footballer's ankle.
incentive
incline bench
incomplete proteins
incontinence
incremental run
indigestion
indisposition *See* run down.
individual differences
  principle
infancy
inflatable belt *See* elastic belt.
infraspinatus *See* rotator
  cuff.
inguinal hernia *See* hernia.
inguinocrural pain *See* groin.
injury *See* sports injury.
inosine monophosphate
inositol
insoluble fibre *See* fibre.
insomnia
instructor *See* coach.
insulin
insulin-dependent diabetes
  See diabetes.
insulin-independent diabetes
  See diabetes.
insulin rebound
intelligence
intensity of exercise
International Olympic
  Committee
intertrigo *See* chafing.
interval sprinting
interval training
intervertebral disc *See* disc.
intrinsic factor
intrinsic motivation
  See motivation.
inversion
inverted U hypothesis
involuntary muscle
iodine
iodized salt *See* table salt.
IQ *See* intelligence.
iron
irritable bowel syndrome
isokinetic contraction
  See muscle contraction.
isolation stress
isoleucine
isometric contraction
  See muscle contraction.
isometrics
isotonic contractions
  See muscle contraction.

isotonic drink *See* electrolyte
  drink.
Italian football diet

J

javelin thrower's elbow
  See golfer's elbow.
jaw wiring
jiu-jitsu *See* martial arts.
jock itch
jogger's nipple
jogger's trots *See* food transit
  time.
jogging
joint injury
joint mice *See* joint
  injury.
joint stability
joint stiffness
jostling *See* massage.
joule
judo *See* martial arts.
judo elbow
jumper's heel
jumper's knee
jump height
jumping
jumping jack
junk food
juvenile-onset diabetes
  See diabetes.

K

karate *See* martial arts.
kayaking *See* canoeing and
  kayaking.
kelp
ketogenic diet
ketone bodies *See* ketogenic
  diet.
ketosis *See* ketogenic diet.
kidney stones
kinaesthesis
kinesiology
kneading *See* massage.
knee
kneecap
knee disorders *See* knee.
kneeling kickback
knee raises
knockout *See* concussion.
Krebs cycle
kung-fu *See* martial arts.
kwashiorkor

L

laceration
lactase *See* lactose.
lactate *See* lactic acid.
lactate threshold *See* lactic
  acid.

lactic acid
lacto-ovo vegetarian diet
lactose
lactose intolerance
  See lactose.
laetrile
lateral arm raise
lateral pull-down
laxative
lean body mass
lecithin
lectins
leg curl
leg extension
leg lift
leg press
leg raise
lentils
libido
lifting
liniment
linoleic acid
lipid
lipid deposit theory
lipolysis
lipoprotein
liposis
liposuction
liposurgery
liquid protein diet
listeria
listeriosis *See* listeria.
loafer's heart theory
local cross-fibre stroke
  See massage.
locking
locomotives
longevity
long-slow distance
  training
loose bodies *See* joint
  injury.
lordosis
low back stretcher
low carbohydrate diet
low-density lipoprotein
  See lipoproteins.
lower leg lift
low fat diet
low impact activity
lunges
lung volume
luxation
lysine

M

macrobiotic diet
macrocycle *See* cycle
  training.
macromineral
macronutrient

mad cow disease *See* bovine spongiform encephalopathy.
magic formula
magnesium
making weight
malabsorption
male menopause *See* viropause.
mallet finger
malnutrition
maltose
mammaplasty
manganese
manipulation
marasmus
march fracture
march haemoglobinuria *See* haematuria.
marijuana
martial arts
massage
massager
mat burn *See* friction burn.
maturation *See* growth.
maximal heart rate
maximal oxygen consumption
maximum passive range *See* range of movement.
McCutcheon's weeping lubrication theory
meal replacement diet
meal tolerance test
medau
medial epicondylitis *See* golfer's elbow.
medical screening *See* health screening.
medicine ball
Mediterranean diet
medium chain triglycerides *See* fatigue.
megadoses
megavitamin
menarche
meniscus
menopause
menstruation
mental health
mental practice
mesocycle *See* cycle training.
mesomorph
mesotherapy *See* cellulite.
MET *See* metabolic equivalent.
metabolic acidosis *See* acidosis.
metabolic equivalent
metabolism
methaemoglobin *See* nitrates.
methionine

methyl donors
microcycle *See* cycle training.
micromineral *See* minerals.
microtrauma
migraine *See* headache.
milk sugar *See* lactose.
military press
minerals
mitochondrion
mixers *See* emulsifiers.
mobility
mode of exercise
molybdenum
monosaccharide
monosodium glutamate
monounsaturated fat
mood swings
motivation
motivational strategies *See* motivation.
MSG *See* monosodium glutamate.
mud treatment *See* body wraps.
multi-gym
multi-poundage system
multi-set system
multi-weight sets *See* descending sets.
mumie
muscle
muscle balance
muscle-bound
muscle bulk
muscle contraction
muscle fibre types
muscle glycogen loading *See* carbohydrate loading.
muscle group
muscle growth
muscle hernia *See* fascial hernia.
muscle poops *See* fascial hernia.
muscle pull *See* muscle strain.
muscle pumping *See* pumping-up.
muscle soreness
muscle strain
muscle strength *See* strength.
muscle tear *See* muscle strain.
muscle triglyceride
mycoprotein
myocardial infarction *See* heart attack.
myocarditis
myoglobin

N

narcotic
neck extension exercise

neck flexion
neck flexion and extension
neck rotation exercise
neck shrugging
neck stretches
negative calories
negative-change goal
negative-resistance training
negative sit-up test
neohesperidine
nephrolithiasis *See* kidney stones.
netball
neutral fat *See* fat.
niacin
nicotinamide *See* niacin.
nicotine
nicotinic acid *See* niacin.
Nieder press
nitrates
nitrites *See* nitrates.
nitrosamine
non-insulin-dependent diabetes *See* diabetes.
non-haem iron
non-starch polysaccharide
non-steroidal anti-inflammatory drug
'no pain, no gain'
noradrenaline
norepinephrine *See* noradrenaline.
normal active range *See* range of movement.
NOS *See* eating disorder not otherwise specified.
NSAID *See* non-steroidal anti-inflammatory drug
nutrient
nutrient density
Nutron diet

O

obesity
obesity gene
OBLA *See* lactic acid.
octacosanol
oesophagitis
oestrogen
omega-3 fatty acids
omnikinetic resistance machine
one food diets
onset of blood lactate accumulation *See* lactic acid.
opiate
opium *See* opiate.
organic food

orienteering
orotic acid
orthostatic hypotension
    See postural hypotension.
orthostatic proteinuria
    See postural proteinuria.
orthotics
Osgood-Schlatter's disease
osteitis pubis See groin pain.
osteoarthritis
osteophytes See footballer's
    ankle.
osteoporosis (brittle bone
    disease)
os trigonum
over distance training
overload principle
overpronation See pronation.
overreaching
overstrain
overtraining
overuse injury
overweight
oxalic acid
oxygen
oxygen cost
oxygen debt
oxygen poisoning
oxymyoglobin
    See myoglobin.
ozone

P
PABA
pain
pain cycle
palpitation
pancreas
pancreatitis See pancreas.
pangamic acid
pantothenic acid
para-aminobenzoic acid
    See PABA.
paracetamol
parahaemolyticus food
    poisoning
paratenon See peritendinitis.
parathormone See parathyroid
    hormone.
parathyroid glands See
    parathyroid hormone.
parathyroid hormone
PAR-Q
passive exercise
patella See kneecap.
patellar tendinitis
    See jumper's knee.
patellofemoral disorders
    See knee.
patellofemoral malalignment
pattering

paunch See pot belly.
peak experience
peaking
pear-shaped obesity See gynoid
    fat distribution.
pec deck
pecs See pectoral muscles.
pectin
pectoral muscles
pectoral stretch
pellagra
pelvic floor exercises
pelvic floor lift
pelvic floor muscles
pelvic tilt
pep pills See amphetamines.
pep talk
peptic ulcer
peptide hormones
perceived exertion
performance plateau
    See plateau.
periodization
periosteum
periostitis See periosteum.
peritendinitis
peritonitis
pernicious anaemia
personality
perspiration See sweating.
phantom
pH control agents
phenylalanine
phenylbutazone
phenylketonuria
phenylpropanolamine
phonophoresis See ultrasound.
phosphagen
phosphagen system
phosphatidylcholine
    See lecithin.
phosphocreatine
    See phosphagen system.
phospholipids
phosphorus
Physical Activity Level
Physical Activity Ratio
physical fitness
physical recreation
physical work capacity
physiological limit
physiotherapy
phytic acid
phytochemical
pica
Pilates
piles See haemorrhoids.
pitcher's elbow See thrower's
    elbow.
pituitary
placebo

plantar fasciitis
plastic surgery
plateau
play
plumpness
plyometrics
PMR See progressive muscle
    relaxation.
PNF See proprioceptive
    neuromuscular facilitation.
polyunsaturated fat
polyunsaturates See
    polyunsaturated fat.
ponderal index See body size.
pooling
postural hypotension
postural proteinuria
posture
potassium
pot belly
power clean
power lifting
power sport
PPA
    See phenylpropanolamine.
praise
preacher curls
pre-activity meal See pre-
    competition meal.
pre-competition meal
pre-exhaustion system
pre-fatigue method
pregnancy
premenstrual tension
prepatellar bursitis
    See housemaid's knee.
preservatives
press See military press.
press-up
pressure training
priapism
prime mover
principle of progression
    See progression.
Pritikin diet
probenecid
Profile Of Mood States
programme setting
progression
progressive muscle relaxation
progressive resistance exercise
prolapsed intervertebral disc
pronation
pronator
proprioceptive
    neuromuscular facilitation
prostaglandin
protective muscle spasm
protective protein theory
protein
protein efficiency ratio

protein-sparing modified fast
protein supplement
proteinuria
prozac
P/S
pseudo-allergy See food intolerance.
PSMF See protein sparing modified fast.
psyche
psyched-out See psyche.
psyching-up See psyche.
psychoneuromuscular theory
pteroyl-L-glutamic acid See folic acid.
PTH See parathormone.
puberty
pull-up See chin-up.
pulse
pulse raiser
pumping-up
punch-drunk syndrome
purging
push-up See press up.
pyramid system
pyrexia See fever.
pyridoxine See vitamin B_6.
pyrosis See heartburn.

Q
Q-angle
quadriceps
quad stretch
Quetelet index See body mass index.
Quorn See mycoprotein.

R
radial pulse See pulse.
range of motion See range of movement.
range of movement
rate–pressure product
rating of perceived exertion See perceived exertion.
Ratzeburg method
RDA See Recommended Dietary Allowance.
reaction time
rebound hypoglycaemia See insulin rebound.
Recommended Daily Amounts See Recommended Dietary Allowance.
Recommended Daily Intake See Recommended Dietary Allowance.
Recommended Dietary Allowance
recommended dietary goals

reconstructive surgery See plastic surgery.
recovery
recovery period
rectus femoris See quadriceps.
recumbent leg press See fixed-weight machine.
reference man and woman
Reference Nutrient Intake See Dietary Reference Values.
rehabilitation
relative strength See strength.
relative weight
relaxation
relaxin
renal stones See kidney stones.
renin
rennin
repetition maximum
repetitions
repetition training
repetitive strain injury
replacement drink
resistance
resistance exercise
resistance stage See general adaptation syndrome.
resistant starch
respiration
respiratory acidosis See acidosis.
respiratory quotient
rest
rest–pause training
retinol See vitamin A.
reversibility principle
Revolutionary Three in One Diet See aromatherapy.
rheumatoid arthritis
riboflavin See vitamin B_2.
RICE
rickets
rider's strain
rock-climbing See climbing.
Rockport Fitness Walking Test
rope jumping
rotation diet
rotator cuff
rowing
Royal Canadian 5BX and XBX Programs
rubber suit
rugby
ruler drop test See reaction time.
run down
runner's haematuria See haematuria.

runner's haemolysis See haematuria.
runner's high
runner's knee
runner's toe See black nail.
rupture See hernia.

S
saccharin
SAD See seasonal affective disorder
Safe Intake See Dietary Reference Values.
SAID principle
salicylates
salicylic acid See salicylates.
salicylism See salicylates.
salmonellosis
salt
salt depletion
salt replacement
salt substitute
salt tablet
saponins
Sargent jump test
saturated fat
sauna baths
sauna suit See rubber suit.
Scarsdale diet
sciatica
sciatic nerve See sciatica.
scintigraphy
SCUBA diving
scurvy
seasonal affective disorder
second wind
secretin
segmenting
selenium
self-concept
self-confidence
self-efficacy See self-confidence.
self-esteem
self-image See self-concept.
self-starvation syndrome See anorexia nervosa.
self-talk See self-confidence.
semi-vegetarian
serotonin
SERP See Sport Emotional Reaction Profile.
serratus anterior See boxer's muscle.
set
set point theory
set system
sex and exercise
sex differences
shallow-water blackout See oxygen poisoning.

shaping
Sheldon's constitutional
  theory *See* somatotype.
shigellosis
shin fracture
shin splints
shin stretcher
shock
shock exercises
short leg
short wave diathermy
  See diathermy.
shoulder lifts
shoulder shrugs
shuttle test
sickle cell disease
side bends
side leg raises
side twist
simple carbohydrate
single sugar
sit-and-reach test
sitting tucks
sit-up
skeletal muscle
skeleton
skier's thumb
skiing
ski jump
skill
skin
skinfold measurements
skin patches *See* slimming
  patch.
sleep
slide training
slimming patch
slimming pills
slipped disc
slow-twitch fibre *See* muscle
  fibre type.
small intestine *See* alimentary
  canal.
smoking
smooth muscle *See* muscle.
snack
snow-blindness
soccer
soccer toe *See* black nail.
SOD *See* superoxide
  dismutase.
sodium
sodium bicarbonate
soft tissue injury
soft workouts
solanine
soluble fibre *See* fibre.
somatotype
spare tyre
spasm
Specific Adaptations to

Imposed Demands
  principle *See* SAID principle.
specific-training principle
speed
speed–accuracy trade off
speed chute
speed play *See* fartlek training.
SPF *See* sun-protection factor
spinner's finger
spleen
split routine
spondylolithesis
  See spondylolysis.
spondylolysis
sport
Sport Emotional Reaction
  Profile
sporting behaviour
sport psychologist
sports clothes *See* clothing.
sports injury
sports medicine
sports science
spot-reducing *See* spot theory
  of fat reduction.
spotter
spot theory of fat reduction
sprain
spreads
sprint
sprue *See* coeliac disease.
squash
squat
squat thrust
stability *See* joint stability.
stage training *See* circuit
  training.
stamina *See* endurance.
standing toe-touch test
staphylococcal food poisoning
starch
starch blockers
starch gum *See* dextrin.
starch sugar *See* dextrin.
star jumps *See* stride jumps.
starvation
state anxiety *See* anxiety.
static stretching *See*
  stretching.
stationary leg change
steadiness
steady state exercise
steam treatment
step aerobics
stepper
stepping-stone test
step test
steroid
stevioside
stick test *See* reaction time.
stiffness

stimulants
stitch
stomach curl
stomach muscles
  See abdominal muscles.
stomach stapling
stomach ulcer *See* peptic ulcer.
storage fat
strain *See* muscle strain.
strength
strength endurance
strength training
stress
stress fracture
stress hormone
stress incontinence
stress inoculation training
stretch-and-curl
stretching
stretch reflex
stretch stress
stride jumps
stride stretch
stroke
stroke volume
strychnine
subluxation *See* dislocation.
sucrose
sudden death
sudden immersion injury
sugar
sugar fix
sugar-free food
sugar malabsorption
sulphites
sulphur
sulphur dioxide *See* sulphites.
sunburn
sun-protection factor
sunstroke
supercompensation *See*
  carbohydrate loading.
superoxide dismutase
super-set system
supination
supinator
supplements
suppleness
suprascapularis *See* rotator
  cuff.
supraspinatus *See* rotator cuff.
surfer's ear *See* swimmer's ear.
SWD *See* diathermy.
sweating
swimmer's ear
swimmer's shoulder
swimming
syncope *See* fainting.
Syndrome X
synergist
synergy

T

table salt
tachycardia
tae kwon do *See* martial arts.
t'ai chi
tannins
tapering down
taping
tempolauf
tendinitis
tendinosis
tendon
tendon injuries
tennis
tennis elbow
tennis leg
tennis toe *See* black nail.
tenpin bowling *See* bowling.
TENS *See* transcutaneous
    electrical nerve
    stimulation.
testosterone
tetanus
tetany
texturizers
thaumatin
thermic effect of food *See* diet
    induced thermogenesis.
thermogenesis
thiamin *See* vitamin B₁.
thinness-demand sport
thirst
thought-stopping
threonine
thrombosis
thrower's elbow
thrower's fracture
throwing
thrush *See* candida.
thyroid hormone
thyroid stimulating
    hormone
thyroxine *See* thyroid
    hormone.
tidal volume *See* lung
    volume.
time of meals
time-trial
timing
TMG *See* methyl donors.
tocopherol *See* vitamin E.
tooth decay
torn cartilage *See* meniscus.
torticollis
total body stretch
total hip machine *See* fixed-
    weight machine.
total thermal load
toxicity
trace element

trainability principle
training
training diary
training duration
training effects
training frequency
training heart rate
training impulse
training intensity
training shoes
training threshold
training unit
transcutaneous electrical
    nerve stimulation
trans fat *See* unsaturated fat.
transfer
transition period
trapezius
traveller's diarrhoea
travel sickness
treadmill
triacylglycerol
triceps *See* triceps brachii.
triceps brachii
triceps extension
triceps surae *See* soleus.
trigger finger
trigger point
triglyceride *See* fat.
trimethylglycine *See* methyl
    donors.
triple-jumper's heel
tri-sets
trunk lifts
trunk rotation
trunk stretcher
trunk twists
tryptophan
turf toe syndrome
twister
type A behaviour
type B behaviour
Type I diabetes *See* diabetes.
Type II diabetes *See* diabetes.
Type I fibre *See* muscle fibre
    types.
Type II fibre *See* muscle fibre
    types.
tyramine
tyrosine

U

ulcer *See* peptic ulcer.
ulnar compression syndrome
    See compression
    neuropathy.
ultrasound
ultraviolet light
undereating
underload principle
underweight

unfitness
unhappy triad
unilateral muscular
    hypertrophy
United States Recommended
    Daily Allowance
unsaturated fat
upright rowing
US RDA *See* United States
    Recommended Daily
    Allowance.

V

valgus
valine
Valsalva's manoeuvre
vanadium
variable resistance exercise
varices *See* varicose veins.
varicose veins
varus
vastus intermedius
    See quadriceps.
vastus lateralis *See* quadriceps.
vastus medialis
    See quadriceps.
vegan
vegetarian
ventilation rate *See* lung
    volume.
versa-ball
vertical jump test *See* Sargent
    jumptest.
very low calorie diet
very low-density lipoprotein
    See lipoprotein.
viropause
visceral fat deposition
visualization
vital capacity
vitamin
vitamin A
vitamin B complex
vitamin B₁
vitamin B₂
vitamin B₃ *See* niacin.
vitamin B₅ *See* pantothenic
    acid.
vitamin B₆
vitamin B₁₂
vitamin B₁₅ *See* pangamic
    acid.
vitamin B₁₇ *See* laetrile.
vitamin C
vitamin D
vitamin deficiency disease
vitamin E
vitamin F *See* linoleic acid.
vitamin K
vitamin supplementation
volleyball

W

waist–hip ratio
walking
warm down *See* cool down.
warm-up
water
water balance
water intoxication
water replacement
water retention *See* fluid
   retention.
water tablets
weight belt
weight cycling
weight-gain diet
weight-lifter's headache
   See headache.
weight-loss maintenance
weight training

weight-training machine
whiplash injury
whirlpool treatment
white adipose tissue
white fibre *See* muscle fibre
   types.
wind *See* flatulence.
winding
windmills
Work Related Upper Limb
   Disorder *See* repetitive
   strain injury.
wrestler's bridge
wrist curl
wryneck *See* torticollis.

X

xanthines
xerophthalmia
X-ray

xylitol
xylose

Y

yang *See* macrobiotic diet.
Yerkes-Dodson curve
ying *See* macrobiotic diet.
yoga
yogacise *See* yoga.
Yo-Yo diet
young runner's heel

Z

Zatopek phenomenon
   See tapering down.
Zen macrobiotic diet
zero fat diet
zinc
zinc oxide ointment
zone of optimal functioning